LIBRARY
LOYOLA UNIVERSITY MEDICAL C
W9-CUH-527

Cardiovascular Physiology

Robert M. Berne, M.D., DSc. (Hon.)
Alumni Professor of Physiology
Department of Physiology
University of Virginia School of Medicine
Charlottesville, Virginia

Matthew N. Levy, M.D.
Chief of Investigative Medicine
Mount Sinai Medical Center;
Professor of Physiology and Biomedical Engineering
Case Western Reserve University
Cleveland, Ohio

SIXTH EDITION
with **251** *illustrations*

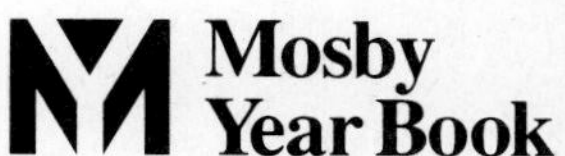

St. Louis Baltimore Boston Chicago London Philadelphia Sydney Toronto

WG
102
B525c6
1992

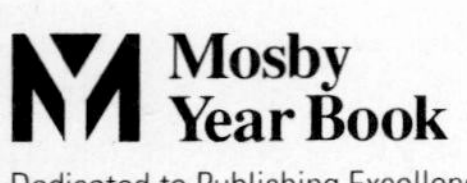

Editor: Kimberly Kist
Assistant Editor: Penny Rudolph
Project Manager: John A. Rogers
Production Editor: Shauna Burnett Sticht
Designer: David Zielinski

Copyright © 1992 by Mosby–Year Book, Inc.

A Mosby imprint of Mosby–Year Book, Inc.

All rights reserved. No part of this publication may be reproduced, stored in a retrieval system, or transmitted, in any form or by any means, electronic, mechanical, photocopying, recording, or otherwise, without prior permission from the publisher.

Previous editions copyrighted 1967, 1972, 1977, 1981, 1986

Printed in the United States of America

Mosby–Year Book, Inc.
11830 Westline Industrial Drive
St. Louis, Missouri 63146

Library of Congress Cataloging-in-Publication Data

Berne, Robert M., 1918-
Cardiovascular physiology / Robert M. Berne, Matthew N. Levy. — 6th ed.
p. cm.
Includes bibliographical references and index.
ISBN 0-8016-6314-8
1. Cardiovascular system—Physiology. I. Levy, Matthew N., 1922- II. Title.
[DNLM: 1. Cardiovascular System—physiology. WG 102 B525c]
QP102.B47 1991
612.1—dc20
DNLM/DLC
for Library of Congress 91-34898
CIP

92 93 94 95 96 C/DC 9 8 7 6 5 4 3 2 1

To our grandchildren, Alex, Ari, Christopher, Maggie, Molly, Sarah, Todd, and Tracy.

Preface

This book is designed primarily for medical and graduate students. With this fundamental purpose in mind, an attempt has been made to emphasize general concepts and to ignore isolated facts, except where they are deemed essential. In accordance with this principle, little documentation is afforded for many of the assertions made, and only a few references have been included in the bibliographies at the end of each chapter. Review articles have been given preference over scientific papers, and articles have been selected primarily for their appropriateness for the beginning student, for the depth of the interpretation included in their discussion sections, for their timeliness, and for the comprehensiveness of their bibliographies.

Because many of the broad principles of cardiovascular physiology are complex and confusing to the student, simplified models have been employed throughout the book. Unquestionably, there are advantages and disadvantages to this pedagogical device. In formulating a model, the instructor retains those elements and properties of the system under consideration that are deemed germane and discards those other components of the system that are not deemed relevant. Furthermore, for those elements to be included in the model, the behavior of certain components is assumed to be less complex than is actually the case. One justification for such simplification is that this behavior is reasonably accurate over a limited range of values. However, once the underlying basis of the system is understood, the complicating details can then be added to approximate more closely the true system. Although models can be very useful when employed properly, they can also lead to erroneous conclusions when misused. Therefore the reader must constantly be aware of the assumptions inherent in a given model and must decide whether a more detailed model is necessary at times to understand the problem under consideration.

In a sense, normal physiology serves as a framework that students of medicine must comprehend before they can understand the derangements caused by disease or toxic agents. There is no intensive consideration of pathological physiology in this text. However, many examples of abnormal function are provided to illustrate more lucidly the behavior of the system under consideration and to indicate the direction in which students will be proceeding in their continuing efforts to understand the effects of many disease processes.

In revising and updating this book, we have profited greatly from the many helpful criticisms and suggestions received from the readers, as well as from our own experience with the book in teaching cardiovascular physiology to medical and graduate students. Several chapters have been extensively revised, particularly Chapter 2, Electrical Activity of the Heart, in which the sections on specific ion channels have been substantially expanded. To avert a significant lengthening of this entire chapter, the section on the basis of electrocardiography has been condensed. The mechanisms involved in contraction and relaxation of cardiac and vascular smooth muscle have been updated, as has the role of the endothelium in the regulation of vascular resistance. A number of old figures have been deleted and new figures added to facilitate comprehension of the material.

The summaries that highlight the key points presented in each chapter are a new feature of this monograph. Within the chapter, italics have been used to emphasize important facts and concepts, and bold face has been used for definitions.

Throughout the book we have attempted to incorporate the most recent information and to indicate which subjects are still controversial. Emphasis has been placed on control mechanisms; thus, to present the clearest view of the various mechanisms involved in the regulation of the circulatory system, the component parts of the system are discussed individually. However, because the body functions as a whole, in the last chapter we have tried to coordinate the various components to show how the cardiovascular system operates in an integrated fashion to respond to a physiological stimulus (exercise) and to a pathophysiological stimulus (hemorrhage).

We wish to thank our readers for their constructive comments and hope that they will continue to provide the input necessary for us to improve future editions. We also wish to thank the numerous investigators and publishers who have granted us permission to use illustrations from their publications. In most cases these illustrations have been altered somewhat to increase their didactic utility. In some cases unpublished data from our own studies have been presented. These investigations were supported by grants HL-10384 and HL-10591 from the U.S. Public Health Service, to which we are indebted.

And last, but by no means least, we thank Frances Langley for her patience and skill in helping us to put our pedagogic ıl ideas into useful illustrations.

Robert M. Berne
Matthew N. Levy

Contents

1 The Circuitry

The circulatory, endocrine, and nervous systems constitute the principal coordinating and integrating systems of the body. Whereas the nervous system is primarily concerned with communications and the endocrine glands with regulation of certain body functions, the circulatory system serves to transport and distribute essential substances to the tissues and to remove by-products of metabolism. The circulatory system also shares in such homeostatic mechanisms as regulation of body temperature, humoral communication throughout the body, and adjustments of oxygen and nutrient supply in different physiological states.

The cardiovascular system that accomplishes these chores is made up of a pump, a series of distributing and collecting tubes, and an extensive system of thin vessels that permit rapid exchange between the tissues and the vascular channels. The primary purpose of this text is to discuss the function of the components of the vascular system and the control mechanisms (with their checks and balances) that are responsible for alteration of blood distribution necessary to meet the changing requirements of different tissues in response to a wide spectrum of physiologic and pathologic conditions.

Before considering the function of the parts of the circulatory system in detail, it is useful to consider it as a whole in a purely descriptive sense. The heart consists of two pumps in series: one to propel blood through the lungs for exchange of oxygen and carbon dioxide (the **pulmonary circulation**) and the other to propel blood to all other tissues of the body (the **systemic circulation**). Unidirectional flow through the heart is achieved by the appropriate arrangement of effective flap valves. Although the cardiac output is intermittent, continuous flow to the periphery occurs by distension of the aorta and its branches during ventricular contraction **(systole)** and elastic recoil of the walls of the large arteries with forward propulsion of the blood during ventricular relaxation **(diastole).** Blood moves rapidly through the aorta and its arterial branches. The branches become narrower and their walls become thinner and change histologically toward the periphery. From a predominantly elastic structure, the aorta, the peripheral arteries become more muscular until at the arterioles the muscular layer predominates (Fig. 1-1).

In the large arteries frictional resistance is relatively small, and pressures are only slightly less than in the aorta. However, the small arter-

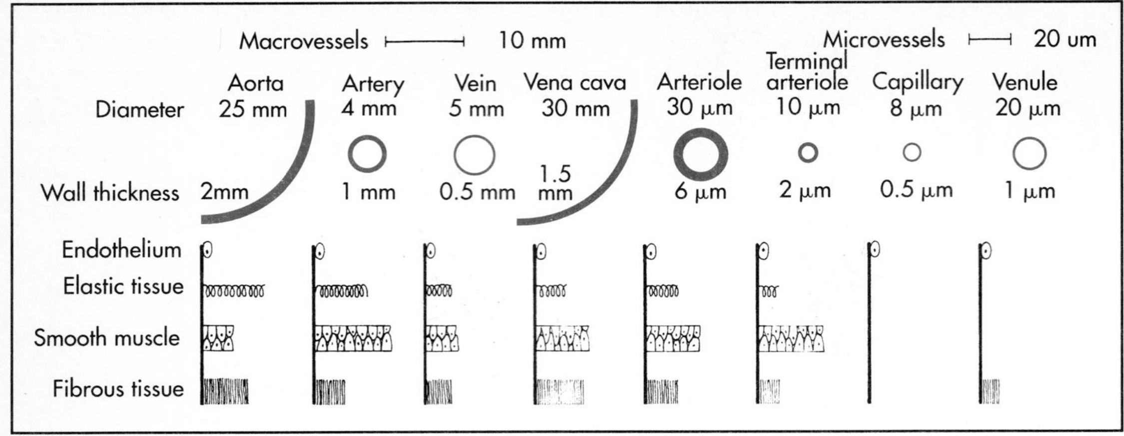

Fig. 1-1 ■ Internal diameter, wall thickness, and relative amounts of the principal components of the vessel walls of the various blood vessels that compose the circulatory system. Cross sections of the vessels are not drawn to scale because of the huge range from aorta and venae cavae to capillary. (Redrawn from Burton, A.C.: Physiol. Rev. 34:619, 1954.)

ies offer moderate resistance to blood flow and this resistance reaches a maximum level in the arterioles, sometimes referred to as the stopcocks of the vascular system. Hence the pressure drop is significant in the small arteries and is greatest across the arterioles (Fig. 1-2). Adjustment in the degree of contraction of the circular muscle of these small vessels permits regulation of tissue blood flow and aids in the control of arterial blood pressure.

In addition to a sharp reduction in pressure across the arterioles, there is also a change from pulsatile to steady flow as pressure continues to decline from the arterial to the venous end of the capillaries. The pulsatile arterial blood flow, caused by the intermittency of cardiac ejection, is damped at the capillary level by the combination of distensibility of the large arteries and frictional resistance in the arterioles. Many capillaries arise from each arteriole so that the total cross-sectional area of the capillary bed is very large, despite the fact that the cross-sectional area of each capillary is less than that of each arteriole. As a result, blood flow becomes quite slow in the capillaries, analogous to the decrease in flow rate seen at the wide regions of a river. Because the capillaries consist of short tubes whose walls are only one cell thick and because flow rate is slow, conditions in the capillaries are ideal for the exchange of diffusible substances between blood and tissue.

On its return to the heart from the capillaries, blood passes through venules and then through veins of increasing size with a progressive decrease in pressure until the blood reaches the right atrium (Fig. 1-2). As the heart is approached, the number of veins decreases, the thickness and composition of the vein walls change (see Fig. 1-1), the total cross-sectional area of the venous channels diminishes, and the velocity of blood flow increases (see Fig. 1-2). Also note that most of the circulating blood is located in the venous vessels (see Fig. 1-2).

Data from a 20 kg dog (Table 1-1) indicate that the number of vessels increases about 3 billion fold, and the total cross-sectional area

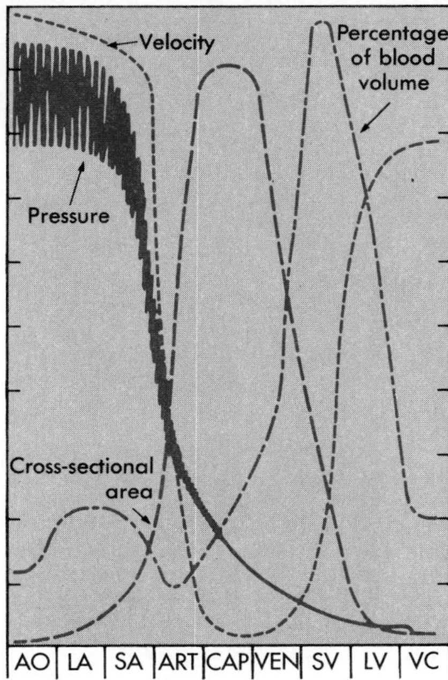

Fig. 1-2 ■ Pressure, velocity of flow, cross-sectional area, and capacity of the blood vessels of the systemic circulation. *The important features are the inverse relationship between velocity and cross-sectional area, the major pressure drop across the arterioles, the maximal cross-sectional area and minimal flow rate in the capillaries, and the large capacity of the venous system.* The small but abrupt drop in pressure in the venae cavae indicates the point of entrance of these vessels into the thoracic cavity and reflects the effect of the negative intrathoracic pressure. To permit schematic representation of velocity and cross-sectional area on a single linear scale, only approximations are possible at the lower values. *AO,* Aorta; *LA,* large arteries; *SA,* small arteries; *ART,* arterioles; *CAP,* capillaries; *VEN,* venules; *SV,* small veins; *LV,* large veins; *VC,* venae cavae.

Table 1-1 ■ **Vascular dimensions in a 20 kg dog**

Vessels	Number	Total cross-sectional area (cm^2)	Total blood volume (%)
Systemic			
Aorta	1	2.8	
Arteries	40-110,000	40	11
Arterioles	2.8×10^6	55	
Capillaries	2.7×10^9	1357	5
Venules	1×10^7	785	
Veins	660,000-110	631	67
Venae cavae	2	3.1	
Pulmonary			
Arteries and arterioles	$1\text{-}1.5 \times 10^6$	137	3
Capillaries	2.7×10^9	1357	4
Venules and veins	2×10^6 -4	210	5
Heart			
Atria	2		5
Ventricles	2		

Data from Milnor, W.R.: Hemodynamics, Baltimore, 1982, Williams & Wilkins.

increases about 500-fold between the aorta and the capillaries. The volume of blood in the capillaries is only 5% of the total blood volume compared with 11% in the aorta, arteries, and arterioles and 67% in the veins and venules. In contrast, blood volume in the pulmonary vascular bed is about equally divided among the arterial, capillary, and venous vessels. The cross-sectional area of the venae cavae is larger than that of the aorta (although not evident from Fig. 1-2 because cross-sectional areas of venae cavae and aorta are so close to zero with a scale that includes the capillaries), and hence the flow is slower than that in the aorta.

Blood entering the right ventricle via the right atrium is pumped through the pulmonary arterial system at a mean pressure about one seventh that in the systemic arteries. The blood then passes through the lung capillaries, where carbon dioxide is released and oxygen

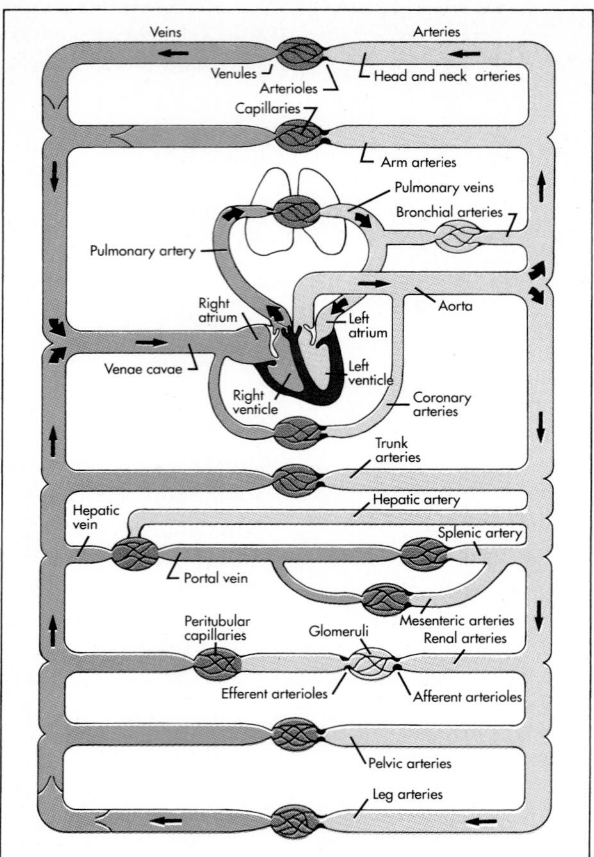

Fig. 1-3 ■ Schematic diagram of the parallel and series arrangement of the vessels composing the circulatory system. The capillary beds are represented by thin lines connecting the arteries (on the right) with the veins (on the left). The crescent-shaped thickenings proximal to the capillary beds represent the arterioles (resistance vessels). (Redrawn from Green, H.D.: In Glasser, O., editor: Medical physics, vol. 1, Chicago, 1944, Year Book Medical Publishers, Inc.)

taken up. The oxygen-rich blood returns via the pulmonary veins to the left atrium and ventricle to complete the cycle. Thus in the normal intact circulation the total volume of blood is constant, and an increase in the volume of blood in one area must be accompanied by a decrease in another. However, the velocity at which the blood circulates through the different regions of the body is determined by the output of the left ventricle and by the contractile state of the arterioles (resistance vessels) of these regions. The circulatory system is composed of conduits arranged in series and in parallel (Fig. 1-3).

2 Electrical Activity of the Heart

The experiments on "animal electricity" conducted by Galvani and Volta two centuries ago led to the discovery that electrical phenomena were involved in the spontaneous contractions of the heart. In 1855 Kölliker and Müller observed that when they placed the nerve of a nerve-muscle preparation in contact with the surface of a frog's heart, the muscle twitched with each cardiac contraction.

The electrical events that normally take place in the heart initiate its contraction. Disorders in electrical activity can induce serious and sometimes lethal rhythm disturbances.

■ TRANSMEMBRANE POTENTIALS

The electrical behavior of single cardiac muscle cells has been investigated by inserting microelectrodes into the interior of the cell. The potential changes recorded from a typical ventricular muscle fiber are illustrated in Fig. 2-1, *A*. When two electrodes are placed in an electrolyte solution near a strip of quiescent cardiac muscle, no potential difference (point *a*) is measurable between the two electrodes. At point *b* one of the electrodes, a microelectrode, was inserted into the interior of a cardiac muscle fiber (see Fig. 2-1). Immediately the galvanometer recorded a potential difference (V_m) across the cell membrane; the potential of the interior of the cell was about 90 mV lower than that of the surrounding medium. Such electronegativity of the interior of the resting cell with respect to the exterior is also characteristic of skeletal and smooth muscle, of nerve, and indeed of most cells within the body.

At point *c* a propagated action potential was transmitted to the cell impaled with the microelectrode. Very rapidly the cell membrane became depolarized; actually, the potential difference was reversed (positive overshoot), so that the potential of the interior of the cell exceeded that of the exterior by about 20 mV. The rapid upstroke of the action potential is designated phase 0. Immediately after the upstroke, there was a brief period of partial repolarization (phase 1), followed by a *plateau* (phase 2) that persisted for about 0.1 to 0.2 s. The potential then became progressively more negative (phase 3), until the resting state of polarization was again attained (at point *e*). Rapid repolarization (phase 3) is a much slower rate of change than is depolarization (phase 0). The interval from the end of repolarization until the beginning of the next action potential is designated phase 4.

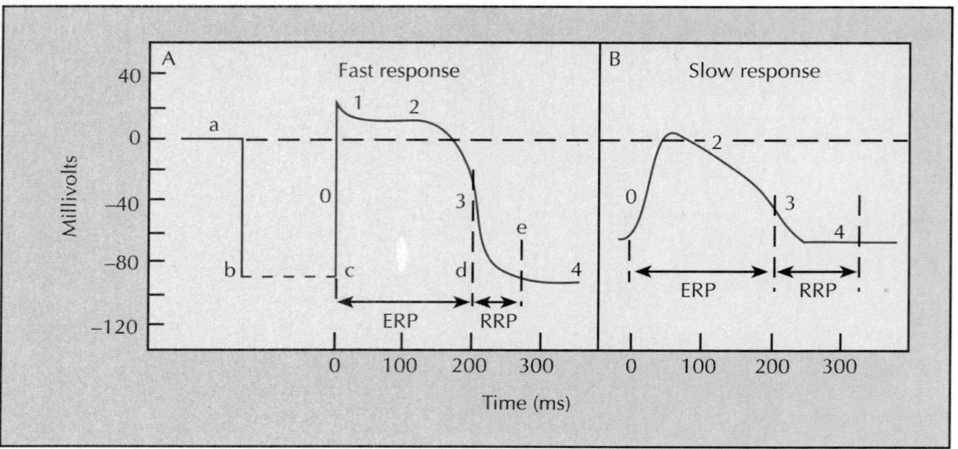

Fig. 2-1 ■ Changes in transmembrane potential recorded from a fast response, *A*, and slow response, *B*, cardiac fiber in isolated cardiac tissue immersed in an electrolyte solution. **A,** At time *a* the microelectrode was in the solution surrounding the cardiac fiber. At time *b* the microelectrode entered the fiber. At time *c* an action potential was initiated in the impaled fiber. Time *c* to *d* represents the effective refractory period *(ERP),* and time *d* to *e* represents the relative refractory period *(RRP).* **B,** An action potential recorded from a slow response cardiac fiber. Note that compared to the fast response fiber, the resting potential of the slow fiber is less negative, the upstroke (phase *0*) of the action potential is less steep, the amplitude of the action potential is smaller, phase *1* is absent, and the relative refractory period (RRP) extends well into phase *4,* after the fiber has fully repolarized.

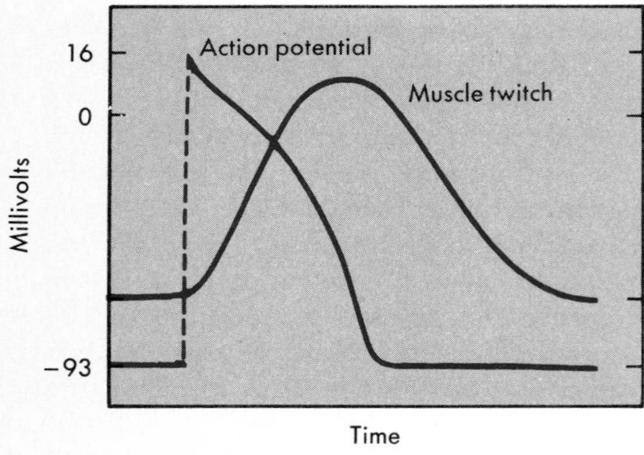

Fig. 2-2 ■ Time relationships between the mechanical tension developed by a thin strip of ventricular muscle and the changes in transmembrane potential. (Redrawn from Kavaler, F., Fisher, V.J., and Stuckey, J.H.: Bull. N.Y. Acad. Med. 41:592, 1965.)

The time relationships between the electrical events and the actual mechanical contraction are shown in Fig. 2-2. Rapid depolarization (phase 0) precedes force development and completion of repolarization coincides approximately with peak force. The duration of contraction tends to parallel the duration of the action potential. Also as the frequency of cardiac contraction is increased, the durations of the action potential and the mechanical contraction decrease.

Principal Types of Cardiac Action Potentials

Two main types of action potentials are observed in the heart, as shown in Fig. 2-1. One type, the **fast response,** occurs in the normal myocardial fibers in the atria and ventricles and in the specialized conducting fibers **(Purkinje fibers).** The other type of action

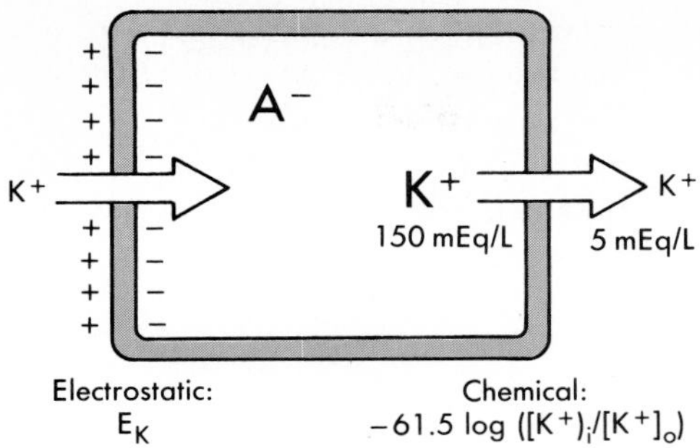

Fig. 2-3 ■ The balance of chemical and electrostatic forces acting on a resting cardiac cell membrane, based on a 30:1 ratio of the intracellular to extracellular K^+ concentrations, and the existence of a nondiffusible anion (A^-) inside but not outside the cell.

Table 2-1 ■ **Intracellular and extracellular ion concentrations and equilibrium potentials in cardiac muscle cells**

Ion	Extracellular concentrations (mM)	Intracellular concentrations (mM)*	Equilibrium potential (mV)
Na^+	145	10	70
K^+	4	135	−94
Ca^{++}	2	10^{-4}	132

Modified from Ten Eick, R.E., Baumgarten, C.M., and Singer, D.H.: Prog. Cardiovasc. Dis. 24:157, 1981.
*The intracellular concentrations are estimates of the free concentrations in the cytoplasm.

potential, the *slow response,* is found in the **sinoatrial (SA) node,** the natural pacemaker region of the heart, and in the **atrioventricular (AV) node,** the specialized tissue involved in conducting the cardiac impulse from atria to ventricles. Furthermore, fast responses may be converted to slow responses either spontaneously or under certain experimental conditions. For example, in a myocardial fiber, a gradual shift of the resting membrane potential from its normal level of about −90 mV to a value of about −60 mV will convert subsequent action potentials to the slow response. Such conversions may occur spontaneously in those regions of the heart to which the blood supply has been severely curtailed.

As shown in Fig. 2-1, not only is the resting membrane potential of the fast response considerably more negative than that of the slow response, but also the slope of the upstroke (phase 0), the amplitude of the action potential, and the extent of the overshoot of the fast response are greater than in the slow response. The amplitude of the action potential and the steepness of the upstroke are important determinants of propagation velocity. Hence, in cardiac tissue characterized by the slow response, conduction velocity is much slower and impulses are more likely to be blocked than in tissues displaying the fast response. Slow conduction and a tendency toward block increase the likelihood of certain rhythm disturbances.

Ionic Basis of the Resting Potential

The various phases of the cardiac action potential are associated with changes in the permeability of the cell membrane, mainly to sodium, potassium, and calcium ions. Changes in cell membrane permeability alter the rate of ion passage across the membrane. The permeability of the membrane to a given ion defines the net quantity of the ion that will diffuse across each unit area of the membrane per unit concentration difference across the membrane. Changes in permeability are accomplished by the opening and closing of **ion channels** that are specific for the individual ions.

Just as with all other cells in the body, the concentration of potassium ions inside a cardiac muscle cell, $[K^+]_i$, greatly exceeds the concentration outside the cell, $[K^+]_o$, as shown in Fig. 2-3. The reverse concentration gradient exists for Na ions and for unbound Ca ions. Estimates of the extracellular and intracellular concentrations of Na^+, K^+, and Ca^{++}, and of the equilibrium potentials (defined below) for these ions, are compiled in Table 2-1.

The resting cell membrane is relatively permeable to K^+, but much less so to Na^+ and Ca^{++}. Because of the high permeability to K^+, there tends to be a net diffusion of K^+ from the inside to the outside of the cell, in the direction of the concentration gradient, as shown on the right side of the cell in Fig. 2-3.

Any flux of K^+ that occurs during phase 4 takes place through certain specific K^+ **channels.** Several types of K^+ channels exist in cardiac cell membranes. Some of these channels are regulated (i.e., opened and closed) by the transmembrane potential, whereas others are regulated by some chemical signal (e.g., the intracellular Ca^{++} concentration). The specific K^+ channel through which K^+ passes during phase 4 is a voltage regulated channel that conducts the K^+ current, called I_{K1}, which is an **inwardly rectifying K^+ current,** as explained below. Many of the anions (labeled A^-) inside the cell, such as the proteins, are not free to diffuse out with the K^+ (see Fig. 2-3). Therefore, as the K^+ diffuses out of the cell and leaves the A^- behind, the deficiency of cations causes the interior of the cell to become electronegative.

Therefore, two opposing forces are involved in the movement of K^+ across the cell membrane. A chemical force, based on the concentration gradient, results in the net outward diffusion of K^+. The counterforce is an electrostatic one; the positively charged K ions are attracted to the interior of the cell by the negative potential that exists there, as shown on the left side of the cell in Fig. 2-3. If the system came into equilibrium, the chemical and the electrostatic forces would be equal.

This equilibrium is expressed by the **Nernst equation** for potassium:

$$E_K = -61.5 \log([K^+]_i / [K^+]_o) \qquad (1)$$

The right-hand term represents the chemical potential difference at the body temperature of 37° C. The left-hand term, E_K, represents the electrostatic potential difference that would exist across the cell membrane if K^+ were the only diffusible ion. E_K is called the **potassium equilibrium potential.**

An experimental disturbance in the equilibrium between electrostatic and chemical forces imposed by **voltage clamping** would cause K^+ to move through the K^+ channels. If the transmembrane potential (V_m) were clamped at a level negative to E_K, the electrostatic forces would exceed the diffusional forces, and K^+ would be attracted into the cell; (i.e., the K^+ current would be **inward**). Conversely, if V_m were clamped at a level positive to E_K, the diffusional forces would exceed the electrostatic forces, and K^+ would leave the cell; (i.e., the K^+ current would be **outward**).

When the measured concentrations of $[K^+]_i$ and $[K^+]_o$ for mammalian myocardial cells are substituted into the Nernst equation, the calculated value of E_K equals about −90 to −100 mV (Table 2-1). This value is close to, but slightly more negative than, the resting potential actually measured in myocardial cells. Therefore, a small potential tends to drive K^+ out of the resting cell.

The balance of forces acting on the Na ions is entirely different from that acting on the K ions in resting cardiac cells. The intracellular Na^+ concentration, $[Na^+]_i$, is much lower than the extracellular concentration, $[Na^+]_o$. At 37° C, the **sodium equilibrium potential,** E_{Na}, expressed by the Nernst equation is:

$$-61.5 \log([Na^+]_i / [Na^+]_o) \qquad (2)$$

For cardiac cells, E_{Na} is about 40 to 70 mV (Table 2-1). At equilibrium, therefore, an electrostatic force of 40 to 70 mV, oriented with the inside of the cell more positive than the outside, would be necessary to counterbalance the chemical potential for Na^+. However, the actual polarization of the resting cell membrane is just the opposite. The resting membrane potential of myocardial fibers is about −90 mV. Hence both chemical and electrostatic forces act to pull extracellular Na^+ into the cell. The influx of Na^+ through the cell membrane is small, however, because the permeability of the resting membrane to Na^+ is very low. Nevertheless, it is mainly this small inward current of positively charged Na ions that causes the potential on the inside of the resting cell membrane to be slightly less negative than the value predicted by the Nernst equation for K^+.

The steady inward leak of Na^+ would gradually depolarize the resting cell membrane were it not for the metabolic pump that continuously extrudes Na^+ from the cell interior and pumps in K^+. The metabolic pump involves the enzyme, Na^+ K^+-activated ATPase, which is located in the cell membrane itself. Because the pump must move Na^+ against both a chemical and an electrostatic gradient, operation of the pump requires the expenditure of metabolic energy. Increases in $[Na^+]_i$ or in $[K^+]_o$ accelerate the activity of the pump. The quantity of Na^+ extruded by the pump exceeds the quantity of K^+ transferred into the cell by a 3:2 ratio. Therefore, the pump itself tends to create a potential difference across the cell membrane, and thus it is termed an **electrogenic pump.** If the pump is partially inhibited, as by digitalis, the concentration gradients for Na^+ and K^+ are partially dissipated, and the resting membrane potential becomes less negative than normal.

The dependence of the transmembrane potential, V_m, on the intracellular and extracellular concentrations of K^+ and Na^+ and on the conductances (g_K and g_{Na}) of these ions is described by the **chord conductance equation:**

$$V_m = \frac{g_K}{g_K + g_{Na}} E_K + \frac{g_{Na}}{g_K + g_{Na}} E_{Na} \qquad (3)$$

For a given ion (X), the conductance (g_x) is defined as the ratio of the current (i_X) carried by that ion to the difference between the V_m and the Nernst equilibrium potential (E_X) for that ion; that is,

$$g_X = \frac{i_x}{V_m - E_x} \qquad (4)$$

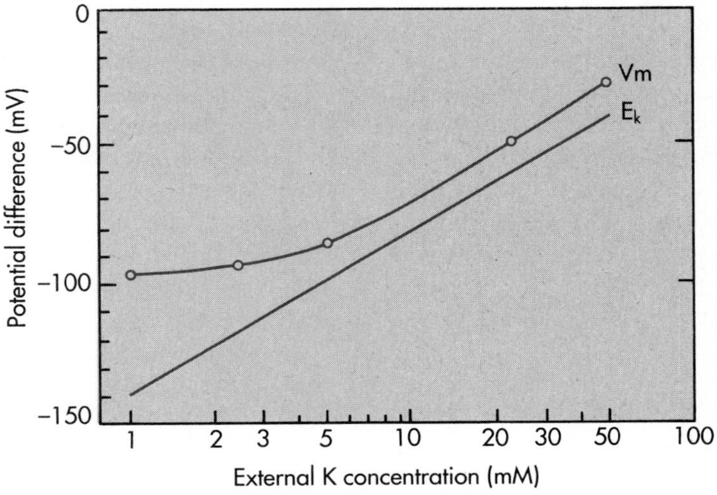

Fig. 2-4 ▪ Transmembrane potential of a cardiac muscle fiber varies inversely with the potassium concentration of the external medium *(colored curve).* The straight black line represents the change in transmembrane potential predicted by the Nernst equation for E_K. (Redrawn from Page, E.: Circulation 26:582, 1962. By permission of the American Heart Association, Inc.)

The chord conductance equation reveals that the relative, not the absolute, conductances to Na^+ and K^+ determine the resting potential. In the resting cardiac cell, g_K is about 100 times greater than g_{Na}. Therefore, the chord conductance equation reduces essentially to the Nernst equation for K^+.

When the ratio $[K^+]_i/[K^+]_o$ is decreased experimentally by raising $[K^+]_o$, the measured value of V_m (red line, Fig. 2-4) approximates that predicted by the Nernst equation for K^+ (black line). For extracellular K^+ concentrations of about 5 mM and above, the measured values correspond closely with the predicted values. The measured levels are slightly less than those predicted by the Nernst equation because of the small but finite value of g_{Na}. For values of $[K^+]_o$ below about 5 mM, g_K decreases as $[K^+]_o$ is diminished. As g_K decreases, the effect of the Na^+ gradient on the transmembrane potential becomes relatively more important, as predicted by equation 3. This change in g_K accounts for the greater deviation of the measured V_m from that predicted by the Nernst equation for K^+ at low levels of $[K^+]_o$ (see Fig. 2-4). Also, in accordance with equation 3, changes in $[Na^+]_o$ have relatively little effect on resting V_m (Fig. 2-5), because of the low value of g_{Na}.

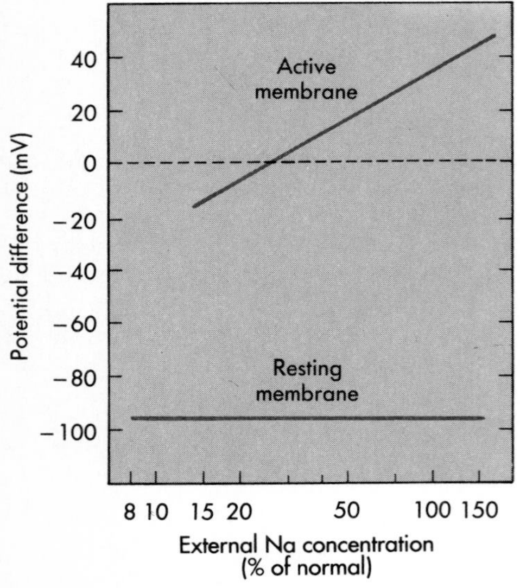

Fig. 2-5 ■ Concentration of sodium in the external medium is a critical determinant of the amplitude of the action potential in cardiac muscle *(upper curve)* but has relatively little influence on the resting potential *(lower curve)*. (Redrawn from Weidmann, S.: Elektrophysiologie der Herzmuskelfaser, Bern, 1956, Verlag Hans Huber.)

Ionic Basis of the Fast Response

Genesis of the Upstroke. Any process that abruptly changes the resting membrane potential to a critical value (called the **threshold**) will result in a propagated action potential. The characteristics of fast-response action potentials are shown in Fig. 2-1, *A*. The rapid depolarization (phase 0) is related almost exclusively to the inrush of Na^+ by virtue of a sudden increase in g_{Na}. The **amplitude** of the action potential (the potential change during phase 0) varies linearly with the logarithm of $[Na^+]_o$, as shown in Fig. 2-5. When $[Na^+]_o$ is reduced from its normal value of about 140 mM to about 20 mM, the cell is no longer excitable.

The physical and chemical forces responsible for these transmembrane movements of Na^+ are explained in Fig. 2-6. When the resting membrane potential, V_m, is suddenly changed to the threshold level of about −65 mV, the properties of the cell membrane change dramatically. Specific **fast channels** for Na^+ exist in the membrane. These channels can be blocked specifically by the puffer fish toxin, **tetrodotoxin.** Also, many of the drugs used to treat certain cardiac rhythm disturbances act principally on these fast Na^+ channels.

Na^+ moves through these channels in a manner that suggests that the flux is controlled by two types of "gates" in each channel. One of these gates, the **m** gate, tends to open the channel as V_m becomes less negative and is therefore called an **activation gate.** The other,

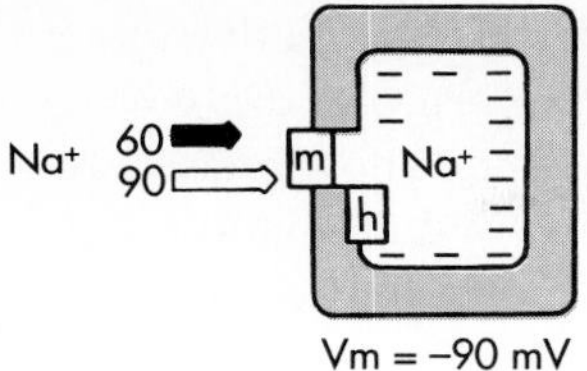

A, During phase 4, the chemical (60 mV) and electrostatic (90 mV) forces favor influx of Na^+ from the extracellular space. Influx is negligible, however, because the activation **(m)** gates are closed.

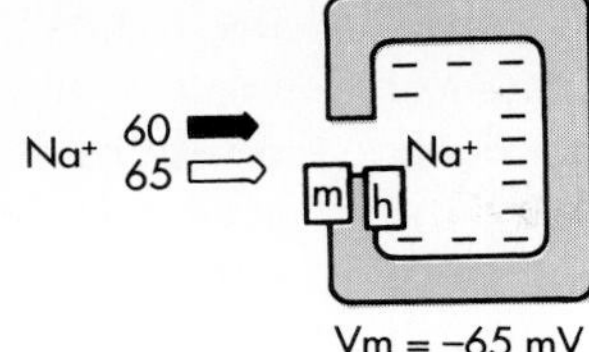

B, If V_m is brought to about −65 V, the **m** gates begin to swing open, and Na^+ begins to enter the cell. This reduces the negative charge inside the cell, and thereby opens still more Na^+ channels, which accelerates the influx of Na^+. The change in V_m also initiates the closure of inactivation **(h)** gates, which operate more slowly than the **m** gates.

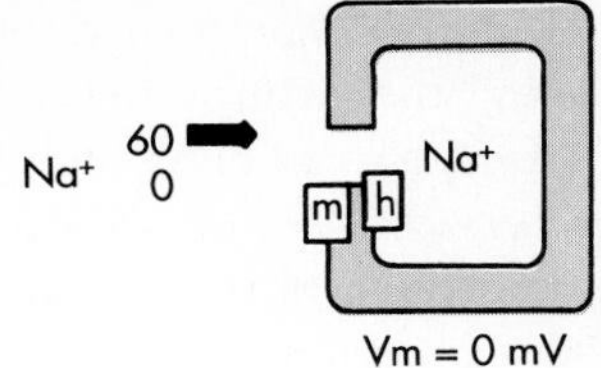

C, The rapid influx of Na^+ rapidly decreases the negativity of V_m. As V_m approaches 0, the electrostatic force attracting Na^+ into the cell is neutralized. Na^+ continues to enter the cell, however, because of the substantial concentration gradient, and V_m begins to become positive.

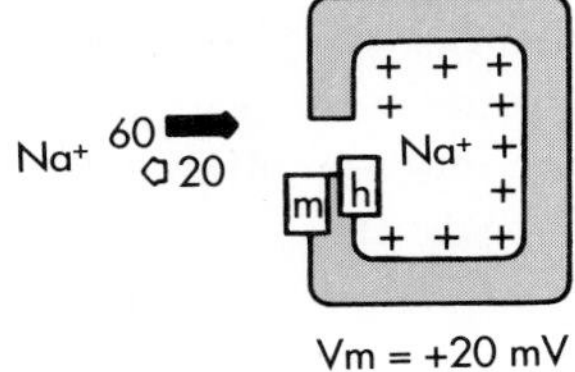

D, When V_m is positive by about 20 mV, Na^+ continues to enter the cell, because the diffusional forces (60 mV) exceed the opposing electrostatic forces (20 mV). The influx of Na^+ is slow, however, because the net driving force is small, and many of the inactivation gates have already closed.

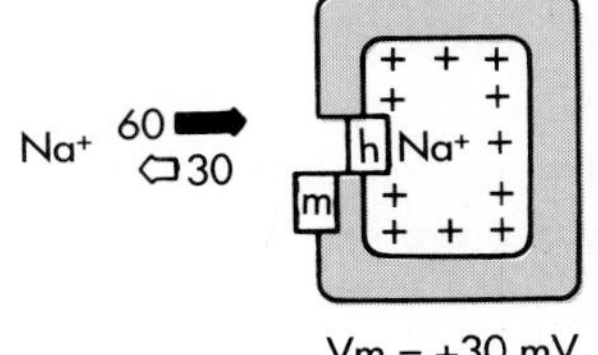

E, When V_m reaches about 30 mV, the **h** gates have now all closed, and Na^+ influx ceases. The **h** gates remain closed until the first half of repolarization, and thus the cell is absolutely refractory during this entire period. During the second half of repolarization, the **m** and **h** gates approach the state represented by panel *A,* and thus the cell is relatively refractory.

Fig. 2-6 ■ The gating of a sodium channel in a cardiac cell membrane during phase 4 *(panel A)* and during various stages of the action potential upstroke *(panels B* to *E*). The positions of the **m** and **h** gates in the fast Na^+ channels are shown at the various levels of V_m. The electrostatic forces are represented by the white arrows and the chemical (diffusional) forces by the black arrows.

the **h** gate, tends to close the channel as V_m becomes less negative and hence is called an **inactivation gate.** The **m** and **h** designations were originally employed by Hodgkin and Huxley in their mathematical model of conduction in nerve fibers.

With the cell at rest, V_m is about −90 mV. At this level, the **m** gates are closed and the **h** gates are wide open, as shown in Fig. 2-6, *A.* The concentration of Na^+ is much greater outside than inside the cell, and the interior of the cell is electrically negative with respect to the exterior. Hence, both chemical and electrostatic forces are oriented to draw Na^+ into the cell.

The electrostatic force in Fig. 2-6, *A,* is a potential difference of 90 mV, and it is represented by the white arrow. The chemical force, based on the difference in Na^+ concentration between the outside and inside of the cell, is represented by the black arrow. For a Na^+ concentration difference of about 130 mM, a potential difference of 60 mV (inside more positive than the outside) would be necessary to counterbalance the chemical, or diffusional, force, according to the Nernst equation for Na^+ (equation 2). Therefore, we may represent the net chemical force favoring the inward movement of Na^+ in Fig. 2-6 (black arrows) as being equivalent to a potential of 60 mV. With the cell at rest the total electrochemical force favoring the inward movement of Na^+ is 150 mV (panel *A*). The **m** gates are closed, however, and the conductance of the resting cell membrane to Na^+ is very low. Hence, virtually no Na^+ moves into the cell; that is, the **inward Na^+ current** is negligible.

Any process that makes V_m less negative tends to open the **m** gates, thereby "activating" the fast Na^+ channels. The activation of the fast channels is therefore called a **voltage-dependent** phenomenon. The precise potential at which the **m** gates swing open varies somewhat from one Na^+ channel to another in the cell membrane. As V_m becomes progressively less negative, more and more **m** gates will open. As the **m** gates open, Na^+ enters the cell (Fig. 2-6, *B*) by virtue of the chemical and electrostatic forces.

The entry of positively charged Na^+ into the interior of the cell neutralizes some of the negative charges inside the cell and thereby diminishes further the transmembrane potential, V_m. The resultant reduction in V_m, in turn, opens more **m** gates, thereby augmenting the inward Na^+ current. This is called a **regenerative process.** As V_m approaches about −65 mV, the remaining **m** gates rapidly swing open in the fast Na^+ channels until virtually all of the **m** gates are open (Fig. 2-6, *B*).

The rapid opening of the *m* gates in the fast Na^+ channels is responsible for the large and

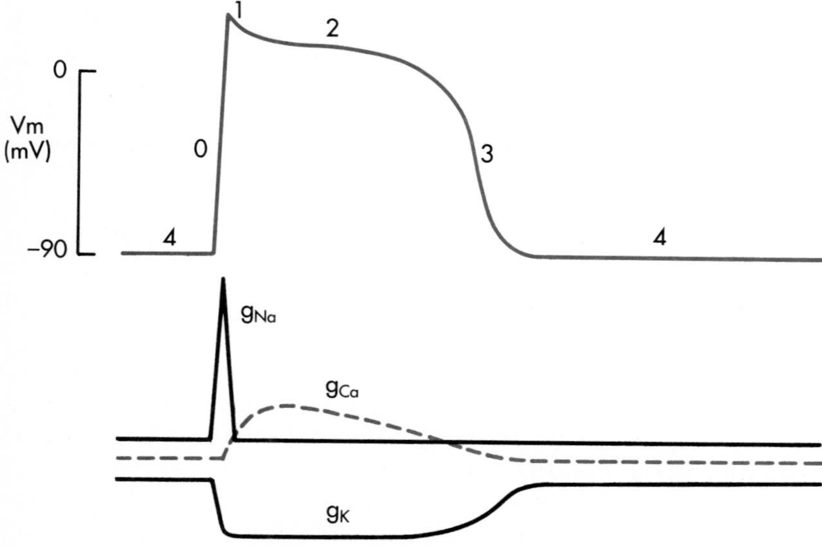

Fig. 2-7 ■ Changes in the conductances of Na^+ (g_{Na}), Ca^{++} (g_{Ca}), and K^+ (g_K) during the various phases of the action potential of a fast-response cardiac cell. The conductance diagram shows directional changes only.

abrupt increase in Na^+ conductance, g_{Na}, coincident with phase 0 of the action potential (Fig. 2-7). The rapid influx of Na^+ accounts for the rapid rate of change of V_m during phase 0. The maximum rate of change of V_m (that is, the maximum dV_m/dt) varies from 100 to 200 V/s in myocardial cells and from 500 to 1000 V/s in Purkinje fibers. Although the quantity of Na^+ that enters the cell during one action potential alters V_m by over 100 mV, that quantity of Na^+ is too small to change the intracellular Na^+ concentration measurably. The chemical force remains virtually constant, and only the electrostatic force changes throughout the action potential. Hence, the lengths of the black arrows in Fig. 2-6 remain constant at 60 mV, whereas the white arrows change in magnitude and direction.

As Na^+ rushes into the cardiac cell during phase 0, the negative charges inside the cell are neutralized, and V_m becomes progressively less negative. When V_m becomes zero (Fig. 2-6, *C*), an electrostatic force no longer pulls Na^+ into the cell. As long as the fast Na^+ channels are open, however, Na^+ continues to enter the cell because of the large concentration gradient. This continuation of the inward Na^+ current causes the inside of the cell to become positively charged (Fig. 2-6, *D*). This reversal of the membrane polarity is the so-called **overshoot** of the cardiac action potential. Such a reversal of the electrostatic gradient would, of course, tend to repel the entry of Na^+ (Fig. 2-6, *D*). However, as long as the inwardly directed chemical forces exceed these outwardly directed electrostatic forces, the net flux of Na^+ will still be inward, although the rate of influx will be diminished.

The inward Na^+ current finally ceases when the **h** (inactivation) gates close (Fig. 2-6, *E*). The activity of the **h** gates is governed by the value of V_m just as is that of the **m** gates. However, whereas the **m** gates open as V_m becomes less negative, the **h** gates close under this same influence. The opening of the **m** gates occurs very rapidly (in about 0.1 to 0.2 ms), whereas the closure of the **h** gates is slower, requiring 1 ms or more. Phase 0 is finally terminated when the **h** gates have closed and have thereby "inactivated" the fast Na^+ channels. The closure of the **h** gates so soon after the opening of the **m** gates accounts for the quick return of g_{Na} to near its resting value (Fig. 2-7).

The **h** gates then remain closed until the cell has partially repolarized during phase 3 (at about time *d* in Fig. 2-1, *A*). From time *c* to time *d*, the cell is in its **effective refractory period,** and it will not respond to further excitation. This mechanism prevents a sustained, tetanic contraction of cardiac muscle. Tetanus would of course preclude the normal intermittent pumping action of the heart.

About midway through phase 3 (time *d* in Fig. 2-1, *A*), the **m** and **h** gates in some of the fast Na^+ channels have resumed the states shown in Fig. 2-6, *A* . Such channels are said to have **recovered from inactivation.** The cell can begin to respond (but weakly at first) to further excitation (see Fig. 2-17). Throughout the remainder of phase 3, the cell completes its recovery from inactivation. By time *e* in Fig. 2-1, *A*, the **h** gates have reopened and the **m** gates have reclosed in the remaining fast Na^+ channels (see Fig. 2-6, *A*).

Statistical Characteristics of the "Gate" Concept. The patch-clamping technique has made it possible to measure ionic currents through single membrane channels. The individual channels have been observed to open and close repeatedly in a quasirandom sequence. This process is illustrated in Fig. 2-8, which shows the current flow through single Na^+ channels in a cultured myocardial cell. To the left of the arrow, the membrane potential was clamped at −85 mV. At the arrow, the potential was suddenly changed to −45 mV, at which value it was held for the remainder of the record.

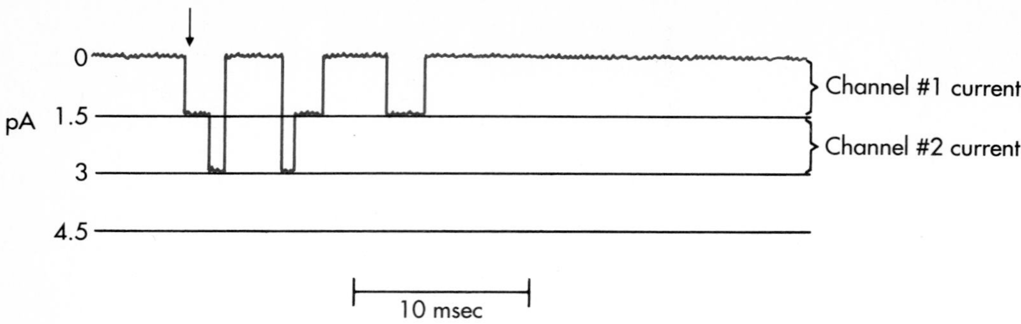

Fig. 2-8 ■ The current flow (in picoamperes) through two individual Na^+ channels in a cultured cardiac cell, recorded by the patch-clamping technique. The membrane potential had been held at −85 mV, but was suddenly changed to −45 mV at the arrow and held at this potential for the remainder of the record. One channel opened three times for about 3 ms each time, which allowed about 1.5 pA of current to flow through the membrane. During the first and second openings, a second channel opened for about 1 ms each time, permitting an additional 1.5 pA of current to flow. (Redrawn from Cachelin, A.B., DePeyer, J.E., Kokubun, S., and Reuter, H.: J. Physiol. 340:389, 1983.)

Fig. 2-8 indicates that immediately after the membrane potential was made less negative, one Na^+ channel opened three times in sequence. It remained open for about 2 or 3 ms each time and was closed for about 4 or 5 ms between openings. In the open state, it allowed 1.5 pA of current to pass. During the first and second openings of this channel, a second channel also opened, but for periods of only 1 ms. During the brief times that both channels were open simultaneously, the total current was 3 pA. After the first channel closed for the third time, both channels remained closed for the rest of the recording, even though the membrane was held at a constant level of relative depolarization.

The overall change in ionic conductance of the entire cell membrane at any given time reflects the number of channels that happens to be open at that time. Because the individual channels open and close in an irregular pattern, the overall membrane conductance represents the statistical probability of the open or closed state of the individual channels. The temporal characteristics of the activation process then represent the time course of the increasing probability that the specific channels will be open, rather than the kinetic characteristics of the activation gates in the individual channels. Similarly, the temporal characteristics of inactivation reflect the time course of the decreasing probability that the channels will be open and not the kinetic characteristics of the inactivation gates in the individual channels.

Genesis of Early Repolarization. In many cardiac cells that have a prominent plateau, phase 1 constitutes an early, brief period of limited repolarization between the end of the upstroke and the beginning of the plateau. Phase 1 reflects the activation of a **transient outward current,** i_{to}, mostly carried by K^+. Activation of these K^+ channels during phase 1 leads to a brief efflux of K^+ from the cell because the interior of the cell is positively charged and because the internal K^+ concentration greatly exceeds the external concentration (Fig. 2-9). This brief efflux of positively

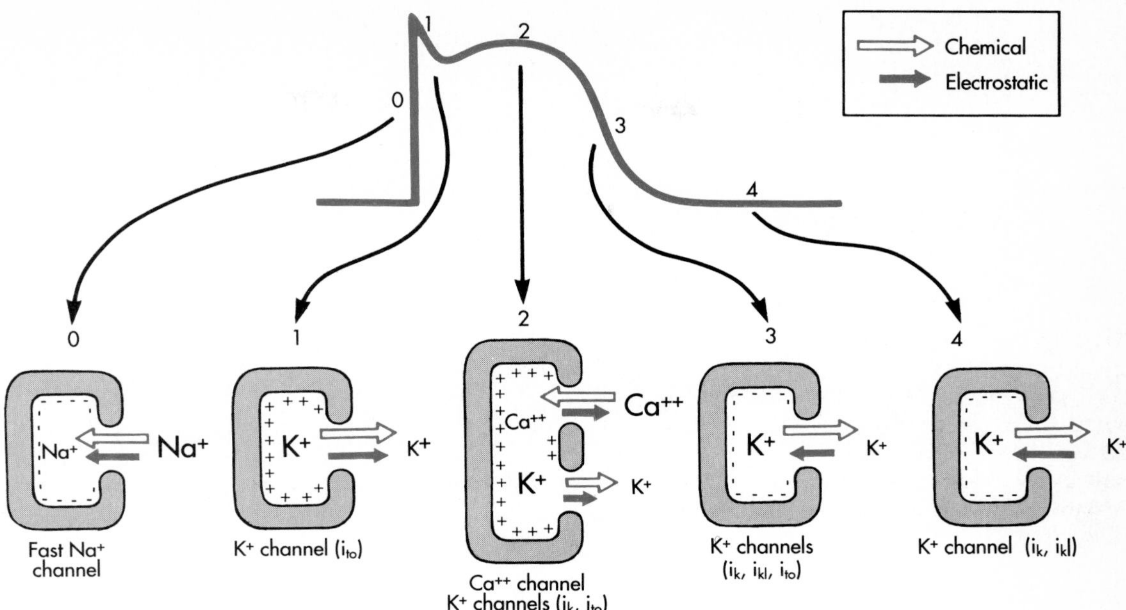

Fig. 2-9 ■ The principal ionic currents and channels that generate the action potential in a cardiac cell.

Phase 0. The chemical and electrostatic forces both favor the entry of Na^+ into the cell through fast Na^+ channels to generate the upstroke.

Phase 1. The chemical and electrostatic forces both favor the efflux of K^+ through i_{to} channels to generate early, partial repolarization.

Phase 2. During the plateau, the net influx of Ca^{++} through Ca^{++} channels is balanced by the efflux of K^+ through i_K, i_{K1}, and i_{to} channels.

Phase 3. The chemical forces that favor the efflux of K^+ through i_K, i_{K1}, and i_{to} channels predominate over the electrostatic forces that favor the influx of K^+ through these same channels.

Phase 4. The chemical forces that favor the efflux of K^+ through i_K and i_{K1} channels exceed very slightly the electrostatic forces that favor the influx of K^+ through these same channels.

charged ions brings about the brief, limited repolarization (phase 1).

Phase 1 is prominent in Purkinje fibers (see Fig. 2-14) and in epicardial fibers from the ventricular myocardium (Fig. 2-10); it is much less developed in endocardial fibers. When the basic cycle length (BCL) at which the epicardial fibers are driven is increased from 300 to 2000 ms, phase 1 becomes more pronounced and the action potential duration is increased substantially. The same increase in basic cycle length has no effect on the early portion of the plateau in endocardial fibers, and it has a smaller effect on the action potential duration than it does in epicardial fibers (Fig. 2-10). In the presence of 4-aminopyridine, which blocks the K^+ channels that carry i_{to}, phase 1 disappears in the epicardial action potentials. However, this compound does not affect the beginning of the plateau in the endocardial action potentials.

Genesis of the Plateau. During the plateau (phase 2) of the action potential, Ca^{++} and some Na^+ enters the cell through channels that activate and inactivate much more slowly than do the fast Na^+ channels. During

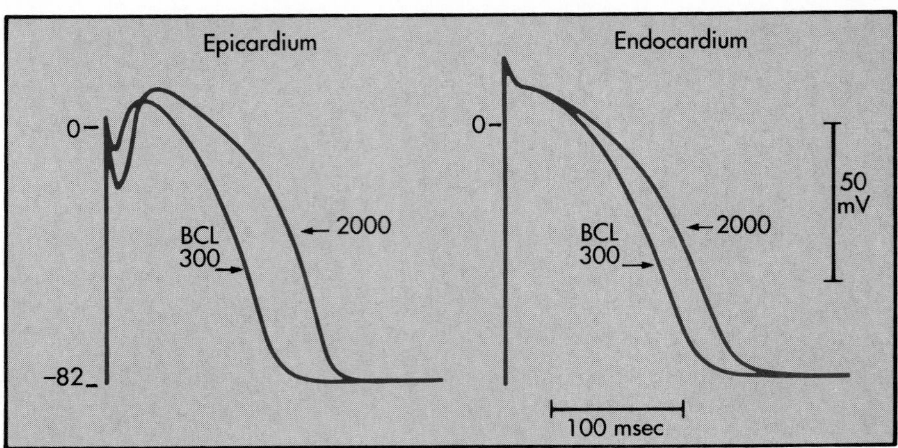

Fig. 2-10 ■ Action potentials recorded from canine epicardial and endocardial strips driven at basic cycle lengths of 300 and 2000 ms. (From Litovsky, S.H., and Antzelevitch, C.: J. Am. Coll. Cardiol., 19:1053, 1989.)

the flat portion of phase 2 (see Fig. 2-9), this influx of positive charge (carried by Ca^{++} and Na^{+}) is balanced by the efflux of an equal amount of positive charge (carried by K^{+}). The K^{+} exits through channels that conduct mainly the i_{to}, i_K, and i_{K1} currents. The i_{to} current is responsible for phase 1, as described previously, but it is not completely inactivated until after phase 2 has expired. The i_K and i_{K1} currents will be described below.

Ca^{++} conductance during the plateau. The slow channels that conduct the inward cationic currents are about 50 to 100 times more permeable to Ca^{++} than to Na^{+}, and therefore they are usually referred to as **calcium channels.** Nevertheless, about 10 to 20 percent of the current may be carried by Na^{+}, because the concentration gradient is so much greater for Na^{+} than for Ca^{++}. The entry of these ions into the cell through the slow channels has been called the **slow inward current,** i_{si}, but now it is more commonly called the **calcium current,** i_{Ca}.

The Ca^{++} channels are voltage-regulated channels that are activated as V_m becomes progressively less negative during the upstroke of the action potential. Two types of Ca^{++} channels (**L-type** and **T-type**) have been identified in cardiac tissues. Some of their important characteristics are illustrated in Fig. 2-11, which displays the Ca^{++} currents generated by voltage-clamping an isolated atrial myocyte. Note that when V_m is suddenly increased to +30 mV from a holding potential of −30 mV (lower panel), an inward Ca^{++} current (denoted by a downward deflection) is activated. Note also that after the inward current reaches its maximum value (in the downward direction), it returns toward zero very gradually; (i.e., the channel inactivates very slowly). Thus, the current that passes through these channels is **long lasting**, and they have therefore been designated as L-type channels. They are the predominant type of Ca^{++} channels in the heart, and are activated during the action potential upstroke when V_m reaches about −10 mV. The L-type channels are blocked by the so-called **Ca^{++} channel blocking drugs,** such as verapamil, nifedipine, and diltiazem.

The T-type (transient) Ca^{++} channels are much less abundant in the heart. They are activated at more negative potentials (about −70 mV) than are the L-type channels. Note in Fig.

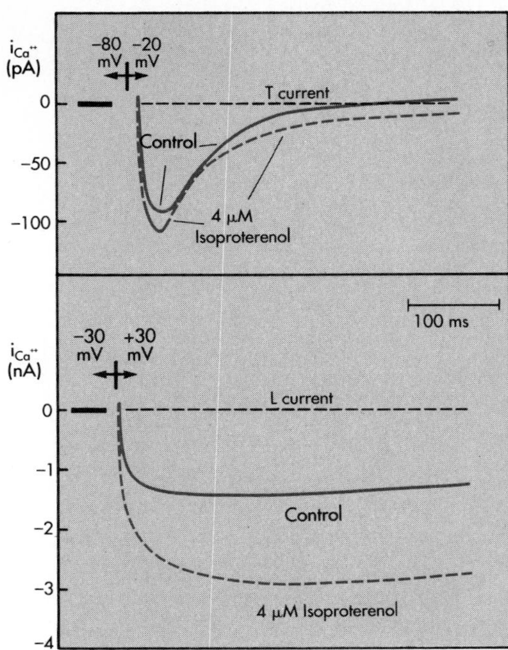

Fig. 2-11 ■ Effects of isoproterenol on the Ca^{++} currents conducted by T-type (upper panel) and L-type (lower panel) Ca^{++} channels in canine atrial myocytes. Upper panel, potential changed from −80 to −20 mV; lower panel, potential changed from −30 to +30 mV. (Redrawn from Bean, B.P.: J. Gen. Physiol., 86:1, 1985.)

2-11 (upper panel) that when V_m is suddenly increased to −20 mV from a holding potential of −80 mV, a Ca^{++} current is activated and then is inactivated very quickly. Note how quickly the current returns to zero even though V_m is maintained at −20 mV. The **transient** nature of this current accounts for the designation of the conducting channels as T-type channels. The T-type channels are not blocked by the commonly used Ca^{++} channel blocking drugs, but they can be blocked experimentally by Ni^{++}.

Opening of the Ca^{++} channels is reflected by an increase in Ca^{++} conductance (g_{Ca}), which begins immediately after the upstroke of the action potential (see Fig. 2-7). At the beginning of the action potential, the intracellular Ca^{++} concentration is much less than the extracellular concentration (Table 2-1). Consequently, with the increase in g_{Ca}, there is an influx of Ca^{++} into the cell throughout the plateau. The Ca^{++} that enters the myocardial cell during the plateau is involved in **excitation-contraction coupling,** as described in Chapter 3.

Various factors may influence g_{Ca}. This conductance may be increased by catecholamines, such as isoproterenol and norepinephrine. This is probably the principal mechanism by which catecholamines enhance cardiac muscle contractility.

Catecholamines interact with β-adrenergic receptors located in the cardiac cell membranes. This interaction stimulates the membrane bound enzyme, **adenylyl cyclase,** which raises the intracellular concentration of **cyclic AMP.** This change enhances the activation of the L-type Ca^{++} channels in the cell membrane (see Fig. 2-11, lower panel) and thus augments the influx of Ca^{++} into the cells from the interstitial fluid. However, catecholamines do not affect the Ca^{++} current through the T-type channels (upper panel).

The Ca^{++} channel blocking drugs decrease g_{Ca}. By reducing the amount of Ca^{++} that enters the myocardial cells during phase 2, these drugs diminish the strength of the cardiac contraction (Fig. 2-12).

K^+ conductance during the plateau. During the plateau of the action potential, the concentration gradient for K^+ between the inside and outside of the cell is virtually the same as it is during phase 4, but the V_m is positive. Therefore the chemical and electrostatic forces greatly favor the efflux of K^+ from the cell (see Fig. 2-9). If g_K were the same during the plateau as it is during phase 4, the efflux of K^+ during phase 2 would greatly exceed the influx of Ca^{++} and Na^+, and a sustained pla-

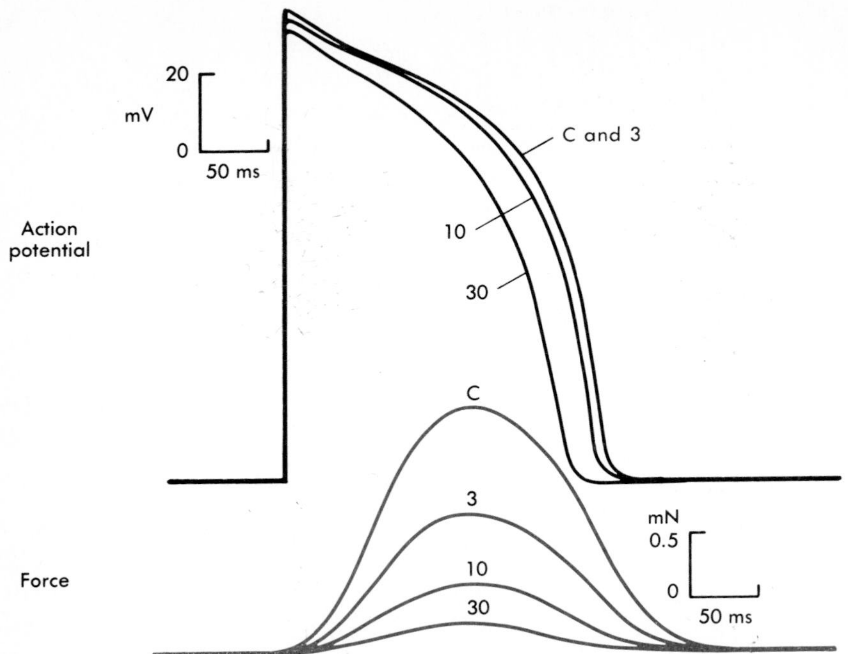

Fig. 2-12 ■ The effects of diltiazem, a Ca^{++} channel blocking drug, on the action potentials (in millivolts) and isometric contractile forces (in millinewtons) recorded from an isolated papillary muscle of a guinea pig. The tracings were recorded under control conditions *(C)* and in the presence of diltiazem, in concentrations of 3, 10, and 30 μmol/L. (Redrawn with permission from Hirth, C., Borchard, U., and Hafner, D.: Journal of Molecular and Cellular Cardiology 15:799, Copyright 1983 by Academic Press, Inc. [London], Limited.)

teau could not be achieved. However, as Vm attains positive values near the end of phase 0, g_K suddenly decreases (see Fig. 2-7).

This reduction in g_K at positive values of V_m is called **inward rectification,** which is a characteristic of the i_{K1} current. The current-voltage relationship of the K^+ channels that conduct i_{K1} has been determined by voltage-clamping cardiac cells (Fig. 2-13). Note that for the cell depicted in the figure, the current-voltage curve intersects the voltage axis at a V_m of −70 mV. The absence of ionic current flow at the point of intersection indicates that the electrostatic forces must have been equal to the chemical (diffusional) forces (see Fig. 2-3) at this potential. Thus, in this ventricular cell, the Nernst equilibrium potential (E_k) for K^+ must have been −70 mV.

When the membrane potential was clamped at levels negative to −70 mV in this cardiac cell (see Fig. 2-13), the electrostatic forces exceeded the chemical forces and an **inward** K^+ current was induced (as denoted by the negative values of K^+ current over this range of voltages). Note also that for V_m negative to −70 mV, the curve has a steep slope, even at the point of intersection (at which $V_m = E_k$). Thus, when V_m equals or is negative to E_K, a small change in V_m induces a large change in K^+ current; that is, g_K is large. During phase 4,

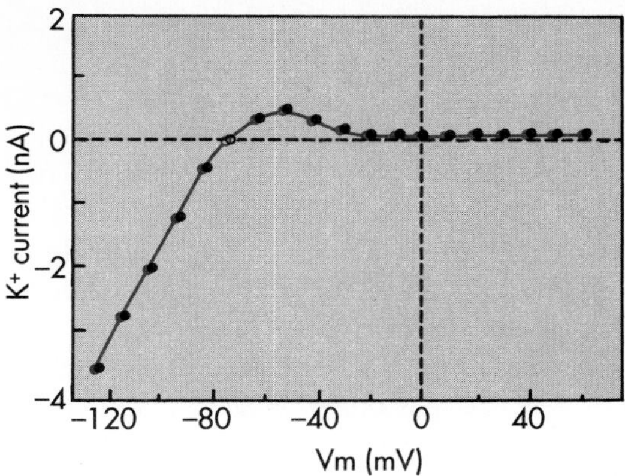

Fig. 2-13 ■ The K^+ currents recorded from a rabbit ventricular myocyte when the potential was changed from a holding potential of −80 mV to various test potentials. Positive values along the vertical axis represent outward currents; negative values represent inward currents. The V_m coordinate of the point of intersection (open circle) of the curve with the X axis is the reversal potential; it denotes the equilibrium potential at which the chemical and electrostatic forces are equal. (Redrawn from Giles, W.R., and Imaizumi, Y.: J. Physiol. (London) 405:123, 1988.)

the V_m of a myocardial cell is approximately equal to E_k; it is actually slightly less negative (see Fig. 2-4). The substantial g_K that prevails during phase 4 of the cardiac action potential (see Fig. 2-7) is accounted for mainly by the i_{K1} channels.

When the transmembrane potential was clamped at levels positive to −70 mV (see Fig. 2-13), the chemical forces exceeded the electrostatic forces. Therefore, the net K^+ currents were **outward** (as denoted by the positive values along the corresponding section of the Y axis). Note that for V_m values positive to −70 mV, the curve is relatively flat. Thus, a given change in voltage causes only a small change in ionic current; (i.e., g_K is small). Thus, g_K is small for outwardly directed K^+ currents, but it is substantial for inwardly directed K^+ currents; i.e., the i_{K1} current is **inwardly rectified**.

Another factor that contributes to the low g_K during the plateau is **delayed rectification,** which is a characteristic of the i_K channels. These K^+ channels are activated by the voltages that prevail toward the end of phase 0, but activation proceeds very slowly, over several hundreds of milliseconds. Hence, activation of these channels tends to increase g_K very slowly and slightly during phase 2. The reduction in g_K achieved by the inward rectification of the i_{K1} current predominates over the tendency for the i_K current to increase g_K throughout the plateau.

The diminished g_K associated with inward rectification prevents an excessive loss of K^+ from the cell during the plateau. The small outward K^+ current that does occur is sufficient to balance the slow inward currents of Ca^{++} and Na^+; hence, V_m remains relatively constant during phase 2.

The effects of altering this balance between the inward currents of Ca^{++} and Na^+ and the outward current of K^+ are demonstrated by the administration of a calcium channel blocking drug. Fig. 2-12 shows that with increasing concentrations of diltiazem, the voltage of the plateau becomes less positive, and the duration of the plateau diminishes.

Genesis of Final Repolarization. The process of final repolarization (phase 3) starts at the end of phase 2, when the efflux of K^+ from the cardiac cell begins to exceed the influx of Ca^{++} and Na^+. At least three outward K^+ currents (i_{to}, i_K, and i_{K1}) reflect the return of g_K to its resting level at the end of the plateau (see Fig. 2-7), and they bring about the rapid repolarization (phase 3) of the cardiac cell (see Fig. 2-9).

The **transient outward current** (i_{to}) not only accounts for phase 1, as previously described, but it also helps determine the duration of the plateau; hence it also helps initiate repolarization. For example, the transient outward current is much more pronounced in atrial than in ventricular myocytes. In atrial cells, therefore, the outward K^+ current exceeds the slow inward Ca^{++} current early in the plateau, whereas the outward and inward currents remain equal for a much longer time in ventricular myocytes. Hence, the plateau of the action potential is much less pronounced in atrial than in ventricular myocytes (see Fig. 2-21).

The **delayed rectifier** K^+ **current** (i_K) is activated near the end of phase 0, but activation is very slow. Hence, the outward i_K current tends to increase throughout the plateau. Concurrently, the Ca^{++} channels are inactivated after the beginning of the plateau, and therefore the slow inward currents of Ca^{++} and Na^+ are decreasing. As the efflux of K^+ begins to exceed the influx of Ca^{++} and Na^+, V_m becomes progressively less positive, and repolarization is initiated.

The **inwardly rectified** K^+ **current,** i_{K1}, contributes substantially to the process of repolarization. As the net efflux of cations causes V_m to become more negative during phase 3, the conductance of the channels that carry the i_{K1} current progressively increases. This is reflected by the hump that is evident in the flat portion of the current-voltage curve at V_m values between −20 and −70 mV. Thus, as V_m passes through this range of values, the outward K^+ current increases, and thereby accelerates repolarization.

Restoration of Ionic Concentrations. The excess Na^+ that had entered the cell mainly during phases 0 and 2 is eliminated by a Na^+/K^+ ATPase, which ejects Na^+ in exchange for the K^+ that had exited mainly during phases 2 and 3. This ion pump exchanges Na^+ for K^+ in a ratio of 3:2.

Similarly, most of the excess Ca^{++} that had entered the cell during phase 2 is eliminated by a Na^+/Ca^{++} exchanger, which exchanges 3 Na^+ for 1 Ca^{++}. However, a small fraction of the Ca^{++} is eliminated by an ATP driven Ca^{++} pump (see page 61).

Ionic Basis of the Slow Response

Fast-response action potentials (see Fig. 2-1, *A*) may be considered to consist of three principal components, a spike (phases 0 and 1), a plateau (phase 2), and a period of repolarization (phase 3). In the slow response (see Fig. 2-1, *B*), the first component is absent, and the second and third components account for the entire action potential. In the fast response, the spike is produced by the influx of Na^+ through the fast channels. These channels can be blocked by certain compounds, such as tetrodotoxin. When the fast Na^+ channels are blocked, slow responses may be generated in the same fibers under appropriate conditions.

The Purkinje fiber action potentials shown

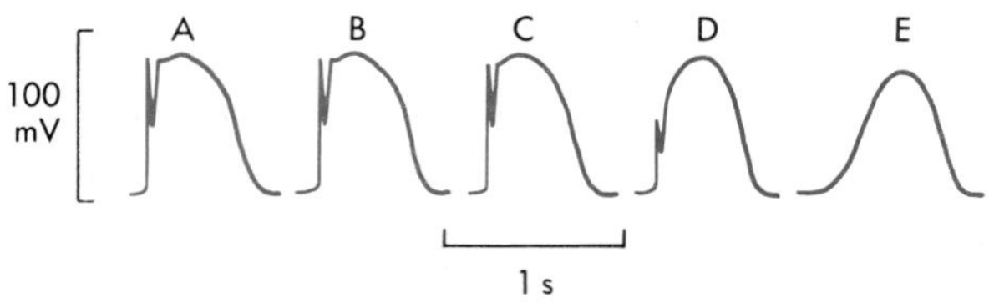

Fig. 2-14 ■ Effect of tetrodotoxin on the action potential recorded in a calf Purkinje fiber perfused with a solution containing epinephrine and 10.8 mM K^+. The concentration of tetrodotoxin was 0 M in **A,** 3×10^{-8} M in **B,** 3×10^{-7} M in **C,** and 3×10^{-6} M in **D** and **E; E** was recorded later than **D.** (Redrawn from Carmeliet, E., and Vereecke, J.: Pflügers Arch. 313:300, 1969.)

in Fig. 2-14 clearly exhibit the two response types. In the control tracing (panel *A*), a prominent notch separates the spike from the plateau. This notch at the beginning of the plateau represents a well-developed phase 1 (see Fig. 2-10), and is ascribable to the transient outward K^+ current, i_{to}. Action potential *A* is a typical fast response action potential. In action potentials *B* to *E*, progressively larger quantities of tetrodotoxin were added to the bathing solution to produce a graded blockade of the fast Na^+ channels. It is evident that the spike becomes progressively less prominent in action potentials *B* to *D*, and it disappears entirely in *E*. Thus, the tetrodotoxin had a pronounced effect on the spike, and only a negligible influence on the plateau. With elimination of the spike (panel *E*), the action potential resembles a typical slow response.

Certain cells in the heart, notably those in the SA and AV nodes, are normally slow response fibers. In such fibers, depolarization is achieved by the slow inward current of Ca^{++} and Na^+ through the Ca^{++} channels. These ionic events closely resemble those that occur during the plateau of fast-response action potentials.

■ CONDUCTION IN CARDIAC FIBERS

An action potential traveling down a cardiac muscle fiber is propagated by local circuit currents, similar to the process that occurs in nerve and skeletal muscle fibers. In Fig. 2-15, consider that the left half of the cardiac fiber already has been depolarized, whereas the right half is still in the resting state. The fluids normally in contact with the external and internal surfaces of the membrane are essentially solutions of electrolytes and thus are good conductors of electricity. Hence, current (in the abstract sense) will flow from regions of higher to those of lower potential, denoted by the plus and minus signs, respectively. In the external fluid, current will flow from right to left between the active and resting zones, and it will flow in the reverse direction intracellularly. In electrolyte solutions, the true current is carried by a movement of cations in one direction and anions in the opposite direction. At the cell exterior, for example, cations will flow from right to left, and anions from left to right (see Fig. 2-15). In the cell interior, the opposite migrations will occur. These local currents will tend to depolarize the region of the resting fiber adjacent to the border.

Conduction of the Fast Response

In the fast response, the fast Na^+ channels will be activated when the transmembrane potential is suddenly brought to the threshold value of about -70 mV. The inward Na^+ current will then depolarize the cell very rapidly at that site. This portion of the fiber will become part of the depolarized zone, and the border will be displaced accordingly (to the right in Fig. 2-15). The same process will then begin at the new border. This process will be repeated over and over, and the border will move continuously down the fiber as a wave of depolarization.

At any given point on the fiber, the greater the **amplitude** of the action potential and the greater the **rate of change of potential** (dV_m/dt) during phase 0, the more rapid the conduction down the fiber. The amplitude of the action potential equals the difference in

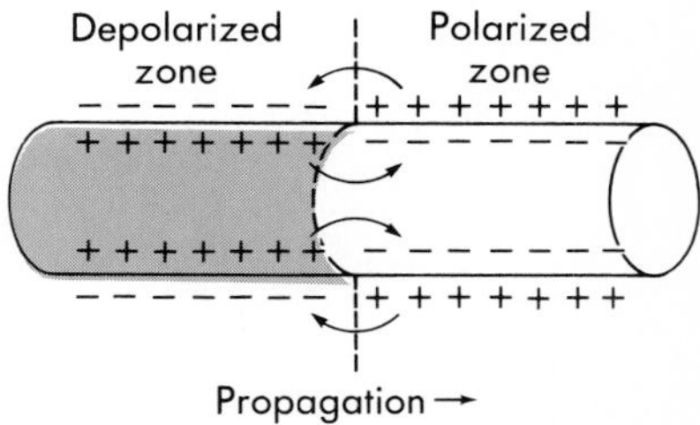

Fig. 2-15 ■ The role of local currents in the propagation of a wave of excitation down a cardiac fiber.

potential between the fully depolarized and the fully polarized regions of the cell interior (see Fig. 2-15). The magnitude of the local currents is proportional to this potential difference. Because these local currents shift the potential of the resting zone toward the threshold value, they are the local stimuli that depolarize the adjacent resting portion of the fiber to its threshold potential. The greater the potential difference between the depolarized and polarized regions (that is, the greater the amplitude of the action potential), the more efficacious the local stimuli, and the more rapidly the wave of depolarization is propagated down the fiber.

The **rate of change potential** (dV_m/dt) during phase 0 is also an important determinant of the conduction velocity. The reason can be appreciated by referring again to Fig. 2-15. If the active portion of the fiber depolarizes very gradually, the local currents across the border between the depolarized and polarized regions would be very small. Thus, the resting region adjacent to the active zone would be depolarized very slowly, and consequently each new section of the fiber would require more time to reach threshold.

The level of the resting membrane potential is also an important determinant of conduction velocity. This factor operates through its influence on the amplitude and maximum slope of the action potential. The resting potential may vary for several reasons: (1) it can be altered experimentally by varying $[K^+]_o$ (see Fig. 2-4), (2) in cardiac fibers that are intrinsically automatic V_m becomes progressively less negative during phase 4 (see Fig. 2-21, *B*), and (3) during a premature contraction, repolarization may not have been completed when the next excitation arrives (see Fig. 2-17). In general, the less negative the level of V_m, the less the velocity of impulse propagation, regardless of the reason for the change in V_m.

The V_m level affects conduction velocity because the inactivation, or **h**, gates (see Fig. 2-6) in the fast Na^+ channels are voltage dependent. The less negative the V_m, the greater is the number of **h** gates that tend to close. During the normal process of excitation, depolarization proceeds so rapidly during phase 0

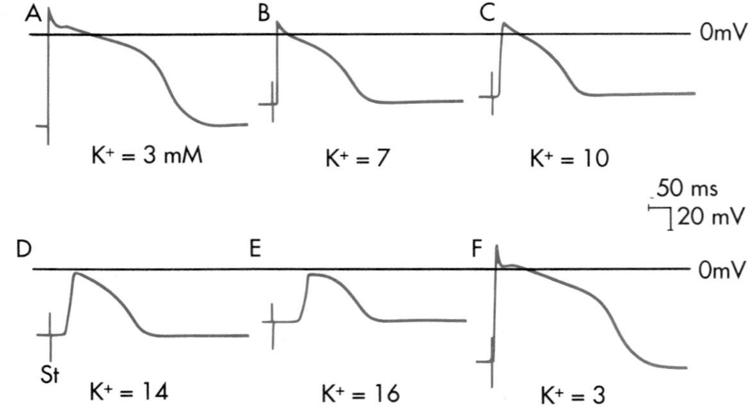

Fig. 2-16 ■ The effect of changes in external potassium concentration on the transmembrane action potentials recorded from a Purkinje fiber. The stimulus artifact (St) appears as a biphasic spike to the left of the upstroke of the action potential. The horizontal lines near the peaks of the action potentials denote 0 mV. (From Myerburg, R.J., and Lazzara, R. In Fisch, E., editor: Complex electrocardiography, Philadelphia, 1973, F.A. Davis Co.)

that the comparatively slow **h** gates do not close until the end of that phase. If partial depolarization is produced by a more gradual process, however, such as by elevating the level of external K^+, then the **h** gates have ample time to close and thereby inactivate some of the Na^+ channels. When the cell is partially depolarized, many of the Na^+ channels will already be inactivated, and only a fraction of these channels will be available to conduct the inward Na^+ current during phase 0.

The results of an experiment in which the resting V_m of a bundle of Purkinje fibers was varied by altering the value of $[K^+]_0$ are shown in Fig. 2- 16 . When $[K^+]_0$ was 3 mM (panels *A* and *F*), the resting V_m was −82 mV and the slope of phase 0 was steep. At the end of phase 0, the overshoot attained a value of 30 mV. Hence, the amplitude of the action potential was 112 mV. The tissue was stimulated at some distance from the impaled cell, and the stimulus artifact (St) appears as a diphasic deflection just before phase 0. The time from this artifact to the beginning of phase 0 is inversely proportional to the conduction velocity.

When $[K^+]_0$ was increased to 16 mM (panels *B* to *E*), the resting V_m became progressively less negative. Concomitantly, the amplitudes and durations of the action potentials and the steepness of the upstrokes all diminished. As a consequence, the conduction velocity diminished progressively, as indicated by the distances from the stimulus artifacts to the upstrokes.

At the $[K^+]_0$ levels of 14 and 16 mM (panels *D* and *E*), the resting V_m had attained levels sufficient to inactivate all the fast Na^+ channels. The action potentials in panels *D* and *E* are characteristic slow responses, presumably mediated by the slow inward current of Ca^{++} and Na^+. When the $[K^+]_0$ concentration of 3 mM was reestablished (panel *F*), the action potential was again characteristic of the normal fast response (as in panel *A*).

Conduction of the Slow Response

Local circuits (see Fig. 2-15) are also responsible for propagation of the slow response. However, the characteristics of the conduction process differ quantitatively from those of the fast response. The threshold potential is about −40 mV for the slow response, and conduction is much slower than for the fast response. The conduction velocities of the slow responses in the SA and AV nodes are about 0.02 to 0.1 m/s. The fast response conduction velocities are about 0.3 to 1 m/s for myocardial cells and 1 to 4 m/s for the specialized conducting fibers in the atria and ventricles. Slow responses are more likely to be blocked than are fast responses. Also, the former cannot be conducted at such rapid repetition rates.

■ CARDIAC EXCITABILITY

Currently, more detailed knowledge of cardiac excitability is being acquired because of the rapid development of artificial pacemakers and other electrical devices for correcting serious disturbances of rhythm. The excitability characteristics of cardiac cells differ considerably, depending on whether the action potentials are fast or slow responses.

Fast Response

Once the fast response has been initiated, the depolarized cell will no longer be excitable until about the middle of the period of final repolarization (see Fig. 2-1, *A*). The interval from the beginning of the action potential until the fiber is able to conduct another action potential is called the **effective refractory period.** In the fast response, this period extends from the beginning of phase 0 to a point in phase 3 where repolarization has reached about −50 mV (time *c* to time *d* in Fig. 2-1, *A*). At about this value of V_m the electrochemical gates (**m** and **h**) for many of the fast Na^+ channels have been reset.

Full excitability is not regained until the car-

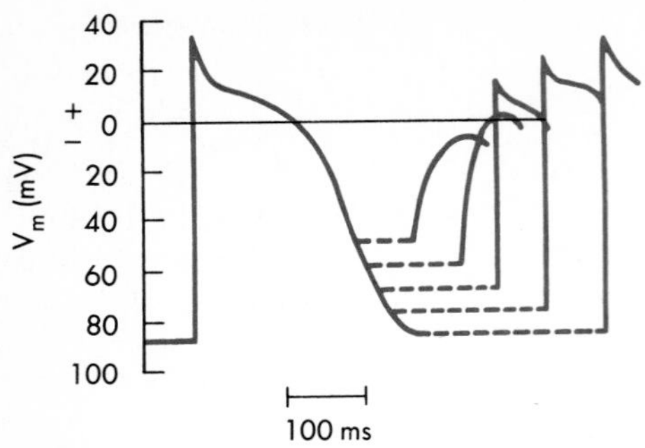

Fig. 2-17 ■ The changes in action potential amplitude and slope of the upstroke as action potentials are initiated at different stages of the relative refractory period of the preceding excitation. (Redrawn from Rosen, M.R., Wit, A.L., and Hoffman, B.F.: Am. Heart J. 88:380, 1974.)

diac fiber has been fully repolarized (time *e* in Fig. 2-1, *A*). During period *d* to *e* in the figure, an action potential may be evoked, but only when the stimulus is stronger than that which could elicit a response during phase 4. Period *d* to *e* is called the **relative refractory period.**

When a fast response is evoked during the relative refractory period of a prior excitation, its characteristics vary with the membrane potential that exists at the time of stimulation. The nature of this voltage dependency is illustrated in Fig. 2-17. As the fiber is stimulated later and later in the relative refractory period, the amplitude of the response and the rate of rise of the upstroke increase progressively. Presumably, the number of fast Na^+ channels that have recovered from inactivation increases as repolarization proceeds during phase 3. As a consequence of the greater amplitude and upstroke slope of the evoked response, the propagation velocity increases as the cell is stimulated later in the relative refractory period. Once the fiber is fully repolarized, the response is constant no matter what time in phase 4 the stimulus is applied. By the end of phase 3, the **m** and **h** gates of all channels are in their final positions and no further change in excitability occurs.

Slow Response

The relative refractory period during the slow response frequently extends well beyond phase 3 (see Fig. 2-1, *B*). Even after the cell has completely repolarized, it may be difficult to evoke a propagated response for some time.

Action potentials evoked early in the relative refractory period are small and the upstokes are not very steep (Fig. 2-18). The amplitudes and upstroke slopes gradually improve as action potentials are elicited later and later in the relative refractory period. The recovery of full excitability is much slower than for the fast response. Impulses that arrive early in its relative refractory period are conducted much more slowly than those that arrive late in that period. The lengthy refractory periods also lead to conduction blocks. Even when slow responses recur at a low repetition rate, the fiber may be able to conduct only a fraction of those impulses.

Effects of Cycle Length

Changes in cycle length alter the action potential duration of cardiac cells and thus change their refractory periods. Consequently, the changes in cycle length are often important factors in the initiation or termination of certain arrhythmias. The changes in action potential durations produced by stepwise reductions in cycle length from 2000 to 200 ms in a Purkinje fiber are shown in Fig. 2-19. Note that as the cycle length is diminished, the action potential duration decreases.

This direct correlation between action potential duration and cycle length is ascribable to changes in g_K that involve at least two types of K^+ channels, namely, those that conduct the **delayed rectifier K^+ current,** i_K, and those that conduct the **transient outward K^+ current,** i_{to}.

The i_K current activates slowly and it re-

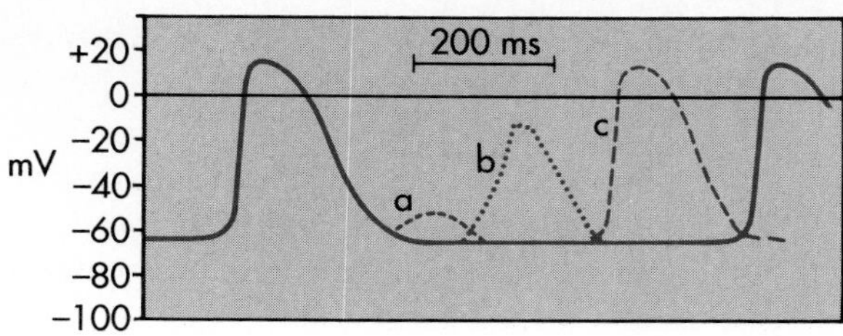

Fig. 2-18 ■ The effects of excitation at various times after the initiation of an action potential in a slow response fiber. In this fiber, excitation very late in phase 3 (or early in phase 4) induces a small, nonpropagated (local) response **(A).** Later in phase 4, a propagated response **(B)** may be elicited; its amplitude is small and the upstroke is not very steep. This response **(B)** will be conducted very slowly. Still later in phase 4, full excitability will be regained, and the response **(C)** will display its normal characteristics. (Modified from Singer, D.H., et al. Prog. Cardiovasc. Dis. 24:97, 1981.)

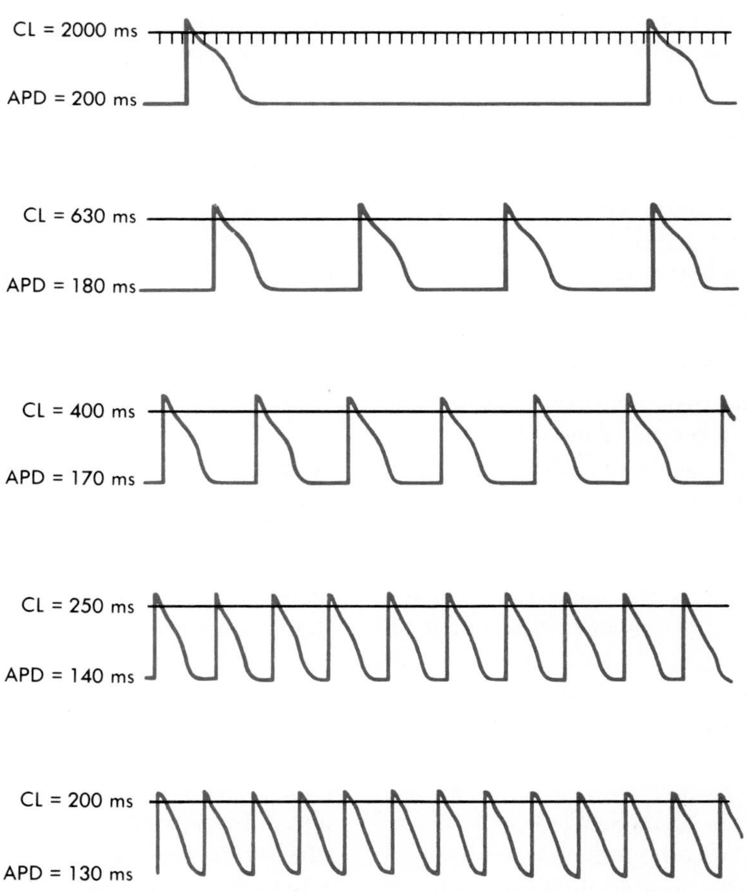

Fig. 2-19 ■ The effect of changes in cycle length *(CL)* on the action potential duration *(APD)* of canine Purkinje fibers. (Modified from Singer, D., and Ten Eick, R.E.: Am. J. Cardiol. 28:381, 1971.)

mains activated for hundreds of milliseconds before it is inactivated, and it also inactivates very slowly. Consequently, as the basic cycle length is diminished, each action potential tends to occur earlier in the inactivation period of the i_K current initiated by the preceding action potential. Therefore the shorter the basic cycle length, the greater will be the outward K^+ current during phase 2, and hence the briefer will be the action potential.

The i_{to} current also influences the relation between cycle length and action potential duration. Experiments on ventricular myocytes have demonstrated that a given increase in basic cycle length will prolong the action potential to a greater extent in epicardial than in endocardial fibers (see Fig. 2-10). The i_{to} current is much more prominent in epicardial than in endocardial fibers. Furthermore, after the myocyte preparations have been treated with 4-aminopyridine, which blocks i_{to}, the cycle length dependent changes in action potential duration do not differ in epicardial and endocardial myocytes.

■ NATURAL EXCITATION OF THE HEART

The nervous system controls various aspects of the behavior of the heart, including the frequency at which it beats and the vigor of each contraction. However, cardiac function certainly does not require intact nervous pathways. Indeed, a patient with a completely denervated heart (a cardiac transplant patient) can function well and can adapt to stressful situations.

The properties of **automaticity** (the ability to initiate its own beat) and of **rhythmicity** (the regularity of such pacemaking activity) are intrinsic to cardiac tissue. The heart will continue to beat even when it is completely removed from the body. If the coronary vasculature is artificially perfused, rhythmic cardiac contraction will persist for considerable periods of time. Apparently, at least some cells in the walls of all four cardiac chambers are capable of initiating beats; such cells probably reside in the nodal tissues or specialized conducting fibers of the heart.

The region of the mammalian heart that ordinarily generates impulses at the greatest frequency is the SA node; it is called the **natural pacemaker** of the heart.

Detailed mapping of the electrical potentials on the surface of the right atrium has revealed that two or three sites of automaticity, located 1 or 2 cm from the SA node itself, serve along with the SA node as an **atrial pacemaker complex.** At times, all of these loci initiate impulses simultaneously. At other times, the site of earliest excitation shifts from locus to locus, depending on such conditions as the level of autonomic neural activity.

Other regions of the heart that initiate beats under special circumstances are called **ectopic foci,** or **ectopic pacemakers.** Ectopic foci may become pacemakers when (1) their own rhythmicity becomes enhanced, (2) the rhythmicity of the higher order pacemakers becomes depressed, or (3) all conduction pathways between the ectopic focus and those regions with greater rhythmicity become blocked.

When the SA node and the other components of the atrial pacemaker complex are excised or destroyed, pacemaker cells in the AV junction usually are the next most rhythmic, and they become the pacemakers for the entire heart. After some time, which may vary from minutes to days, automatic cells in the atria usually become dominant. In the dog, the most common site for the ectopic atrial pacemaking region is at the junction between the inferior vena cava and the right atrium. Purkinje fibers in the specialized conduction system of the ventricles also possess automaticity. Characteristically, they fire at a very slow rate. When the AV junction is unable to conduct the cardiac impulse from the atria to the ventricles, such **idioventricular pacemakers** in the Purkinje fiber network initiate the ventric-

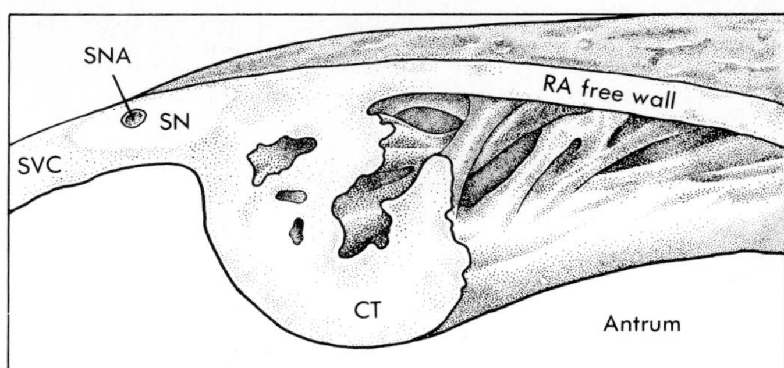

Fig. 2-20 ■ The location of the SA node near the junction between the superior vena cava and the right atrium. *SN,* SA node; *SNA,* sinoatrial artery; *SVC,* superior vena cava; *RA,* right atrium; *CT,* crista terminalis. (Redrawn from James, T.N.: Am. J. Cardiol. 40:965, 1977.)

ular contractions. Such ventricular contractions occur at a frequency of only 30 to 40 beats per minute.

Sinoatrial Node

The SA node is the phylogenetic remnant of the sinus venosus of lower vertebrate hearts. In humans it is about 8 mm long and 2 mm thick. It lies in the groove where the superior vena cava joins the right atrium (Fig. 2-20). The sinus node artery runs lengthwise through the center of the node.

The SA node contains two principal types of cells: (1) small, round cells, which have few organelles and myofibrils, and (2) slender, elongated cells, which are intermediate in appearance between the round and the ordinary atrial myocardial cells. The round cells are probably the pacemaker cells, whereas the transitional cells probably conduct the impulses within the node and to the nodal margins.

A typical transmembrane action potential recorded from a cell in the SA node is depicted in Fig. 2-21, *B*. Compared with the transmembrane potential recorded from a ventricular myocardial cell (Fig. 2-21, *A*), the resting potential of the SA node cell is usually less, the upstroke of the action potential (phase 0) is less steep, a plateau is not sustained, and repolarization (phase 3) is more gradual. These are all characteristic of the slow response. Under

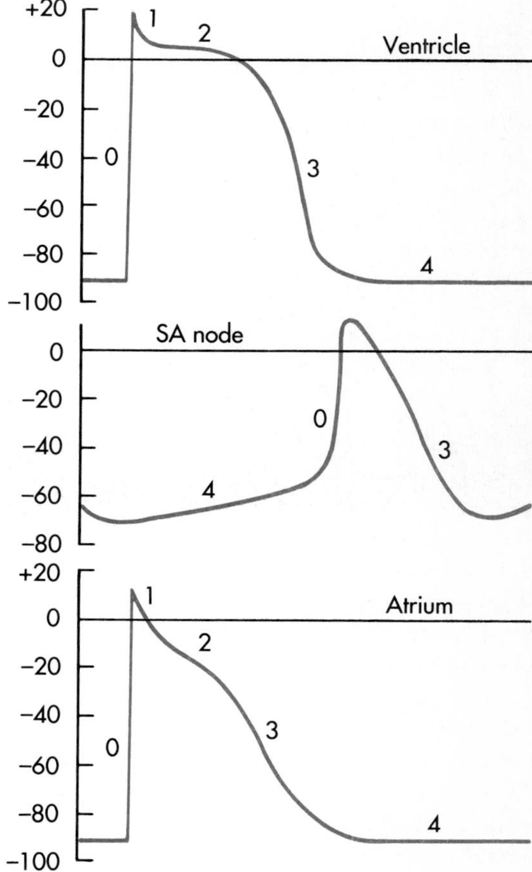

Fig. 2-21 ■ Typical action potentials (in millivolts) recorded from cells in the ventricle, **A,** SA node, **B,** and atrium, **C.** Sweep velocity in **B** is one half that in **A** or **C.** (From Hoffman, B.F., and Cranefield, P.F.: Electrophysiology of the heart, New York, 1960. Used by permission of McGraw-Hill Book Co.)

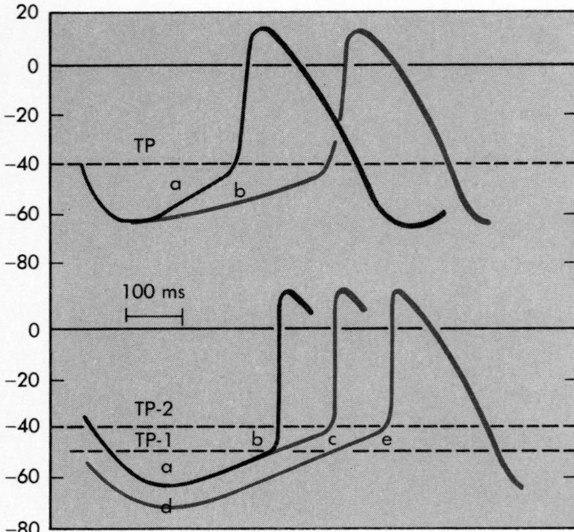

Fig. 2-22 ▪ Mechanisms involved in changes of frequency of pacemaker firing. In section **A** a reduction in the slope of the pacemaker potential from *a* to *b* will diminish the frequency. In section **B** an increase in the threshold (from *TP-1* to *TP-2*) or an increase in the magnitude of the resting potential (from *a* to *d*) will also diminish the frequency. (Redrawn from Hoffman, B.F., and Cranefield, P.F.: Electrophysiology of the heart, New York, 1960. Used by permission of McGraw-Hill Book Co.)

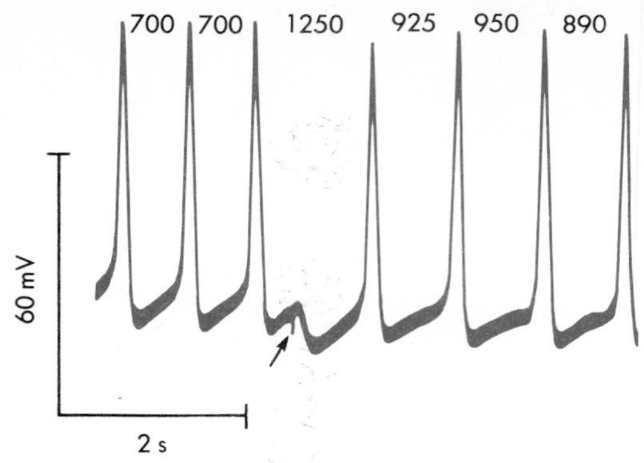

Fig. 2-23 ▪ Effect of a brief vagal stimulus *(arrow)* on the transmembrane potential recorded from an SA node pacemaker cell in an isolated cat atrium preparation. The cardiac cycle lengths, in milliseconds, are denoted by the numbers at the top of the figure. (Modified from Jalife, J., and Moe, G.K.: Circ. Res. 45:595, 1979.)

ordinary conditions, tetrodotoxin has no influence on the SA nodal action potential. This indicates that the upstroke of the action potential is not produced by an inward current of Na^+ through the fast channels.

However, the principal distinguishing feature of a pacemaker fiber resides in phase 4. In nonautomatic cells the potential remains constant during this phase, whereas in a pacemaker fiber there is a slow depolarization, called the **pacemaker potential,** throughout phase 4. Depolarization proceeds at a steady rate until a threshold is attained, and then an action potential is triggered.

The discharge frequency of pacemaker cells may be varied by a change in (1) the rate of depolarization during phase 4, (2) the threshold potential, or (3) the resting potential (Fig. 2-22). With an increase in the rate of depolarization (*b* to *a* in Fig. 2-22, *A*) the threshold potential will be attained earlier, and the heart rate will increase. A rise in the threshold potential (from *TP-1* to *TP-2* in Fig. 2-22, *B*) will delay the onset of phase 0 (from time *b* to time *c*), and the heart rate will be reduced accordingly. Similarly, when the maximum diastolic potential is increased (from *a* to *d*), more time will be required to reach threshold *TP-2* when the slope of phase 4 remains unchanged, and the heart rate will diminish.

Ordinarily, the frequency of pacemaker firing is controlled by the activity of both divisions of the autonomic nervous system. Increased sympathetic nervous activity, through the release of norepinephrine, raises the heart rate principally by increasing the slope of the pacemaker potential. Increased vagal activity, through the release of acetylcholine, diminishes the heart rate by hyperpolarizing the

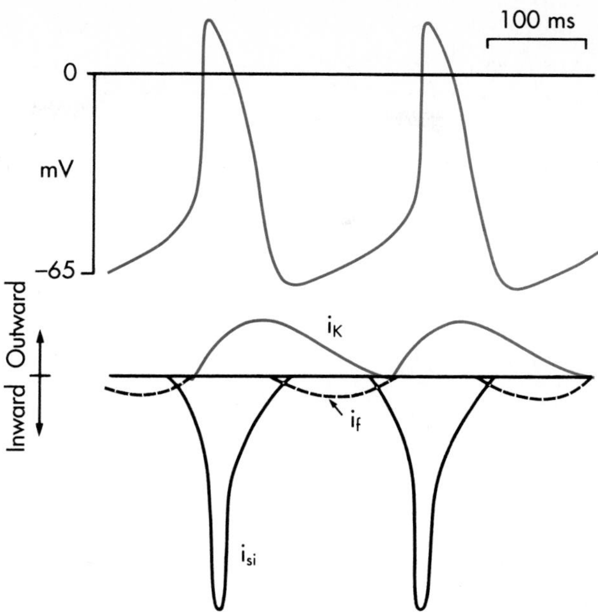

Fig. 2-24 ■ The transmembrane potential changes *(top half)* that occur in SA node cells are produced by three principal currents *(bottom half)*: (1) the slow inward current, i_{si}; (2) a hyperpolarization-induced inward current, i_f; and (3) an outward K^+ current, i_K. (Redrawn from Brown, H.F.: Physiol. Rev. 61:644, 1981.)

pacemaker cell membrane and by reducing the slope of the pacemaker potential (Fig. 2-23).

Changes in autonomic neural activity often also induce a **pacemaker shift,** where the site of initiation of the cardiac impulse may shift to a different locus within the SA node or to a different component of the atrial pacemaker complex.

Ionic Basis of Automaticity

Several ionic currents contribute to the slow depolarization that occurs during phase 4 in automatic cells in the heart. In the pacemaker cells of the SA node, the diastolic depolarization is ascribable to at least three ionic currents: (1) an inward current, i_f, induced by hyperpolarization; (2) the slow inward current, i_{si}; and (3) an outward K^+ current, i_K (Fig. 2-24).

The inward current, i_f, is carried mainly by Na^+; the current is conducted through specific channels that differ from the fast Na^+ channels. This current becomes activated during the repolarization phase of the action potential, as the membrane potential becomes more negative than about −50 mV. The more negative the membrane potential becomes at the end of repolarization, the greater will be the activation of the i_f current.

The second current responsible for diastolic depolarization is the slow inward current, i_{si}. This current, comprised mainly of Ca^{++}, becomes activated toward the end of phase 4, as the transmembrane potential reaches a value of about −55 mV (see Fig. 2-3).

This Ca^{++} current is carried mainly by T-type Ca^{++} channels, because this channel type activates at such transmembrane poten-

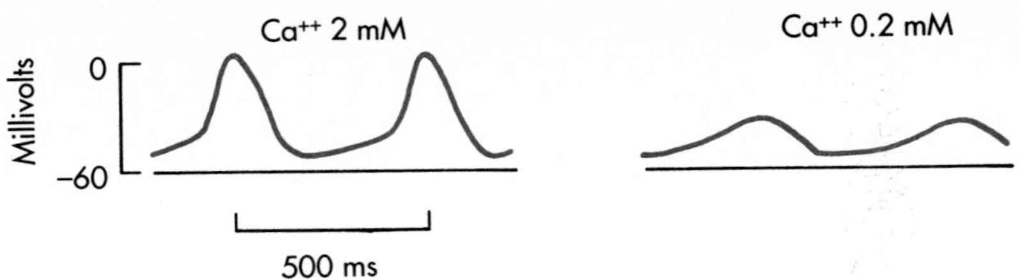

Fig. 2-25 ■ Transmembrane action potentials recorded from an SA node pacemaker cell in an isolated rabbit atrium preparation. The concentration of Ca^{++} in the bath was changed from 2 to 0.2 mM. (Modified from Kohlhardt, M., Figulla, H.-R., and Tripathi, O.: Basic Res. Cardiol. 71:17, 1976.)

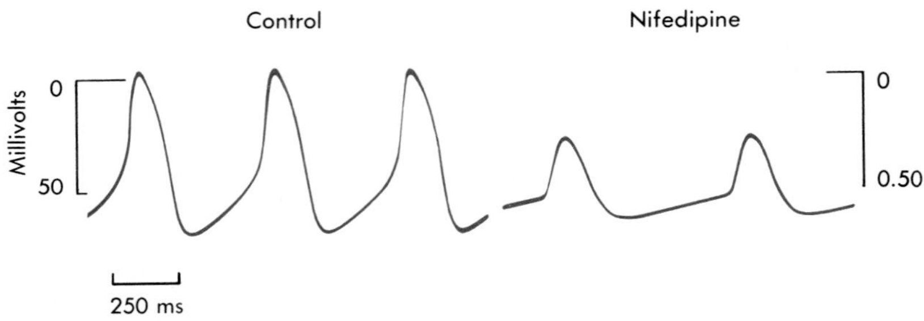

Fig. 2-26 ■ The effects of nifedipine (5.6×10^{-7} M), a Ca^{++} channel blocking drug, on the transmembrane potentials recorded from a rabbit's SA node cell. (From Ning, W., and Wit, A.L.: Am. Heart J. 106:345, 1983.)

tials (see Fig. 2-11). Once the Ca^{++} channels become activated, the influx of Ca^{++} into the cell increases. The influx of Ca^{++} accelerates the rate of diastolic depolarization, which then leads to the upstroke of the action potential. A decrease in the external Ca^{++} concentration (Fig. 2-25) or the addition of calcium channel blocking agents (Fig. 2-26) diminishes the amplitude of the action potential and the slope of the pacemaker potential in SA node cells.

The progressive diastolic depolarization mediated by the two inward currents, i_f and i_{si}, is opposed by a third current, an outward K^+ current, i_K. This efflux of K^+ tends to repolarize the cell after the upstroke of the action potential. The outward K^+ current continues well beyond the time of maximum repolarization, but it diminishes throughout phase 4 (see Fig. 2-24). Hence, the opposition of i_K to the depolarizing effects of the two inward currents (i_{si} and i_f) gradually decreases.

The ionic basis for automaticity in the AV node pacemaker cells is probably identical to that in the SA node cells. Similar mechanisms probably also account for automaticity in Purkinje fibers, except that the slow inward current is not involved. Hence, the slow diastolic depolarization is mediated principally by the imbalance between the hyperpolarization-induced inward current, i_f and the outward K^+ current, i_K.

The autonomic neurotransmitters affect automaticity by altering the ionic currents across the cell membranes. The adrenergic transmitters increase all three currents involved in SA nodal automaticity. The adrenergically mediated increase in the slope of diastolic depolarization indicates that the augmentations of i_f and i_{si} must exceed the enhancement of i_K.

The hyperpolarization (see Fig. 2-23) induced by the acetylcholine released at the vagus endings in the heart is achieved by an increase in g_K. This change in conductance is mediated through activation of specific K^+ channels that are controlled by the cholinergic receptors. Acetylcholine also depresses the i_f and i_{si} currents.

Overdrive Suppression

The automaticity of pacemaker cells becomes depressed after a period of excitation at a high frequency. This phenomenon is known as **overdrive suppression.** Because of the greater intrinsic rhythmicity of the SA node than of the other latent pacemaking sites in the heart, the firing of the SA node tends to suppress the automaticity in the other loci. If an ectopic focus in one of the atria suddenly began to fire at a high rate in an individual with a normal heart rate of 70 beats per minute, the ectopic center would become the pacemaker for the entire heart. When that rapid ectopic focus suddenly stopped firing, the SA node might remain quiescent briefly because of overdrive suppression. The interval from the end of the period of overdrive until the SA node resumes firing is called the **sinus node recovery time.** In patients with the so-called **sick sinus syndrome,** the sinus node recovery time may be markedly prolonged. The resultant period of asystole might cause syncope.

The mechanism responsible for overdrive suppression appears to be based on the activity of the membrane pump that actively extrudes Na^+ from the cell, in partial exchange for K^+. During each depolarization, a certain quantity of Na^+ enters the cell. The more frequently it is depolarized, therefore, the more Na^+ that enters the cell per minute. At high excitation frequencies the Na^+ pump becomes more active in extruding this larger quantity of Na^+ from the cell interior. The quantity of Na^+ extruded by the pump exceeds the quantity of K^+ that enters the cell; the ratio is 3:2. This enhanced activity of the pump hyperpolarizes the cell, because of the net loss of cations from the cell interior. Because of the hyperpolarization, the pacemaker potential requires more time to reach the threshold, as shown in Fig. 2-22, *B.* Furthermore, when the overdrive suddenly ceases, the Na^+ pump may not decelerate instantaneously, but may continue to operate at an accelerated rate for some time. This excessive extrusion of Na^+ opposes the gradual depolarization of the pacemaker cell during phase 4, thereby suppressing its intrinsic automaticity temporarily.

Atrial Conduction

From the SA node, the cardiac impulse spreads radially throughout the right atrium (Fig. 2-27) along ordinary atrial myocardial fibers, at a conduction velocity of approximately 1 m/s. A special pathway, the **anterior interatrial myocardial band** (or **Bachmann's bundle**), conducts the impulse from the SA node directly to the left atrium. Three tracts, the **anterior, middle,** and **posterior internodal pathways,** have been described. These tracts consist of a mixture of ordinary myocardial cells and specialized conducting fibers. Some authorities assert that these pathways constitute the principal routes for conduction of the cardiac impulse from the SA to the AV node.

The configuration of the atrial transmembrane potential is depicted in Fig. 2-21, *C.* Compared with the potential recorded from a typical ventricular fiber (see Fig. 2-21, *A*), the plateau (phase 2) is not as well developed and repolarization (phase 3) occurs at a slower rate.

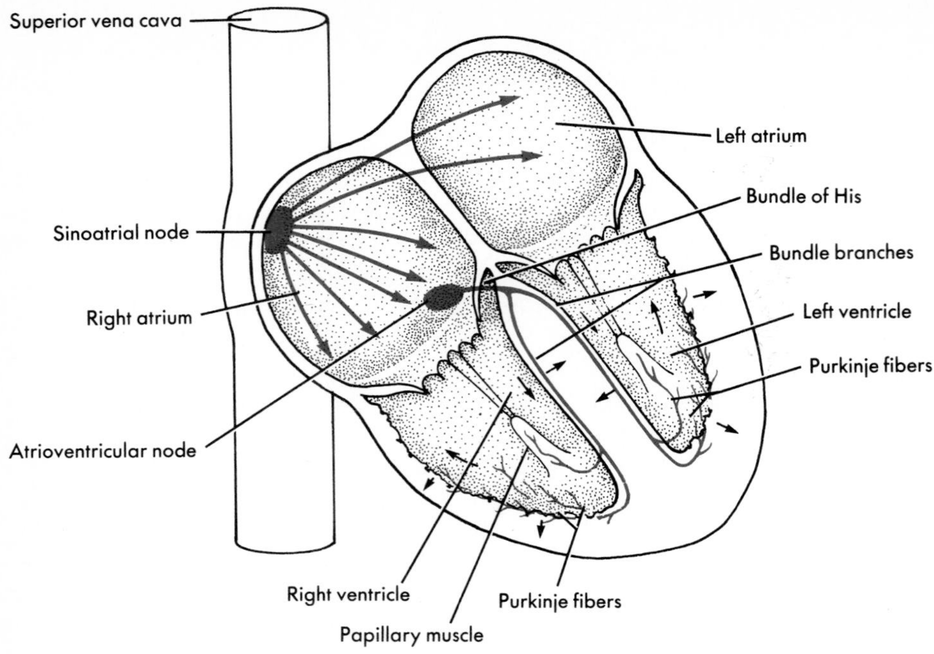

Fig. 2-27 ■ Schematic representation of the conduction system of the heart.

Atrioventricular Conduction

The cardiac action potential proceeds along the internodal pathways in the atrium and ultimately reaches the AV node. This node is approximately 22 mm long, 10 mm wide, and 3 mm thick in adult humans. The node is situated posteriorly on the right side of the interatrial septum near the ostium of the coronary sinus. The AV node contains the same two cell types as the SA node, but the round cells are more sparse and the elongated cells preponderate.

The AV node has been divided into three functional regions: (1) the AN region, the transitional zone between the atrium and the remainder of the node; (2) the N region, the midportion of the AV node; and (3) the NH region, the zone in which nodal fibers gradually merge with the **bundle of His,** which is the upper portion of the specialized conducting system for the ventricles. Normally, the AV node and bundle of His constitute the only pathways for conduction from atria to ventricles. Accessory AV pathways are present in some people, however. Such pathways often serve as a part of a reentry loop (see p. 36), which could lead to serious cardiac rhythm disturbances in these patients.

Several features of AV conduction are of physiological and clinical significance. The principal delay in the passage of the impulse from the atria to the ventricles occurs in the AN and N regions of the AV node. The conduction velocity is actually less in the N region than in the AN region. However, the path length is substantially greater in the AN than in the N region. The conduction times through the AN and N zones account for the delay between the onsets of the **P wave** (the electrical manifestation of the spread of atrial excitation)

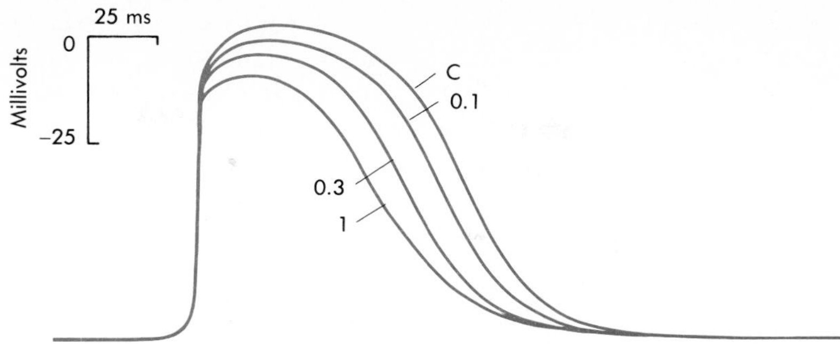

Fig. 2-28 ■ Transmembrane potentials recorded from a rabbit AV node cell under control conditions *(C)* and in the presence of the calcium channel blocking drug, diltiazem, in concentrations of 0.1, 0.3, and 1 μmol/L. (Redrawn from Hirth, C., Borchard, U., and Hafner, D.: J. Mol. Cell. Cardiol. 15:799, 1983.)

and the **QRS complex** (spread of ventricular excitation) in the electrocardiogram (see Fig. 2-34). Functionally, this delay between atrial and ventricular excitation permits optimal ventricular filling during atrial contraction.

In the N region, slow response action potentials prevail. The resting potential is about −60 mV, the upstroke velocity is very low (about 5 V/s), and the conduction velocity is about 0.05 m/s. Tetrodotoxin, which blocks the fast Na^+ channels, has virtually no effect on the action potentials in this region. Conversely, the Ca^{++} channel blocking agents decrease the amplitude and duration of the action potentials (Fig. 2-28) and depress AV conduction. The shapes of the action potentials in the AN region are intermediate between those in the N region and atria. Similarly, the action potentials in the NH region are transitional between those in the N region and bundle of His.

The relative refractory period of the cells in the N region extends well beyond the period of complete repolarization; (i.e., these cells display postrepolarization refractoriness) (see Fig. 2-18). As the repetition rate of atrial depolarizations is increased, conduction through the AV junction slows. Most of that slowing takes place in the N region. Impulses tend to be blocked at stimulus repetition rates that are easily conducted in other regions of the heart. If the atria are depolarized at a high frequency, only one half or one third of the atrial impulses might be conducted through the AV junction to the ventricles. This protects the ventricles from excessive contraction frequencies, wherein the filling time between contractions might be inadequate. Retrograde conduction can occur through the AV node. However, the propagation time is significantly longer and the impulse is blocked at lower repetition rates during conduction in the retrograde than in the antegrade direction. Finally, the AV node is a common site for reentry; the underlying mechanisms will be explained on p. 36.

The autonomic nervous system regulates AV conduction. Weak vagal activity may simply prolong the AV conduction time. Stronger vagal activity may cause some or all of the impulses arriving from the atria to be blocked in the node. The delayed conduction or block occurs largely in the N region of the node. The acetylcholine released by the vagal nerve fibers hyperpolarizes the conducting fibers in the N region (Fig. 2-29). The greater the hyperpolar-

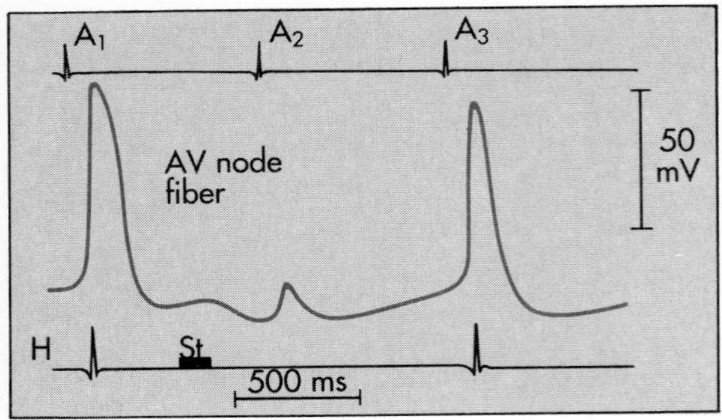

Fig. 2-29 ■ Effects of a brief vagal stimulus *(St)* on the transmembrane potential recorded from an AV nodal fiber from a rabbit. Note that shortly after vagal stimulation, the membrane of the fiber was hyperpolarized. The atrial excitation (A_2) that arrived at the AV node when the cell was hyperpolarized failed to be conducted, as denoted by the absence of a depolarization in the His electrogram *(H)*. The atrial excitations that preceded (A_1) and followed (A_3) excitation A_2 were conducted to the His bundle region. (Redrawn from Mazgalev, T., et al.: Am. J. Physiol., H631, 1986.)

ization at the time of arrival of the atrial impulse, the more impaired the AV conduction will be. In the experiment shown in Fig. 2-29, vagus nerve fibers were stimulated intensely (at St) shortly before the second atrial depolarization (A_2). That atrial impulse arrived at the AV node cell when its cell membrane was maximally hyperpolarized. The absence of a corresponding depolarization of the His bundle shows that the second atrial impulse was not conducted through the AV node. Only a small, nonpropagated response to the second atrial impulse is evident in the recording from the conducting fiber.

The cardiac sympathetic nerves, on the other hand, have a facilitative effect. They decrease the AV conduction time and enhance the rhythmicity of the latent pacemakers in the AV junction. The norepinephrine released at the sympathetic nerve terminals increases the amplitude and slope of the upstroke of the AV nodal action potentials, principally in the AN and N regions of the node.

Ventricular Conduction

The bundle of His passes subendocardially down the right side of the interventricular septum for about 1 cm and then divides into the right and left **bundle branches** (Figs. 2-27 and 2-30). The right bundle branch is a direct continuation of the bundle of His and it proceeds down the right side of the interventricular septum. The left bundle branch, which is considerably thicker than the right, arises almost perpendicularly from the bundle of His and perforates the interventricular septum. On the subendocardial surface of the left side of the interventricular septum, the main left bundle branch splits into a thin **anterior division** and a thick **posterior division.** Clinically, impulse conduction in the right bundle branch, the main left bundle branch, or either division of the left bundle branch may be impaired. Conduction blocks in one or more of these pathways give rise to characteristic electrocardiographic patterns. Block of either of the main bundle branches is known as right or left **bundle branch block.** Block of either division of the left bundle branch is called **left anterior hemiblock** or **left posterior hemiblock.**

The right bundle branch and the two divisions of the left bundle branch ultimately subdivide into a complex network of conducting fibers called **Purkinje fibers,** which ramify over the subendocardial surfaces of both ventricles. In certain mammalian species, such as cattle, the Purkinje fiber network is arranged in discrete, encapsulated bundles (see Fig. 2-30).

Purkinje fibers are the broadest cells in the heart, 70 to 80 μm in diameter, compared with 10 to 15 μm for ventricular myocardial cells. The large diameter accounts in part for the greater conduction velocity in Purkinje

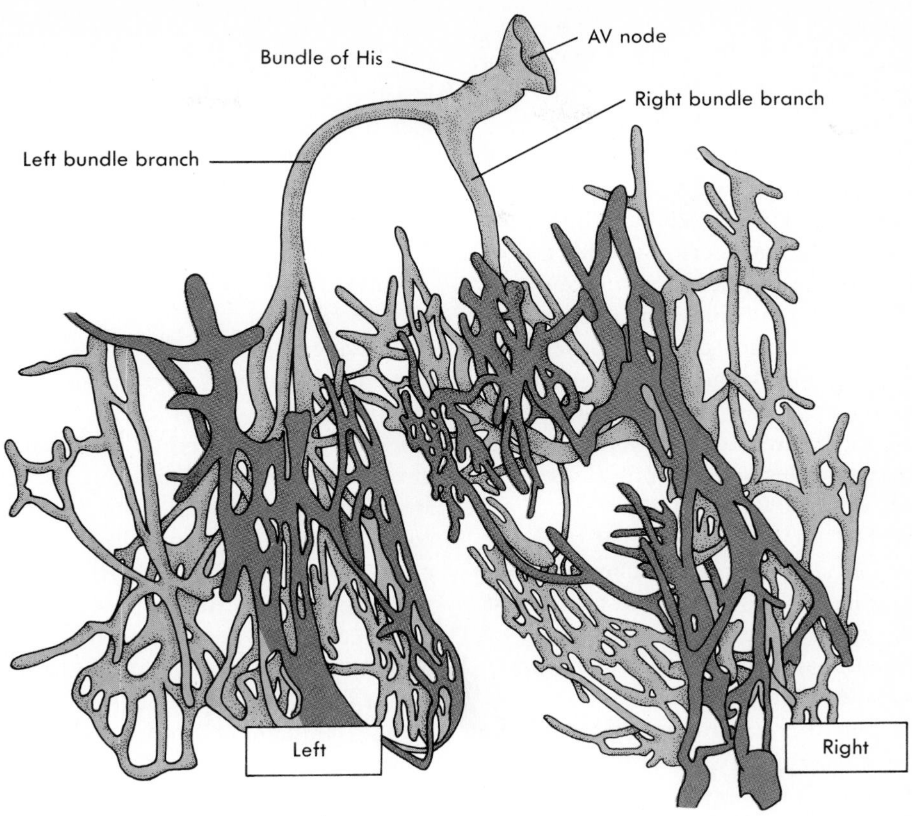

Fig. 2-30 ■ AV and ventricular conduction system of the calf heart. (Redrawn from DeWitt, L.M.: Anat. Rec. 3:475, 1909.)

than in myocardial fibers. Purkinje cells have abundant, linearly arranged sarcomeres, just as do myocardial cells. However, the T-tubular system is absent in the Purkinje cells of many species, but it is well developed in the myocardial cells.

The conduction of the action potential over the Purkinje fiber system is the fastest of any tissue within the heart; estimates vary from 1 to 4 m/s. This permits a rapid activation of the entire endocardial surface of the ventricles.

The action potentials recorded from Purkinje fibers resembles that of ordinary ventricular myocardial fibers (see Fig. 2-21, *A*). In general, phase 1 is more prominent in Purkinje fiber action potentials (see Fig. 2-14) than in those recorded from ventricular fibers (especially endocardial fibers) and the duration of the plateau (phase 2) is longer.

Because of the long refractory period of the Purkinje fibers, many premature activations of the atria are conducted through the AV junction but are blocked by the Purkinje fibers. Therefore, they fail to evoke a premature contraction of the ventricles. This function of protecting the ventricles against the effects of premature atrial depolarizations is especially pronounced at slow heart rates, because the action potential duration and hence the effective refractory period of the Purkinje fibers vary inversely with the heart rate (see Fig. 2-19). At slow heart rates, the effective refractory period of the Purkinje fibers is especially prolonged; as the heart rate increases, the refractory period diminishes. Similar directional changes in the refractory period occur in most of the other cells in the heart with changes in rate. However, in the AV node, the effective refractory period does not change appreciably over the normal range of heart rates, and it actually increases at very rapid heart rates. Therefore, at high rates, it is the AV node that protects the ventricles when impulses arrive at excessive repetition rates.

The spread of the action potential over the ventricles is of major concern in clinical cardiology. Numerous studies have been conducted to determine the precise course of the wave of excitation under normal and abnormal conditions. Such knowledge serves as a basis for the interpretation of the electrocardiogram. However, only the elementary, salient features of ventricular activation will be considered here.

The first portions of the ventricles to be excited are the interventricular septum (except the basal portion) and the papillary muscles. The wave of activation spreads into the substance of the septum from both its left and its right endocardial surfaces. Early contraction of the septum tends to make it more rigid and allows it to serve as an anchor point for the contraction of the remaining ventricular myocardium. Also, early contraction of the papillary muscles prevents eversion of the AV valves during ventricular systole.

The endocardial surfaces of both ventricles are activated rapidly, but the wave of excitation spreads from endocardium to epicardium at a slower velocity (about 0.3 to 0.4 m/s). Because the right ventricular wall is appreciably thinner than the left, the epicardial surface of the right ventricle is activated earlier than that of the left ventricle. Also, apical and central epicardial regions of both ventricles are activated somewhat earlier than their respective basal regions. The last portions of the ventricles to be excited are the posterior basal epicardial regions and a small zone in the basal portion of the interventricular septum.

■ REENTRY

Under certain conditions, a cardiac impulse may reexcite some region through which it had passed previously. This phenomenon, known as **reentry,** is responsible for many clinical disturbances of cardiac rhythm. The reentry may be **ordered** or **random.** In the ordered variety, the impulse traverses a fixed anatomical path, whereas in the random type the path continues to change. The principal example of random reentry is **fibrillation** (p. 49).

The conditions necessary for reentry are illustrated in Fig. 2-31. In each of the four panels, a single bundle *(S)* of cardiac fibers splits into a left *(L)* and a right *(R)* branch. A connecting bundle *(C)* runs between the two branches. Normally, the impulse coming down bundle *S* is conducted along the *L* and *R* branches (panel *A*). As the impulse reaches connecting link *C,* it enters from both sides and becomes extinguished at the point of collision. The impulse from the left side cannot proceed further because the tissue beyond is absolutely refractory because it had just been depolarized from the other direction. The impulse cannot pass through bundle *C* from the right either, for the same reason.

It is obvious from panel *B* that the impulse cannot make a complete circuit if antegrade block exists in the two branches (*L* and *R*) of the fiber bundle. Furthermore, if bidirectional block exists at any point in the loop (for example, branch *R* in panel *C*), the impulse will not be able to reenter.

A necessary condition for reentry is that at some point in the loop, the impulse is able to pass in one direction but not in the other. This phenomenon is called **unidirectional block.**

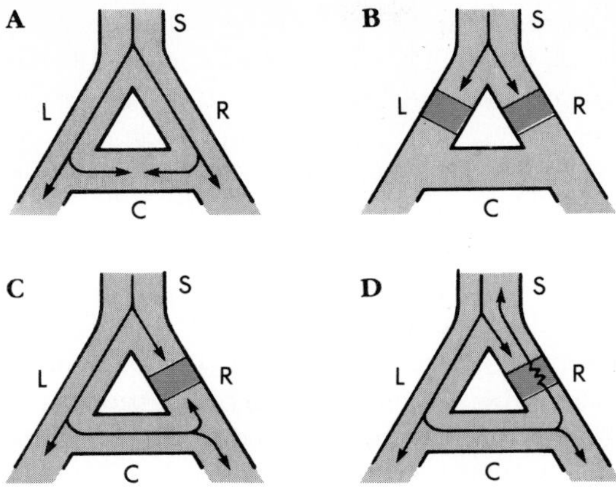

Fig. 2-31 ■ The role of unidirectional block in reentry. In panel **A**, an excitation wave traveling down a single bundle *(S)* of fibers continues down the left *(L)* and right *(R)* branches. The depolarization wave enters the connecting branch *(C)* from both ends and is extinguished at the zone of collision. In panel **B**, the wave is blocked in the *L* and *R* branches. In panel **C**, bidirectional block exists in branch *R*. In panel **D**, unidirectional block exists in branch *R*. The antegrade impulse is blocked, but the retrograde impulse is conducted through and reenters bundle *S*.

As shown in panel *D*, the impulse may travel down branch *L* normally and may be blocked in the antegrade direction in branch *R*. The impulse that had been conducted down branch *L* and through the connecting branch *C* may be able to penetrate the depressed region in branch *R* from the retrograde direction, even though the antegrade impulse had been blocked previously at this same site. The antegrade impulse will arrive at the depressed region in branch *R* earlier than the impulse that traverses a longer path and enters branch *R* from the opposite direction. The antegrade impulse may be blocked simply because it arrives at the depressed region during its effective refractory period. If the retrograde impulse is delayed sufficiently, the refractory period may have ended, and the impulse will be conducted back into bundle *S*.

Unidirectional block is a necessary condition for reentry, but not a sufficient one. It is also essential that the effective refractory period of the reentered region be less than the propagation time around the loop. In panel *D*, if the retrograde impulse is conducted through the depressed zone in branch *R* and if the tissue just beyond is still refractory from the antegrade depolarization, branch *S* will not be reexcited. Therefore, the conditions that promote reentry are those that prolong conduction time or shorten the effective refractory period.

The functional components of reentry loops responsible for specific arrhythmias in intact hearts are diverse. Some loops are very large and involve entire specialized conduction bundles; others are microscopic. The loop may include myocardial fibers, specialized conducting fibers, nodal cells, and junctional tissues, in almost any conceivable arrangement. Also, the cardiac cells in the loop may be normal or deranged.

■ TRIGGERED ACTIVITY

Triggered activity is so named because it is always coupled to a preceding action potential. Consequently, arrhythmias induced by triggered activity are difficult to distinguish from those induced by reentry. Triggered activity is caused by **afterdepolarizations.** Two types of afterdepolarizations are recognized: **early afterdepolarizations (EADs),** and **delayed afterdepolarizations (DADs).** EADs occur at the end of the plateau (phase 2) or about midway through repolarization (phase 3), whereas DADs occur near the very end of repolarization or just after full repolarization (phase 4).

Early Afterdepolarizations

EADs are more likely to occur when the prevailing heart rate is slow; rapid pacing suppresses EADs. In the experiment shown in Fig. 2-32, EADs were induced by cesium in an isolated Purkinje fiber preparation. No afterdepo-

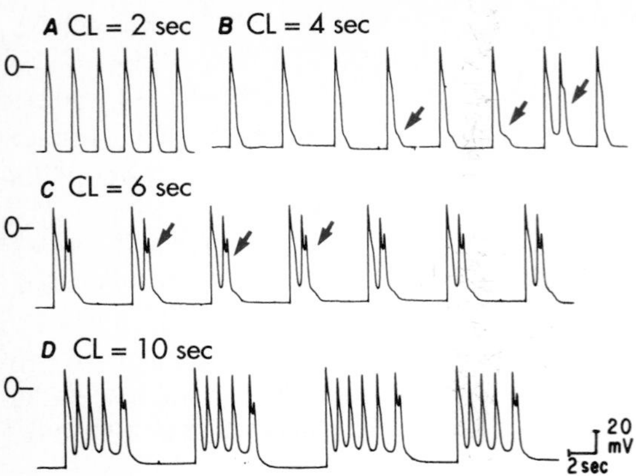

Fig. 2-32 ■ Effect of pacing at different cycle lengths *(CL)* on cesium-induced early afterdepolarizations (EADs) in a canine Purkinje fiber. (Modified with permission from Damiano B.P., and Rosen M.: Circulation 69:1013, 1984, with permission from the American Heart Association, Inc.)

A. EADs not evident.

B. EADs first appear *(arrows)*. Third EAD reaches threshold and triggers an action potential *(third arrow)*.

C. EADs that appear after each driven depolarization trigger an action potential.

D. Triggered action potentials occur in salvos.

larizations were evident when the preparation was driven at a cycle length of 2 s. When the cycle length was increased to 4 s, EADs appeared. Most were subthreshold (first two arrows), but one of the EADs did reach threshold and triggered an action potential. When the cycle length was increased to 6 s, each driven action potential generated an EAD that triggered a second action potential. Furthermore, when the cycle length was increased to 10 s, each driven action potential triggered a salvo of four or five additional action potentials.

EADs may be produced experimentally by interventions that prolong the action potential. Because EADs may be initiated at either of two distinct levels of transmembrane potential, namely at the end of the plateau and about midway through repolarization, two different mechanisms may be involved in generating them.

Considerable information has been obtained about the mechanism responsible for those EADs that appear at the end of the **plateau.** EADs are more likely to occur the more prolonged the action potential. For those action potentials that trigger EADs, the plateau appears to be prolonged enough that those Ca^{++} channels that were activated at the beginning of the plateau and then inactivated would have sufficient time to be activated again before the plateau had expired. This secondary activation would trigger an afterdepolarization.

Less information is available about the cellular mechanisms responsible for those EADs that appear midway through **repolarization.** The mechanism may be very similar to that for the EADs that occur at plateau potentials, as previously described. The difference may involve the specific type of Ca^{++} channels involved in the process. Experiments have adduced convincing evidence that the L-type Ca^{++} channels (see page 21) mediate the EADs that occur at plateau potentials. These channels are activated at levels of V_m that prevail during the plateau. Recent experiments suggest that the EADs which occur at more negative potentials are generated through a similar mechanism, but are mediated instead by T-type Ca^{++} channels. The T-type channels are activated at levels of V_m significantly more negative than the plateau.

Delayed Afterdepolarizations

The salient characteristics of DADs are shown in Fig. 2-33. The transmembrane potentials were recorded from Purkinje fibers that were exposed to a high concentration of acetylstrophanthidin, a digitalis-like substance. In the absence of driving stimuli these fibers were quiescent. In each panel, a sequence of six

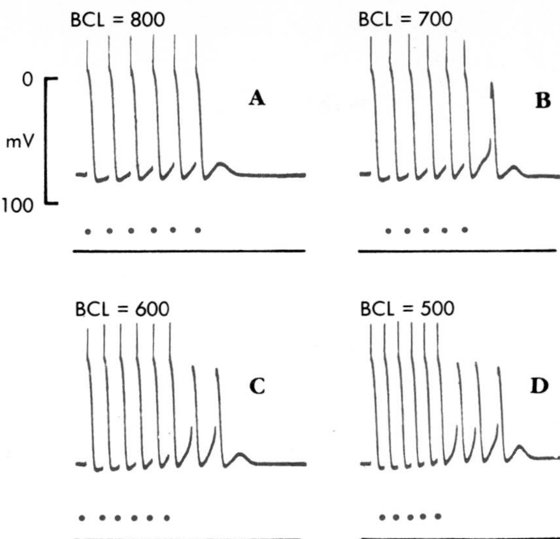

Fig. 2-33 ■ Transmembrane action potentials recorded from isolated canine Purkinje fibers. Acetylstrophanthidin was added to the bath, and sequences of six driven beats (denoted by the dots) were produced at basic cycle lengths *(BCL)* of 800, 700, 600, and 500 ms. Note that delayed afterpotentials occurred after the driven beats, and that these afterpotentials reached threshold after the last driven beat in panels **B** to **D.** (From Ferrier, G.R., Saunders, J.H., and Mendez, C.: Circ. Res. 32:600, 1973. By permission of the American Heart Association, Inc.)

driven depolarizations were induced at various basic cycle lengths.

When the cycle length was 800 ms (panel *A*), the last driven depolarization was followed by a brief DAD that did not reach threshold. Once that afterdepolarization had subsided, the transmembrane potential remained constant until another driving stimulus was given. The upstroke of a DAD can be detected after each of the first five driven depolarizations.

When the basic cycle length was diminished to 700 ms (panel *B*), the DAD that followed the last driven beat did reach threshold, and a nondriven depolarization (or **extrasystole**) ensued. This extrasystole was itself followed by an afterpotential that was subthreshold. Diminution of the basic cycle length to 600 ms (panel *C*) also evoked an extrasystole after the last driven depolarization. The afterpotential that followed the extrasystole did reach threshold, however, and a second extrasystole occurred. A sequence of three extrasystoles followed the six driven depolarizations that were separated by intervals of 500 ms (panel *D*). Slightly shorter basic cycle lengths or slightly greater concentrations of acetylstrophanthidin evoked a continuous sequence of nondriven beats, resembling a **paroxysmal tachycardia** (described on p. 49).

DADs are associated with elevated intracellular Ca^{++} concentrations. The amplitudes of the DADs are increased by interventions that raise intracellular Ca^{++} concentrations. Such interventions include elevated extracellular Ca^{++} concentrations and toxic levels of digitalis glycosides. The elevated levels of intracellular Ca^{++} provoke the oscillatory release of Ca^{++} from the sarcoplasmic reticulum. Hence, in myocardial cells the DADs are accompanied by small changes in developed force. The high intracellular Ca^{++} concentrations also activate certain membrane channels that permit the passage of Na^+ and K^+. The net flux of these cations constitutes a transient inward current, i_{ti}, that is at least partly responsible for the afterdepolarization of the cell membrane. The elevated intracellular Ca^{++} may also activate Na^+/Ca^{++} exchange. This electrogenic exchanger, which brings into the cell three Na^+ for each Ca^{++} it ejects, also creates a net inward current of cations that would contribute to the DAD.

■ ELECTROCARDIOGRAPHY

The electrocardiograph is a valuable instrument, because it enables the physician to infer the course of the cardiac impulse simply by recording the variations in electrical potential at various loci on the surface of the body. By analyzing the details of these potential fluctuations, the physician gains valuable insight concerning (1) the anatomical orientation of the heart, (2) the relative sizes of its chambers, (3) a variety of disturbances of rhythm and conduction, (4) the extent, location, and progress of ischemic damage to the myocardium, (5) the effects of altered electrolyte concentrations, and (6) the influence of certain drugs (notably digitalis and its derivatives). The science of electrocardiography is extensive and complex, but only the elementary basis of electrocardiography will be considered here.

Scalar Electrocardiography

The systems of leads used to record routine electrocardiograms are oriented in certain planes of the body. The diverse electromotive forces that exist in the heart at any moment can be represented by a three-dimensional vector. A system of recording leads oriented in a given plane detects only the projection of the three-dimensional vector on that plane. Furthermore, the potential difference between two recording electrodes represents the projection of the vector on the line between the two leads. Components of vectors projected on such lines are not vectors but are **scalar quantities** (having magnitude, but not direction). Hence, a recording of the changes with time of the differences of potential between two points on the surface of the skin is called a **scalar electrocardiogram.**

Configuration of the Scalar Electrocardiogram. The scalar electrocardiograph detects the changes with time of the electrical potential between some point on the surface of the skin and an indifferent electrode or between pairs of points on the skin surface. The cardiac impulse progresses through the heart in a complex three-dimensional pattern. Hence, the precise configuration of the electrocardiogram varies from individual to individual, and in any given individual the pattern varies with the anatomical location of the leads.

In general, the pattern consists of P, QRS, and T waves (Fig. 2-34). The P-R interval (or more precisely, the P-Q interval) is a measure of the time from the onset of atrial activation to the onset of ventricular activation; it normally ranges from 0.12 to 0.20 s. A considerable fraction of this time involves passage of the impulse through the AV conduction system. Pathological prolongations of this interval are associated with disturbances of AV conduction produced by inflammatory, circulatory, pharmacological, or nervous mechanisms.

The configuration and amplitude of the QRS complex vary considerably among individuals. The duration is usually between 0.06 and 0.10 s. Abnormal prolongation may indicate a block in the normal conduction pathways through the ventricles (such as a block of the left or right bundle branch). During the ST interval the entire ventricular myocardium is depolarized. Therefore, the ST segment lies on the **isoelectric line** under normal conditions. Any appreciable deviation from the isoelectric line is noteworthy and may indicate ischemic damage of the myocardium. The Q-T interval is sometimes referred to as the period of "electrical systole" of the ventricles. Its duration is about 0.4 s, but it varies inversely with the heart rate, mainly because the myocardial cell action potential duration varies inversely with the heart rate (see Fig. 2-19).

In most leads the T wave is deflected in the same direction from the isoelectric line as the major component of the QRS complex, although biphasic or oppositely directed T waves are perfectly normal in certain leads. When the T wave and QRS complex deviate in the same direction from the isoelectric line, it indicates that the repolarization process proceeds in a direction counter to the depolarization process. T waves that are abnormal either

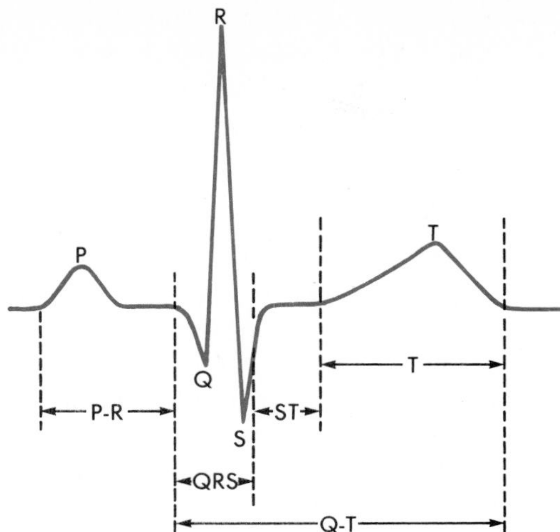

Fig. 2-34 ■ Configuration of a typical scalar electrocardiogram, illustrating the important deflections and intervals.

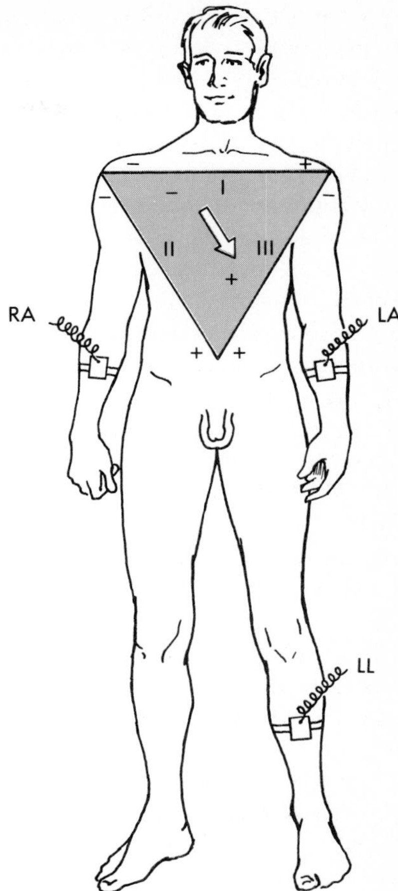

Fig. 2-35 ■ Einthoven triangle, illustrating the galvanometer connections for standard limb leads I, II, and III.

in direction or amplitude may indicate myocardial damage, electrolyte disturbances, or cardiac hypertrophy.

Standard Limb Leads. The original electrocardiographic lead system was devised by Einthoven. In his lead system the **resultant cardiac vector** (the vector sum of all electrical activity occurring in the heart at any given moment) was considered to lie in the center of a triangle (assumed to be equilateral) formed by the left and right shoulders and the pubic region (Fig. 2-35). This triangle, called the **Einthoven triangle,** is oriented in the frontal plane of the body. Hence, only the projection of the resultant cardiac vector on the frontal plane will be detected by this system of leads. For convenience, the electrodes are connected to the right and left forearms rather than to the corresponding shoulders, because the arms represent simple extensions of the leads from the shoulders. Similarly, the leg is taken as an extension of the lead system from the pubis, and the third electrode is connected to the left leg (by convention).

Certain conventions dictate the manner in which these **standard limb leads** are connected to the galvanometer. Lead I records the potential difference between the left arm (LA) and the right arm (RA). The galvanometer connections are such that when the potential at LA (V_{LA}) exceeds the potential at RA (V_{RA}), the galvanometer will be deflected upward from the isoelectric line. In Figs. 2-35 and 2-36 this arrangement of the galvanometer connections for lead I is designated by a (+) at LA and by a (−) at RA. Lead II records the potential difference between RA and LL (left leg) and yields an upward deflection when V_{LL} exceeds V_{RA}. Finally, lead III registers the potential difference between LA and LL and yields an upward deflection when V_{LL} exceeds V_{LA}. These galvanometer connections were arbitrarily chosen so that the QRS complexes will be upright in all three standard limb leads in most normal individuals.

Let the frontal projection of the resultant cardiac vector at some moment be represented by an arrow (tail negative, head positive), as in Fig. 2-35. Then the potential difference, $V_{LA} - V_{RA}$, recorded in lead I will be represented by the component of the vector projected along the horizontal line between LA and RA, as shown in Fig. 2-36. If the vector makes an angle, θ, of 60 degrees with the horizontal (as in the top section of Fig. 2-36), the magnitude of the potential recorded by lead I will equal the vector magnitude times cosine 60 degrees. The deflection recorded in lead I will be upward, because the positive arrowhead lies closer to LA than to RA. The deflection in lead II also will be upright, because the arrowhead lies closer to LL than to RA. The magnitude of the lead II deflection will be greater than that in lead I, because in this example the direction of the vector parallels that

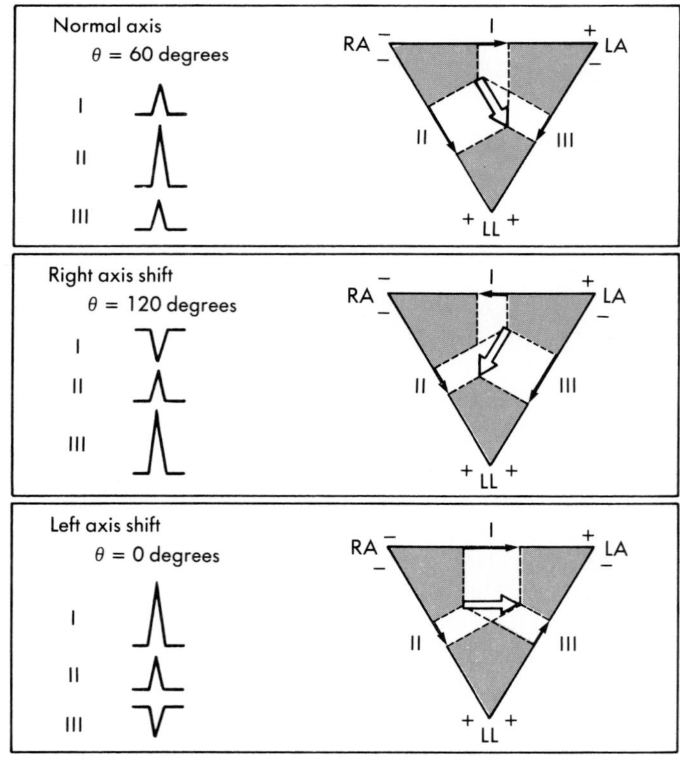

Fig. 2-36 ■ Magnitude and direction of the QRS complexes in limb leads I, II, and III, when the mean electrical axis (θ) is 60 degrees *(top section),* 120 degrees *(middle section),* and 0 degrees *(bottom section).*

of lead II; therefore, the magnitude of the projection on lead II exceeds that on lead I. Similarly, in lead III the deflection will be upright, and in this example, where $\theta = 60$ degrees, its magnitude will equal that in lead I.

If the vector in the top section of Fig. 2-36 is the resultant of the electrical events occurring during the peak of the QRS complex, then the orientation of this vector is said to represent the **mean electrical axis** of the heart in the frontal plane. The positive direction of this axis is taken in the clockwise direction from the horizontal plane (contrary to the usual mathematical convention). For normal individuals the average mean electrical axis is approximately + 60 degrees (as in the top section of Fig. 2-36). Therefore, the QRS complexes are usually upright in all three leads and largest in lead II.

Changes in the mean electrical axis may occur with alterations in the anatomical position of the heart or with changes in the relative preponderance of the right and left ventricles. For example, the axis tends to shift toward the left (more horizontal) in short, stocky individuals and toward the right (more vertical) in tall, thin persons. Also, with left or right ventricular hypertrophy (increased myocardial mass), the axis will shift toward the hypertrophied side.

With appreciable shift of the mean electrical axis to the right (middle section of Fig. 2-36, where $\theta = 120$ degrees), the displacements of the QRS complexes in the standard leads will change considerably. In this case the largest upright deflection will be in lead III and the deflection in lead I will be inverted, because the arrowhead will be closer to RA than to LA. With left axis shift (bottom section of Fig. 2-36, where $\theta = 0$ degrees), the largest upright deflection will be in lead I, and the QRS complex in lead III will be inverted.

As is evident from this discussion, the standard limb leads, I, II, and III, are oriented in the frontal plane at 0, 60, and 120 degrees, respectively, from the horizontal plane. Other limb leads, which are also oriented in the frontal plane, are usually recorded in addition to the standard leads. These "unipolar limb leads" lie along axes at angles of +90, −30, and −150 degrees from the horizontal plane. Such lead systems are described in all textbooks on electrocardiography and will not be considered further here.

To obtain information concerning the projections of the cardiac vector on the sagittal and transverse planes of the body in scalar electrocardiography, the **precordial leads** are usually recorded. Most commonly, each of six selected points on the anterior and lateral surfaces of the chest in the vicinity of the heart is connected in turn to the galvanometer. The other galvanometer terminal is usually connected to a **central terminal,** which is composed of a junction of three leads from LA, RA, and LL, each in series with a 5000 ohm resistor. The voltage of this central terminal remains at a theoretical zero potential throughout the cardiac cycle.

■ ARRHYTHMIAS

Cardiac arrhythmias reflect disturbances of either **impulse propagation** or **impulse initiation.** The principal disturbances of impulse propagation are conduction blocks and reentrant rhythms. Disturbances of impulse initiation include those that arise from the SA node and those that originate from various ectopic foci.

Altered Sinoatrial Rhythms

The frequency of pacemaker discharge varies by the mechanisms described earlier in this chapter (see Fig. 2-22). Changes in SA nodal discharge frequency are usually produced by the cardiac autonomic nerves. Examples of electrocardiograms of sinus tachycardia and sinus bradycardia are shown in Fig. 2-37. The P,

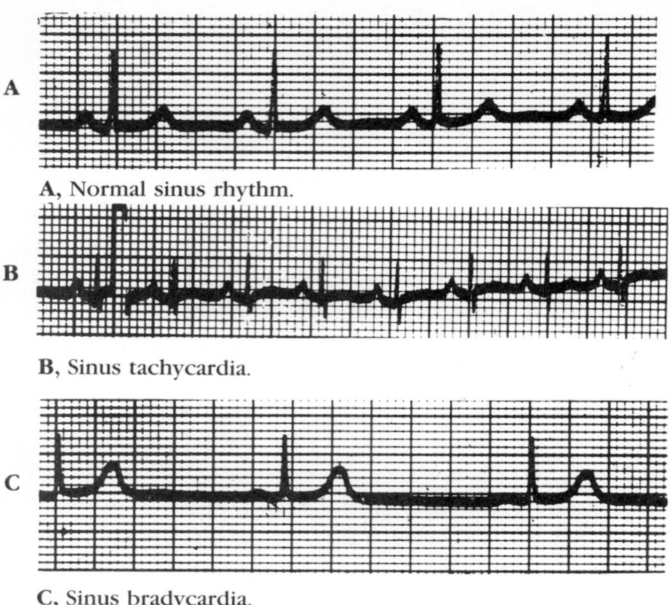

A, Normal sinus rhythm.

B, Sinus tachycardia.

C, Sinus bradycardia.

Fig. 2-37 ■ Sinoatrial rhythms.

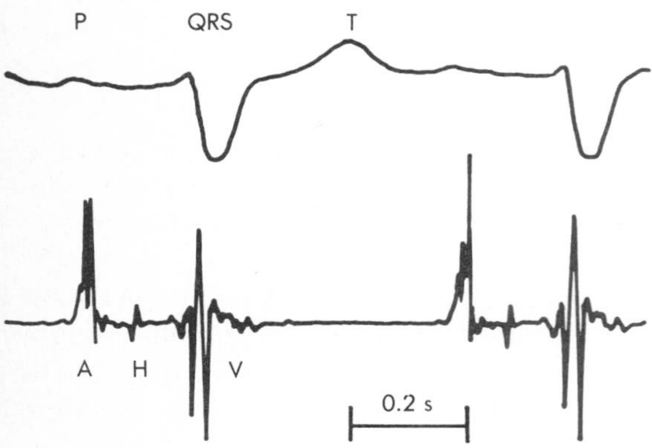

Fig. 2-38 ■ His bundle electrogram (lower tracing, retouched) and lead II of the scalar electrocardiogram (upper tracing). The deflection, *H,* which represents the impulse conduction over the bundle of His, is clearly visible between the atrial, *A,* and ventricular, *V,* deflections. The conduction time from the atria to the bundle of His is denoted by the A-H interval; that from the bundle of His to the ventricles, by the H-V interval. (Courtesy Dr. J. Edelstein.)

QRS, and T deflections are all normal, but the duration of the cardiac cycle (the **P-P interval**) is altered. Characteristically, when sinus bradycardia or tachycardia develops, the cardiac frequency changes gradually and requires several beats to attain its new steady-state value. Electrocardiographic evidence of **respiratory cardiac arrhythmia** is common and is manifested as a rhythmic variation in the P-P interval at the respiratory frequency (p. 88).

Atrioventricular Transmission Blocks

Various physiological, pharmacological, and pathological processes can impede impulse transmission through the AV conduction tissue. The site of block can be localized more precisely by recording the **His bundle electrogram** (Fig. 2-38). To obtain such tracings, an electrode catheter is introduced into a peripheral vein and is threaded centrally until the tip containing the electrodes lies in the AV

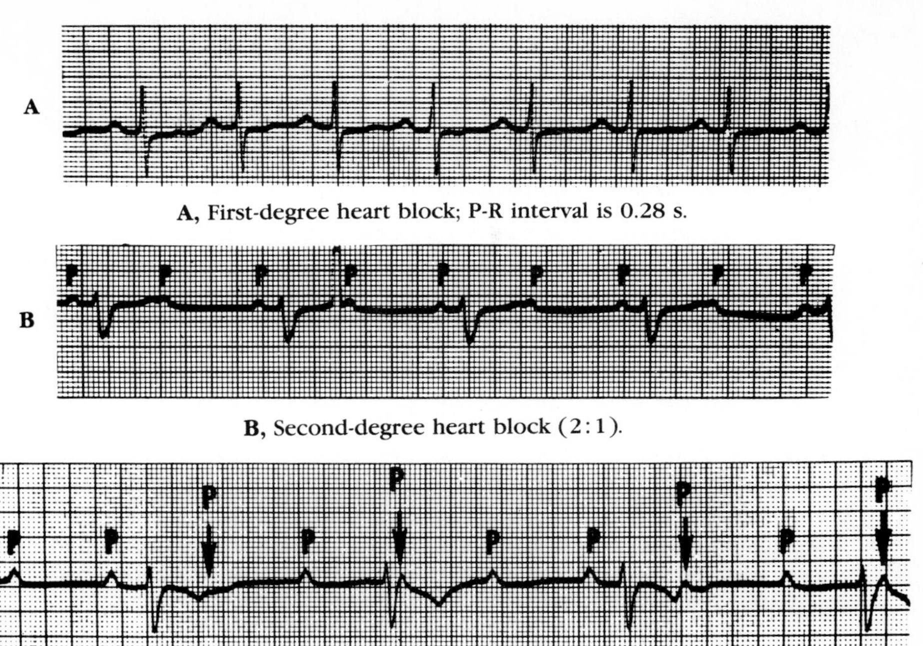

A, First-degree heart block; P-R interval is 0.28 s.

B, Second-degree heart block (2:1).

C, Third-degree heart block; note the dissociation between the P waves and the QRS complexes.

Fig. 2-39 ■ AV blocks.

junctional region between the right atrium and ventricle. When the electrodes are properly positioned, a distinct deflection (Fig. 2-38, *H*) is registered, which represents the passage of the cardiac impulse down the bundle of His. The time intervals required for propagation from the atrium to the bundle of His **(A-H interval)** and from the bundle of His to the ventricles **(H-V interval)** may be measured accurately. Abnormal prolongation of the former or latter interval indicates block above or below the bundle of His, respectively.

Three degrees of AV block can be distinguished, as shown in Fig. 2-39. **First-degree AV block** is characterized by a prolonged P-R interval. In Fig. 2-39, *A,* the P-R interval is 0.28 s; an interval greater than 0.2 s is abnormal. In most cases of first-degree block the A-H interval of the His bundle electrogram is prolonged, and the H-V interval is normal. Hence, the delay is located above the bundle of His, that is, in the AV node.

In **second-degree AV block** all QRS complexes are preceded by P waves, but not all P waves are followed by QRS complexes. The ratio of P waves to QRS complexes is usually the ratio of two small integers (such as 2:1, 3:1, 3:2). Fig. 2-39, *B,* illustrates a typical 2:1 block. His bundle electrograms have demonstrated that the site of block may be above or below the bundle of His. A block below the bundle is more serious than one above the bundle, because it more often evolves into a third-degree block. Hence, an artificial pacemaker is frequently implanted when the block is found to be below the bundle.

Third-degree AV block is often referred to as **complete heart block** because the impulse is unable to traverse the AV conduction pathway from atria to ventricles. His bundle electrograms reveal that the most common sites of complete block are distal to the bundle of His. In complete heart block the atrial and ventricular rhythms are entirely independent. A typical example is displayed in Fig. 2-39, *C,* where the QRS complexes bear no fixed relationship to the P waves. Because of the slow ventricular rhythm (32 beats per minute in this example), circulation is often inadequate, especially during muscular activity. Third-degree block is often associated with syncope (so-called Stokes-Adams attacks) caused principally by insufficient cerebral blood flow. Third-degree block is one of the most common conditions requiring treatment by artificial pacemakers.

Premature Depolarizations

Premature depolarizations occur at times in most normal individuals but are more common under certain abnormal conditions. They may originate in the atria, AV junction, or ventricles. One type of premature depolarization is coupled to a normally conducted depolarization by a constant **coupling interval.** If the normal depolarization is suppressed in some way (for example, by vagal stimulation), the premature depolarization also will be abolished. Such premature depolarizations are called **coupled extrasystoles,** or simply **extrasystoles,** and they probably reflect a reentry phenomenon (see Fig. 2-31). A second type of premature depolarization occurs as the result of enhanced automaticity in some ectopic focus. This ectopic center may fire regularly and be protected from depolarization by the

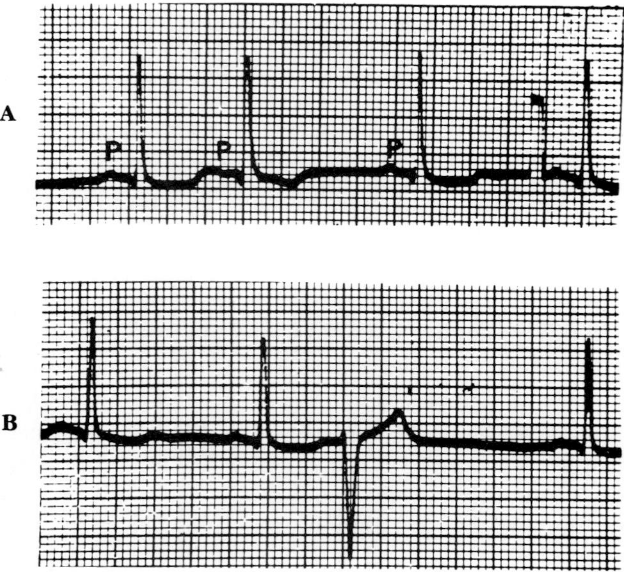

Fig. 2-40 ■ A premature atrial depolarization, **A,** and a premature ventricular depolarization, **B.** The premature atrial depolarization (the second beat in the top tracing) is characterized by an inverted P wave and normal QRS and T waves. The interval following the premature depolarization is not much longer than the usual interval between beats. The brief rectangular deflection just before the last depolarization is a standardization signal. The premature ventricular depolarization, **B,** is characterized by bizarre QRS and T waves and is followed by a compensatory pause.

normal cardiac impulse. If this premature depolarization occurs at a regular interval or at a simple multiple of that interval, the disturbance is called **parasystole.**

A **premature atrial depolarization** is shown in the electrocardiogram in Fig. 2-40, *A*. The normal interval between beats was 0.89 s (heart rate, 68 beats per minute). The premature atrial depolarization (second P wave in the figure) followed the preceding P wave by only 0.56 s. The configuration of the premature P wave differs from the configuration of the other, normal P waves because the course of atrial excitation, originating at some ectopic focus in the atrium, is different from the normal spread of excitation originating at the SA node. The QRS complex of the premature depolarization is usually normal in configuration because the spread of ventricular excitation occurs over the usual pathways.

A **premature ventricular depolarization** appears in Fig. 2-40, *B*. Because the premature excitation originated at some ectopic focus in the ventricles, the impulse spread was aberrant and the configurations of the QRS and T waves were entirely different from the normal deflections. The premature QRS complex followed the preceding normal QRS complex by only 0.47 s. The interval after the premature excitation was 1.28 s, considerably longer than the normal interval between beats (0.89 s). The interval (1.75 s) from the QRS complex just before the premature excitation to the QRS complex just after it was virtually equal to the duration of two normal cardiac cycles (1.78 s).

The prolonged interval that usually follows a premature ventricular depolarization is called a **compensatory pause.** The reason for the compensatory pause after a premature ventricular depolarization is that the ectopic ventricular impulse does not disturb the natural rhythm of the SA node. Either the ectopic ventricular impulse is not conducted retrograde through the AV conduction system or, if it is, the time required is such that the SA node has already fired at its natural interval before the ectopic impulse could have reached it. Likewise, the SA nodal impulse usually does not affect the ventricle, because the AV junction and perhaps also the ventricles are still refractory from the premature excitation. In Fig. 2-40, *B*, the P wave originating in the SA node at the time of the premature depolarization occurred at the same time as the T wave of the premature cycle and therefore cannot easily be identified in the tracing.

Ectopic Tachycardias

When a tachycardia originates from some ectopic site in the heart, the onset and termination are typically abrupt, in contrast to the more gradual changes in heart rate in sinus tachycardia. Because of the sudden appearance and abrupt cessation, such ectopic tachycardias are usually called **paroxysmal tachycardias.** Episodes of ectopic tachycardia may persist for only a few beats or for many hours or days, and the episodes often recur. Paroxysmal tachycardias may occur either as the result of (1) the rapid firing of an ectopic pacemaker, (2) triggered activity secondary to afterpotentials that reach threshold, or (3) an impulse circling a reentry loop repetitively.

Paroxysmal tachycardias originating in the atria or in the AV junctional tissues (Fig. 2-41, *A*) are usually indistinguishable, and therefore both are included in the term **paroxysmal supraventricular tachycardia.** The tachycardia often results from an impulse repetitively circling a reentry loop that includes atrial tissue and the AV junction. The QRS complexes are often normal, because ventricular activation proceeds over the normal pathways.

Paroxysmal ventricular tachycardia originates from an ectopic focus in the ventricles. The electrocardiogram is characterized by repeated, bizarre QRS complexes that reflect the aberrant intraventricular impulse conduction

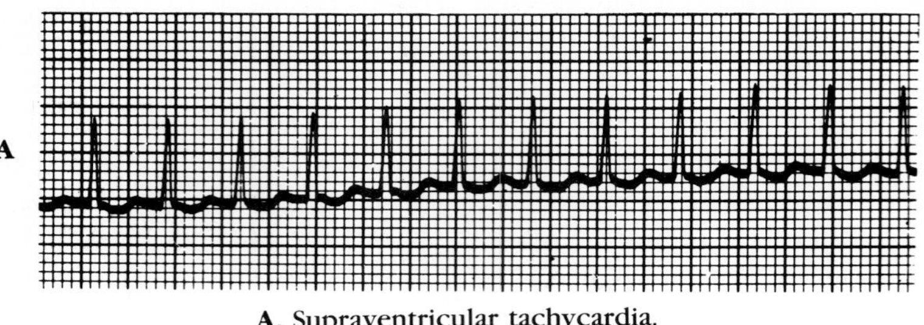

A, Supraventricular tachycardia.

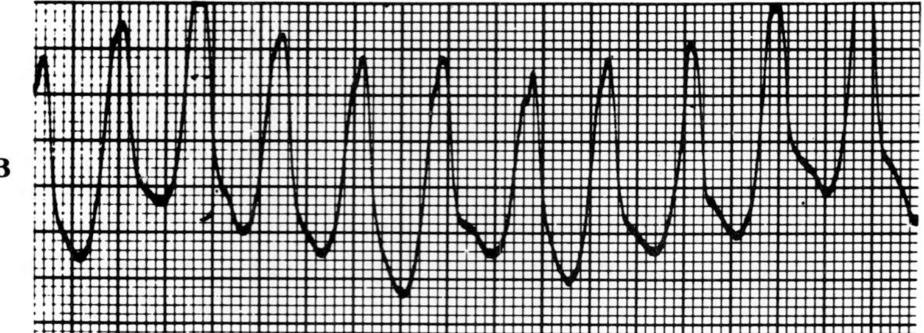

B, Ventricular tachycardia.

Fig. 2-41 ■ Paroxysmal tachycardias.

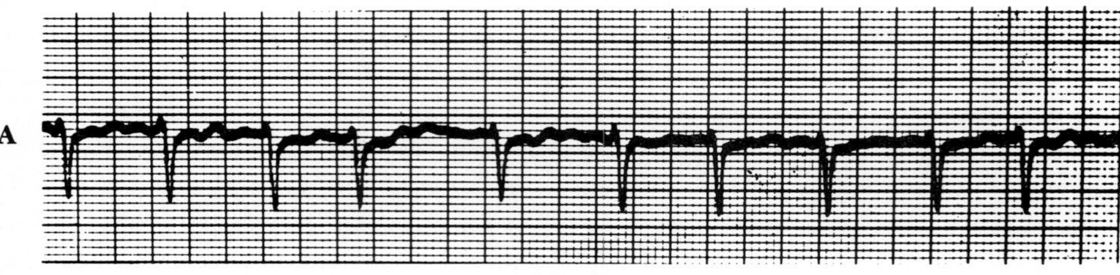

A, Atrial fibrillation.

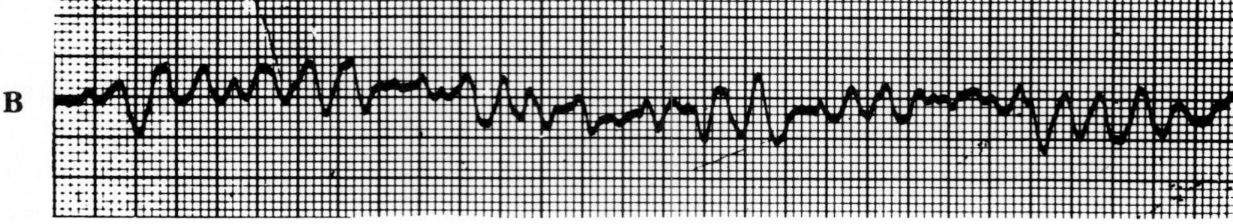

B, Ventricular fibrillation.

Fig. 2-42 ■ Atrial and ventricular fibrillation.

(see Fig. 2-41, *B*). Paroxysmal ventricular tachycardia is much more ominous than supraventricular tachycardia because it is frequently a precursor of ventricular fibrillation, a lethal arrhythmia that will be described in the next section.

Fibrillation

Under certain conditions cardiac muscle undergoes an irregular type of contraction that is entirely ineffectual in propelling blood. Such an arrhythmia is termed **fibrillation** and may involve either the atria or ventricles. Fibrillation probably represents a reentry phenomenon, in which the reentry loop fragments into multiple, irregular circuits.

The tracing in Fig. 2-42, *A*, illustrates the electrocardiographic changes in **atrial fibrillation.** This condition occurs in various types of chronic heart disease. The atria do not contract and relax sequentially during each cardiac cycle and hence do not contribute to ventricular filling. Instead, the atria undergo a continuous, uncoordinated, rippling type of activity. In the electrocardiogram there are no P waves; they are replaced by continuous irregular fluctuations of potential, called **f** waves. The AV node is activated at intervals that may vary considerably from cycle to cycle. Hence, there is no constant interval between QRS complexes and therefore between ventricular contractions. Because the strength of ventricular contraction depends on the interval between beats (as explained on p. 100), the volume and the rhythm of the pulse is very irregular. In many patients the atrial reentry loop and the pattern of AV conduction are more regular. The rhythm is then referred to as **atrial flutter.**

Although atrial fibrillation and flutter are compatible with life and even with full activity, the onset of **ventricular fibrillation** leads to loss of consciousness within a few seconds. The irregular, continuous, uncoordinated twitchings of the ventricular muscle fibers pump no blood. Death ensues unless immediate, effective resuscitation is achieved or unless the rhythm reverts to normal spontaneously, which rarely occurs. Ventricular fibrillation may supervene when the entire ventricle, or some portion of it, is deprived of its normal blood supply. It may also occur as a result of electrocution or in response to certain drugs and anesthetics. In the electrocardiogram (see Fig. 2-42, *B*) irregular fluctuations of potential are manifest.

Fibrillation is often initiated when a premature impulse arrives during the **vulnerable period.** In the ventricles, this period coincides with the downslope of the T wave. During this period, the excitability of the cardiac cells varies. Some fibers are still in their effective refractory periods, others have almost fully recovered their excitability, and still others are able to conduct impulses, but only at very slow conduction velocities. As a consequence, the action potentials are propagated over the chambers in multiple wavelets that travel along circuitous paths and at various conduction velocities. As a region of cardiac cells becomes excitable again, it will ultimately be reentered by one of the wave fronts traveling about the chamber. The process is self-sustaining.

Atrial fibrillation may be reverted to a normal sinus rhythm by drugs that prolong the refractory period. As the cardiac impulse completes the reentry loop, it may then find the myocardial fibers no longer excitable. However, much more dramatic therapy is required in ventricular fibrillation. Conversion to a normal sinus rhythm is accomplished by means of a strong electric current that places the entire myocardium briefly in a refractory state. Techniques have been developed to safely administer the current through the intact chest wall. In successful cases the SA node again takes over as the normal pacemaker for the entire heart.

■ SUMMARY

Transmembrane Action Potentials

The **transmembrane action potentials** that can be recorded from cardiac myocytes comprise five phases (0 to 4):

1. **Phase 0, upstroke.** A suprathreshold stimulus rapidly depolarizes the membrane by activating the fast Na^+ channels.
2. **Phase I, early partial repolarization.** Achieved by the efflux of K^+ through channels that conduct the transient outward current, i_{to}.
3. **Phase 2, plateau.** Achieved by a balance between the influx of Ca^{++} through Ca^{++} channels and the efflux of K^+ through several types of K^+ channels.
4. **Phase 3, final repolarization.** Initiated when the efflux of K^+ exceeds the influx of Ca^{++}. The resulting partial repolarization rapidly increases the K^+ conductance and rapidly restores full repolarization.
5. **Phase 4, resting potential.** The transmembrane potential of the fully repolarized cell is determined mainly by the conductance of the cell membrane to K^+.

Types of Action Potentials

Two principal **types of action potentials** may be recorded from cardiac cells:

1. **Fast response action potential.** Recorded from atrial and ventricular myocardial fibers and from specialized conducting (Purkinje) fibers. The action potential is characterized by a large amplitude, steep upstroke, which is produced by the activation of fast Na^+ channels. The effective refractory period begins at the upstroke of the action potential and it persists until about midway through phase 3. The fiber is relatively refractory during the remainder of phase 3, but it regains full excitability as soon as it is fully repolarized (phase 4).
2. **Slow response action potential.** Recorded from normal SA and AV nodal cells and from abnormal myocardial cells that have been partially depolarized. The action potential is characterized by a less negative resting potential, a smaller amplitude, and a less steep upstroke than is the fast response action potential. The upstroke is produced by the activation of Ca^{++} channels. The fiber becomes absolutely refractory at the beginning of the upstroke, but partial excitability may not be regained until very late in phase 3 or after the fiber is fully repolarized. The fiber remains relatively refractory for a significant time after the fiber has fully repolarized.

Automaticity

Automaticity is characteristic of certain cells in the heart, notably those in the SA and AV nodes and in the specialized conducting system. Automaticity is ascribable to a slow depolarization of the membrane during phase 4. Ultimately, the transmembrane potential achieves threshold; this leads to the upstroke of the action potential and the firing of the automatic cell.

Cardiac Excitation

Normally, the SA node initiates the impulse that induces cardiac contraction. This impulse is propagated from the SA node to the atria, and the wave of excitation ultimately reaches the AV node. Because the cells in the AV node are slow response fibers, the impulse travels very slowly through the AV node. The consequent delay between atrial and ventricular depolarization provides adequate time for atrial contraction to help fill the ventricles.

Disturbances of Impulse Initiation

Impulses may be initiated abnormally (a) by slow diastolic depolarization of automatic cells in ectopic sites, or (b) by afterdepolarizations that reach threshold.

1. **Ectopic foci.** Automatic cells in the atrium,

AV node, or His-Purkinje system may initiate propagated cardiac impulses either because the ordinarily more rhythmic, normal pacemaker cells are suppressed, or because the rhythmicity of the ectopic foci is abnormally enhanced.

2. **Afterdepolarizations.** Under abnormal conditions, afterdepolarizations may appear early in phase 3 of a normally initiated beat, or they may be delayed until near the end of phase 3 or the beginning of phase 4. Such afterdepolarizations may themselves trigger propagated impulses.
   a. **Early afterdepolarization.** More likely to occur when the basic cycle length of the initiating beats is very long and when the cardiac action potentials are abnormally prolonged.
   b. **Delayed afterdepolarizations.** More likely to occur when the basic cycle length of the initiating beats is short and when the cardiac cells are overloaded with Ca^{++}.

Disturbances of Impulse Conduction. Disturbances of impulse conduction consist mainly of simple conduction block and reentry.

1. **Simple conduction block.** Failure of propagation in a cardiac fiber as the result of a disease process (ischemia, inflammation) or a drug.
2. **Reentry.** A cardiac impulse may traverse a loop of cardiac fibers and reenter previously excited tissue when (a) the impulse is conducted slowly around the loop, and (b) the impulse is blocked unidirectionally in some section of the loop.

Electrocardiogram

The *electrocardiogram* is recorded from the surface of the body, and it traces the conduction of the cardiac impulse through the heart. The component waves of the electrocardiogram are:

1. **P wave.** Spread of excitation over the atria.
2. **QRS interval.** Spread of excitation over the ventricles.
3. **T wave.** Spread of repolarization over the ventricles.

The electrocardiogram may be used to detect and analyze certain cardiac arrhythmias, such as altered sinoatrial rhythms, atrioventricular conduction blocks, premature depolarizations, ectopic tachycardias, and atrial and ventricular fibrillation.

■ BIBLIOGRAPHY

Journal articles

Armstrong, C.W.: Sodium channels and gating currents, Physiol. Rev. 61:644, 1981.

Bean, B.P.: Multiple types of calcium channels in heart muscle and neurons, Ann. N.Y. Acad. Sci. 560:334, 1989.

Bonke, F.I.M., Kirchhof, C.J.H.J., Allessie, M.A., and Wit, A.L.: Impulse propagation from the SA-node to the ventricles, Experientia 43:1044, 1987.

Bouman, L.N., and Jongsma, H.J.: Structure and function of the sino-atrial node: A review, Eur. Heart J. 7:94, 1986.

Brown, H.F.: Electrophysiology of the sinoatrial node, Physiol. Rev. 62:505, 1982.

Carafoli, E.: The homeostasis of calcium in heart cells, J. Mol. Cell. Cardiol. 17:203, 1985.

Childers, R.: The AV node: normal and abnormal physiology, Prog. Cardiovasc. Dis. 19:361, 1977.

De Mello, W.C.: Modulation of junctional permeability, Fed. Proc. 43:2692, 1984.

Grant, A.O.: Evolving concepts of cardiac sodium channel function, J. Cardiovasc. Electrophysiol. 1:53, 1990.

Hoffman, B.F., and Rosen, M.R.: Cellular mechanisms for cardiac arrhythmias, Circ. Res. 49:69, 1981.

Horackova, M.: Transmembrane calcium transport and the activation of cardiac contraction, Can. J. Physiol. Pharmacol. 62:874, 1984.

January, C.T., and Fozzard, H.A.: Delayed afterdepolarizations in heart muscle: Mechanisms and relevance. Pharmacol. Rev. 40:219, 1988.

January, C.T., and Shorofsky, S.: Early afterdepolarizations: Newer insights into cellular mechanisms. J. Cardiovasc. Electrophysiol. 1:161, 1990.

Langer, G.A.: Sodium-calcium exchange in the heart, Ann. Rev. Physiol. 44:435, 1982.

Lee, C.O.: Ionic activities in cardiac muscle cells and application of ion-selective microelectrodes, Am. J. Physiol. 241:H459, 1981.

Levy, M.N.: Role of calcium in arrhythmogenesis. Circ. 80:IV-23, 1989.

Maylie, J., and Morad, M.: Ionic currents responsible for the generation of pacemaker current in the rabbit sinoatrial node, J. Physiol. 355:215, 1984.

Meijler, F.L., and Janse, M.J.: Morphology and electrophysiology of the mammalian atrioventricular node. Physiol. Rev. 68:608, 1988.

Noble, D.: The surprising heart: A review of recent progress in cardiac electrophysiology. J. Physiol. (London) 353:1, 1984.

Opthof, T.: Mammalian sinoatrial node. Cardiovasc. Drugs Therap. 1:573, 1988.

Pressler, M.L., and Rardon, D.P.: Molecular basis for arrhythmias: Two nonsarcolemmal ion channels. J. Cardiovasc. Electrophysiol. 1:464, 1990.

Reiter, M.: Calcium mobilization and cardiac inotropic mechanisms. Pharmacol. Rev. 40:189, 1988.

Rosen, M.R.: Links between basic and clinical cardiac electrophysiology. Circ. 77:251, 1988.

Shamoo, A.E., and Ambudkar, I.S.: Regulation of calcium transport in cardiac cells, Can. J. Physiol. Pharmacol. 62:9, 1984.

Singer, D.H., Baumgarten, C.M., and Ten Eick, R.E.: Cellular electrophysiology of ventricular and other dysrhythmias: studies on diseased and ischemic heart, Prog. Cardiovasc. Dis. 24:97, 1981.

Spach, M.S., and Kootsey, J.M.: The nature of electrical propagation in cardiac muscle, Am. J. Physiol. 244:H3, 1983.

Sperelakis, N.: Hormonal and neurotransmitter regulation of Ca^{++} influx through voltage-dependent slow channels in cardiac muscle membrane. Membr. Biochem. 5:131, 1984.

Ten Eick, R.E., Baumgarten, C.M., and Singer, D.H.: Ventricular dysrhythmia: membrane basis, or of currents, channels, gates, and cables, Prog. Cardiovasc. Dis. 24:157, 1981.

Tseng, G.-N., and Boyden, P.A.: Multiple types of Ca^{2+} currents in single canine Purkinje cells. Circ. Res. 65:1735, 1989.

Zelis, R., and Moore, R.: Recent insights into the calcium channels. Circ. 80:IV-14, 1989.

Books and monographs

Blaustein, M.P., and Lieberman, M.: Electrogenic transport: fundamental principles and physiological implications, New York, 1984, Raven Press.

Bouman, L.N., and Jongsma, H.J.: Cardiac rate and rhythm, The Hague, 1982, Martinus Nijhoff Publishers.

Cranefield, P.F., and Aronson, R.S.: Cardiac arrhythmias: The role of triggered activity and other mechanisms, Mt. Kisco, N.Y., 1988, Futura Publishing Company.

Hille, B.: Ionic channels of excitable membranes. Sunderland, Mass., 1984, Sinauer Associates Inc.

Levy, M.N., and Vassalle, M.: Excitation and neural control of the heart, Bethesda, Md., 1982, American Physiological Society.

Mazgalev, T., Dreifus, L.S., and Michelson, E.L.: Electrophysiology of the sinoatrial and atrioventricular nodes, New York, 1988, Alan R. Liss, Inc.

Mullins, L.J.: Ion transport in heart, New York, 1981, Raven Press.

Nathan, R.D.: Cardiac muscle: Regulation of excitation and contraction, Orlando, 1986, Academic Press, Inc.

Noble, D., and Powell, T.: Electrophysiology of single cardiac cells, Orlando, 1987, Academic Press.

Paes de Carvalho, A., Hoffman, B.F., and Lieberman, M.: Normal and abnormal conduction in the heart, Mt. Kisco, N.Y., 1982, Futura Publishing Co., Inc.

Rüegg, J.C.: Calcium in muscle activation, New York, New York, 1986, Springer-Verlag.

Sakmann, B., and Neher, E.: Single channel recording, New York, 1983, Plenum Press.

Sperelakis, N.: Physiology and pathophysiology of the heart ed 2, Hingham, Mass., 1989, Martinus Nijhoff Publishers.

Stein, W.D.: Ion channels: molecular and physiological aspects, Orlando, Fla., 1985, Academic Press, Inc.

Zipes, D.P., and Jalife, J.: Cardiac electrophysiology: From cell to bedside, Philadelphia, 1990, W.B. Saunders Co.

3 The Cardiac Pump

It is nearly impossible to contemplate the pumping action of the heart without being struck by its simplicity of design, its wide range of activity and functional capacity, and the staggering amount of work it performs relentlessly over the lifetime of an individual. To understand how the heart accomplishes its important task, it is first necessary to consider the relationships between the structure and function of its components.

■ STRUCTURE OF THE HEART IN RELATION TO FUNCTION

Myocardial Cell

A number of important morphological and functional differences exist between myocardial and skeletal muscle cells. However, the contractile elements within the two types of cells are quite similar; each skeletal and cardiac muscle cell is made up of **sarcomeres** (from Z line to Z line) containing thick filaments composed of myosin (in the A band) and thin filaments containing actin. The thin filaments extend from the point where they are anchored to the Z line (through the I band) to interdigitate with the thick filaments. As in the case of skeletal muscle, shortening occurs by the sliding filament mechanism. Actin filaments slide along adjacent myosin filaments by cycling of the intervening crossbridges, thereby bringing the Z lines closer together.

Skeletal and cardiac muscle show similar length-force relationships. The sarcomere length has been determined with electron microscopy in papillary muscles and intact ventricles rapidly fixed during systole or diastole. Maximal developed force is observed at resting sarcomere lengths of 2 to 2.4 μm for cardiac muscle. At such lengths, there is optimal overlap of thick and thin filaments, and a maximal number of crossbridge attachments. Stretch of the myocardium also increases contractile force by an unexplained increase in sensitivity of the myofilaments to calcium. Developed force of cardiac muscle is less than the maximum value when the sarcomeres are stretched beyond the optimum length, because of less overlap of the filaments, and hence less cycling of the crossbridges. At resting sarcomere lengths shorter than optimum value, the thin filaments overlap each other, which diminishes contractile force.

In general, the fiber length-force relationship for the papillary muscle also holds true for fibers in the intact heart. This relationship may be expressed graphically, as in Fig. 3-1, by substituting ventricular systolic pressure for force

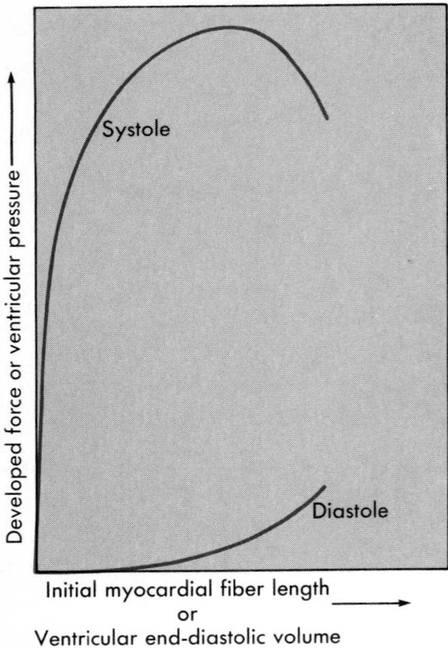

Fig. 3-1 ■ Relationship of myocardial resting fiber length (sarcomere length) or end-diastolic volume to developed force or peak systolic ventricular pressure during ventricular contraction in the intact dog heart. (Redrawn from Patterson, S.W., Piper, H., and Starling, E.H.: J. Physiol. 48:465, 1914.)

and end-diastolic ventricular volume for myocardial resting fiber (and hence sarcomere) length. The lower curve in Fig. 3-1 represents the increment in pressure produced by each increment in volume when the heart is in diastole. The upper curve represents the peak pressure developed by the ventricle during systole at each degree of filling and illustrates the **Frank-Starling relationship** of initial myocardial fiber length (or initial volume) to force (or pressure) development by the ventricle.

Note that the pressure-volume curve in diastole is initially quite flat, indicating that large increases in volume can be accommodated with only small increases in pressure, yet systolic pressure development is considerable at the lower filling pressures. However, the ventricle becomes much less distensible with greater filling, as evidenced by the sharp rise of the diastolic curve at large intraventricular volumes. In the normal intact heart, peak force may be attained at a filling pressure of 12 mm Hg. At this intraventricular diastolic pressure, which is about the upper limit observed in the normal heart, the sarcomere length is 2.2 μm. However, developed force peaks at filling pressures as high as 30 mm Hg in the isolated heart. Even at higher diastolic pressures (>50 mm Hg) the sarcomere length is not greater than 2.6 μm in cardiac muscle. This resistance to stretch of the myocardium at high filling pressures probably resides in the noncontractile constituents of the tissue (connective tissue) and may serve as a safety factor against overloading of the heart in diastole. Usually, ventricular diastolic pressure is about 0 to 7 mm Hg, and the average diastolic sarcomere length is about 2.2 μm. Thus the normal heart operates on the ascending portion of the Frank-Starling curve depicted in Fig. 3-1.

If the heart becomes greatly distended with blood during diastole, as may occur in cardiac failure, it is less efficient; more energy is required (greater wall tension) for the distended heart to eject the same volume of blood per beat than for the normal undilated heart. This is an example of Laplace's law (p. 154), which states that the tension in the wall of a vessel (in this case the ventricles) equals the transmural pressure (pressure across the wall, or distending pressure) times the radius of the vessel or chamber. The Laplace relationship applies to infinitely thin-walled vessels but can be applied to the heart if correction is made for wall thickness. The equation is $\tau = Pr/w$ where τ = wall stress, P = transmural pressure, r = radius and w = wall thickness.

A striking difference in the appearance of cardiac and skeletal muscle is the semblance of a syncytium in cardiac muscle with branching interconnecting fibers (Figs. 3-2 and 3-3). However, the myocardium is not a true anatomical syncytium, because laterally the myocardial fibers are separated from adjacent fibers by their respective sarcolemmas, and the end of each fiber is separated from its neighbor by dense structures, **intercalated disks,** that are continuous with the sarcolemma (Figs. 3-2 to 3-4). Nevertheless, *cardiac muscle functions as a syncytium,* because a wave of depolarization followed by contraction of the entire myocardium (an all-or-none response) occurs when a suprathreshold stimulus is applied to any one focus.

As the wave of excitation approaches the end of a cardiac cell, the spread of excitation to the next cell depends on the electrical conductance of the boundary between the two cells. **Gap junctions (nexi)** with high conductances are present in the intercalated disks between adjacent cells (Figs. 3-2 to 3-4). These gap junctions, which facilitate the conduction of the cardiac impulse from one cell to the next, are made up of **connexons,** which are hexagonal structures that connect the cytosol of adjacent cells. Each connexon consists of 6 polypeptides surrounding a core channel approximately 1.6 to 2.0 nm wide, which serves as a low resistance pathway for cell to cell conductance.

Impulse conduction in cardiac tissues progresses more rapidly in a direction parallel to the long axes of the constituent fibers than in a direction perpendicular to the long axes of those fibers. Gap junctions exist in the borders between myocardial fibers that are in contact with each other longitudinally; they are very sparse or absent in the borders between myocardial fibers that lie side by side.

Another difference between cardiac and fast skeletal muscle fibers is in the abundance of mitochondria **(sarcosomes)** in the two tissues. Fast skeletal muscle, which is called on for relatively short periods of repetitive or sustained contraction and which can metabolize anaerobically and build up a substantial oxygen debt, has relatively few mitochondria in the muscle fibers. In contrast, cardiac muscle, which contracts repetitively for a lifetime and requires a continuous supply of oxygen, is very rich in mitochondria (see Figs. 3-2 to 3-4). Rapid oxidation of substrates with the synthesis of adenosine triphosphate (ATP) can keep pace with the myocardial energy requirements because of the large numbers of mitochondria containing the respiratory enzymes necessary for oxidative phosphorylation.

To provide adequate oxygen and substrate for its metabolic machinery, the myocardium is also endowed with a rich capillary supply, about one capillary per fiber. Thus diffusion distances are short, and oxygen, carbon dioxide, substrates, and waste material can move rapidly between myocardial cell and capillary. With respect to exchange of substances between the capillary blood and the myocardial cells, electron micrographs of myocardium show deep invaginations of the sarcolemma into the fiber at the Z lines (see Figs. 3-2 to 3-4). These sarcolemmal invaginations constitute the **transverse-tubular,** *or* **T-tubular, system.** The lumina of these T-tubules are continuous with the bulk interstitial fluid, and they play a key role in excitation-contraction coupling.

In mammalian ventricular cells, adjacent T-tubules are interconnected by longitudinally running or axial tubules, thus forming an extensively interconnected lattice of "intracellular" tubules (see Fig. 3-4). This T-tubule system is open to the interstitial fluid, is lined with a basement membrane continuous with that of the surface sarcolemma, and contains micropinocytotic-like vesicles. Thus in ventricular cells the myofibrils and mitochondria have ready access to a space that is continuous with the interstitial fluid. The T-tubular system is absent or poorly developed in atrial cells of many mammalian hearts.

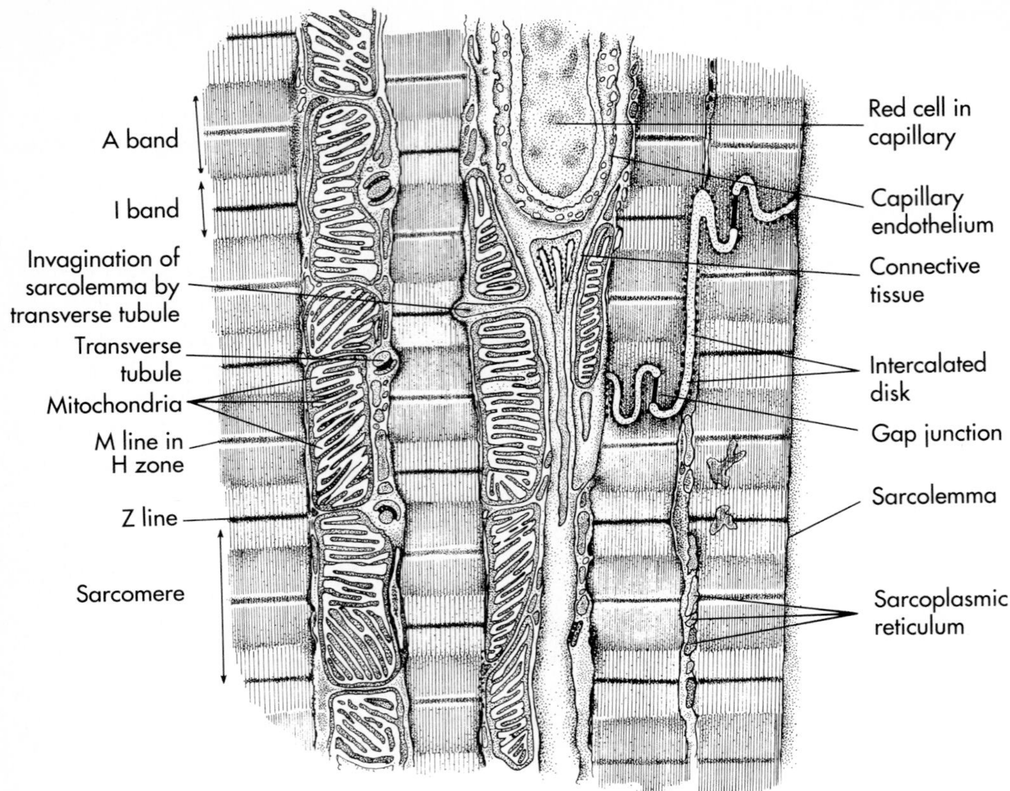

Fig. 3-2 ■ Diagram of an electron micrograph of cardiac muscle showing large numbers of mitochondria and the intercalated disks with nexi (gap junctions), transverse tubules, and longitudinal tubules.

Fig. 3-3 ■ **A,** Low-magnification electron micrograph of a monkey heart (ventricle). Typical features of myocardial cells include the elongated nucleus *(Nu),* striated myofibrils *(MF)* with columns of mitochondria *(Mit)* between the myofibrils, and intercellular junctions (intercalated disks, *ID*). A blood vessel *(BV)* is located between two myocardial cells. **B,** Medium-magnification electron micrograph of monkey ventricular cells, showing details of ultrastructure. The sarcolemma *(SL)* is the boundary of the muscle cells and is thrown into multiple folds where the cells meet at the intercalated disk region *(ID).* The prominent myofibrils *(MF)* show distinct banding patterns, including the A band *(A),* dark Z lines *(Z),* I band regions *(I),* and M lines *(M)* at the center of each sarcomere unit. Mitochondria *(Mit)* occur either in rows between myofibrils or masses just underneath the sarcolemma. Regularly spaced transverse tubules *(TT)* appear at the Z line levels of the myofibrils. **C,** High-magnification electron micrograph of a specialized intercellular junction between two myocardial cells of the mouse. Called a gap junction *(GJ)* or nexus, this attachment consists of very close apposition of the sarcolemmal membranes of the two cells and appears in thin section to consist of seven layers. **D,** Freeze-fracture replica of mouse myocardial gap junction, showing distinct arrays of characteristic intramembranous particles. Large particles *(P)* belong to the inner half of the sarcolemma of one myocardial cell, whereas the "pitted" membrane face *(E)* is formed by the outer half of the sarcolemma of the cell above. (Electron micrographs courtesy Dr. Michael S. Forbes.)

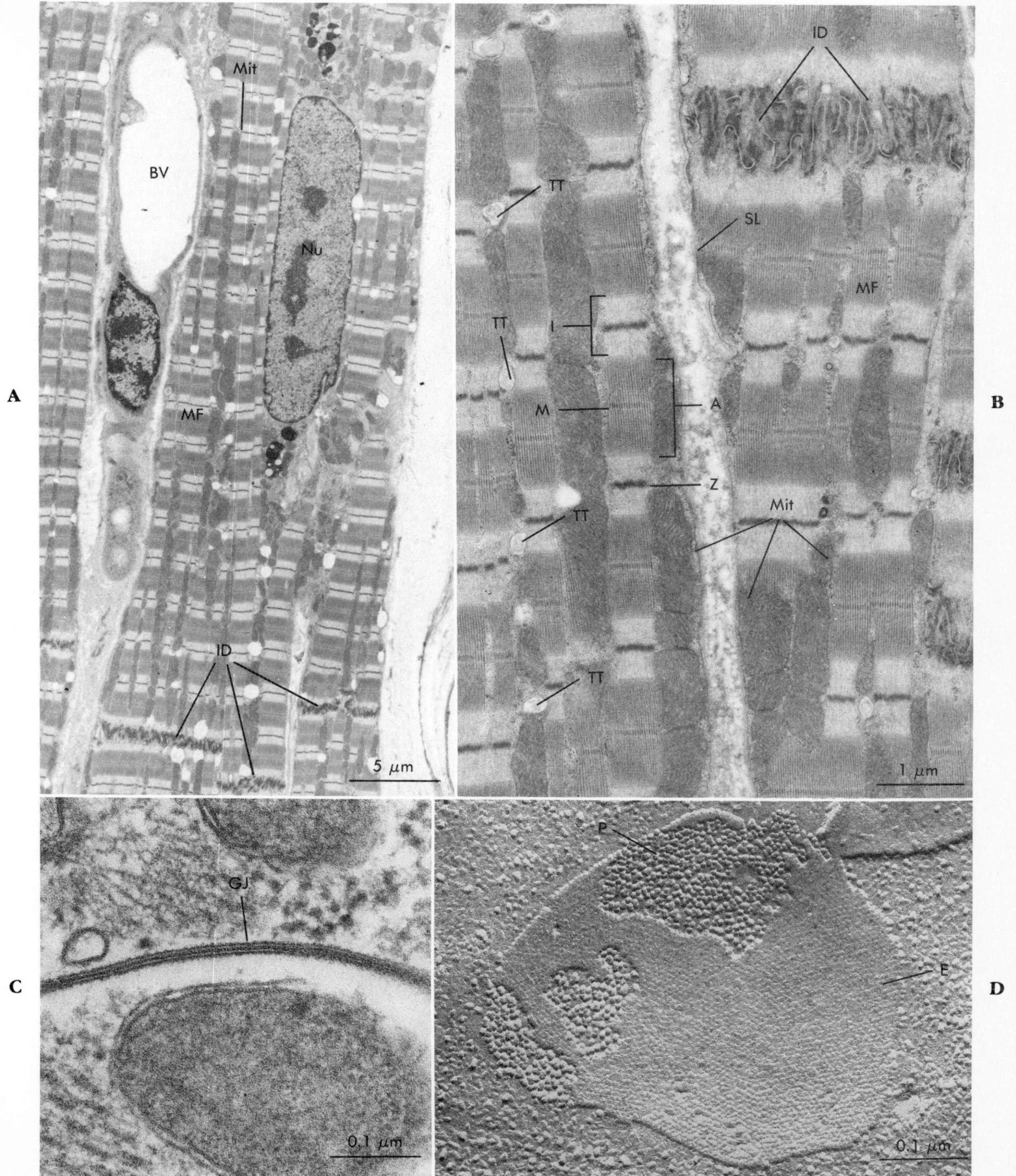

Fig. 3-3 ■ For legend see opposite page.

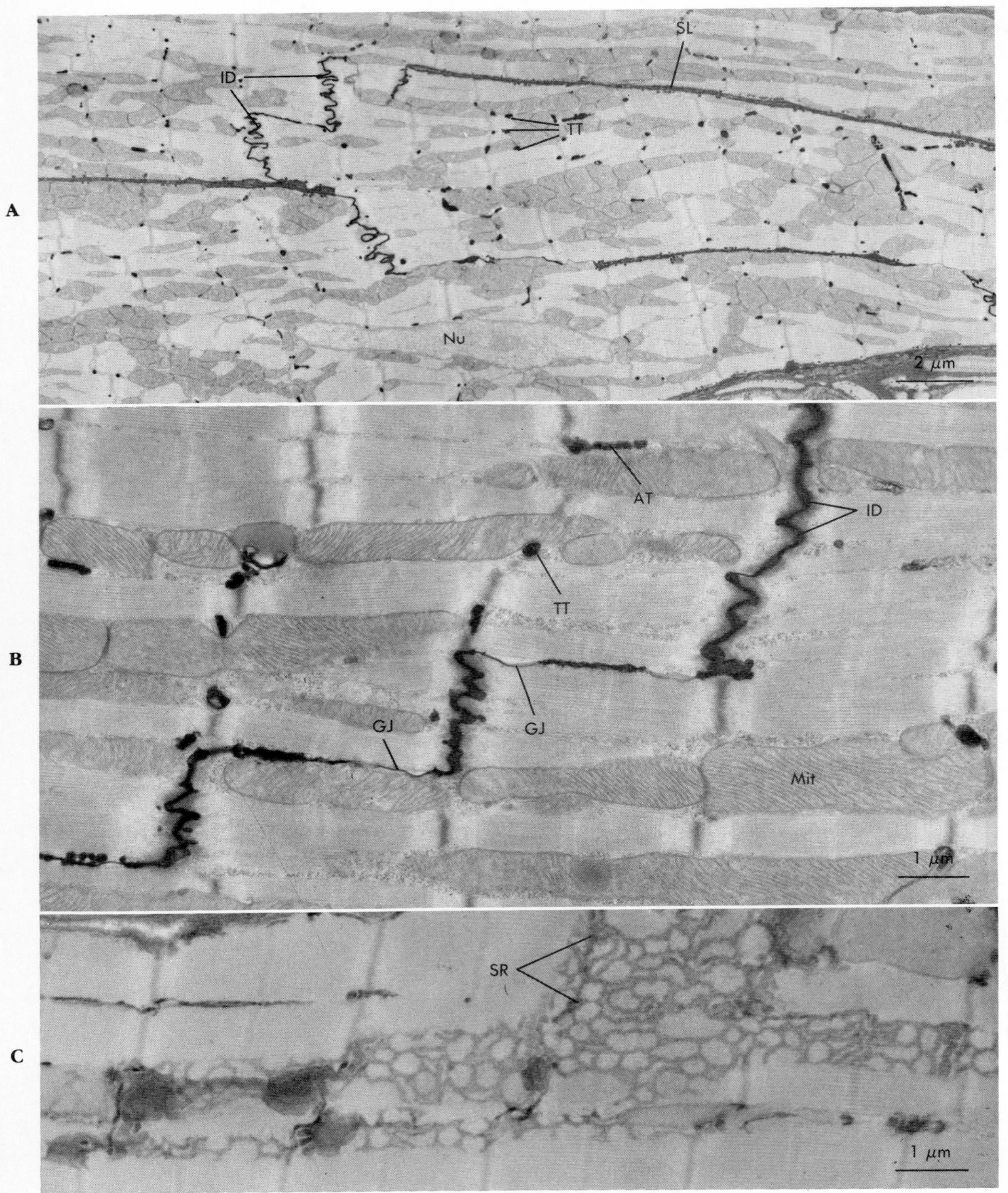

Fig. 3-4 ■ For legend see opposite page.

Fig. 3-4 ■ **A,** Low-magnification electron micrograph of the right ventricular wall of a mouse heart. Tissue was fixed in a phosphate-buffered glutaraldehyde solution and postfixed in ferrocyanide-reduced osmium tetroxide. This procedure has resulted in the deposition of electron-opaque precipitate in the extracellular space, thus outlining the sarcolemmal borders *(SL)* of the muscle cells and delineating the intercalated disks *(ID)* and transverse tubules *(TT)*. *Nu,* Nucleus of the myocardial cell. **B,** Mouse cardiac muscle in longitudinal section, treated as in panel **A.** The path of the extracellular space is traced through the intercalated disk region *(ID),* and sarcolemmal invaginations that are oriented transverse to the cell axis (transverse tubules, *TT*) or parallel to it (axial tubules, *AT*) are clearly identified. Gap junctions *(GJ)* are associated with the intercalated disk. Mitochondria are large and elongated and lie between the myofibrils. **C,** Mouse cardiac muscle. Tissue treated with ferrocyanide-reduced osmium tetroxide so as to identify the internal membrane system (sarcoplasmic reticulum, *SR*). Specific staining of the SR reveals its architecture as a complex network of small-diameter tubules that are closely associated with the myofibrils and mitochondria. (Electron micrographs courtesy Dr. Michael S. Forbes.)

A network of **sarcoplasmic reticulum** (see Fig. 3-4) consisting of small-diameter sarcotubules is also present surrounding the myofibrils; these sarcotubules are believed to be "closed," because colloidal tracer particles (2 to 10 nm in diameter) do not enter them. They do not contain basement membrane. Flattened elements of the sarcoplasmic reticulum are often found in close proximity to the T-tubular system, as well as to the surface sarcolemma, forming "diads."

Excitation-Contraction Coupling. The earliest studies on isolated hearts perfused with isotonic saline solutions indicated the need for optimum concentrations of Na^+, K^+, and Ca^{++}. In the absence of Na^+ the heart is not excitable and will not beat because the action potential depends on extracellular Na ions. In contrast, the resting membrane potential is independent of the Na ion gradient across the membrane (see Fig. 2-5). Under normal conditions the extracellular K^+ concentration is about 4 mM. A reduction in extracellular K^+ has little effect on myocardial excitation and contraction. However, increases in extracellular K^+, if great enough, produce depolarization, loss of excitability of the myocardial cells, and cardiac arrest in diastole. *Ca^{++} is also essential for cardiac contraction;* removal of Ca^{++} from the extracellular fluid results in decreased contractile force and eventually arrest in diastole. Conversely, an increase in extracellular Ca^{++} enhances contractile force, and very high Ca^{++} concentrations induce cardiac arrest in systole (rigor). It is now well documented that free intracellular Ca^{++} is the agent responsible for the contractile state of the myocardium.

Initially a wave of excitation spreads rapidly along the myocardial sarcolemma from cell to cell via gap junctions. Excitation also spreads into the interior of the cells via the T-tubules (see Figs. 3-2 to 3-4), which invaginate the cardiac fibers at the Z lines. (Electrical stimulation at the Z line or the application of ionized Ca to the Z lines in the skinned [sarcolemma removed] cardiac fiber elicits a localized contraction of adjacent myofibrils.) During the plateau (phase 2) of the action potential, Ca^{++} permeability of the sarcolemma increases. Ca^{++} flows down its electrochemical gradient and is largely responsible for the slow inward current (p. 16). Ca^{++} enters the cell through Ca^{++} channels in the sarcolemma and in the invaginations of the sarcolemma, the T-tubules. Opening of the Ca^{++} channels is believed to

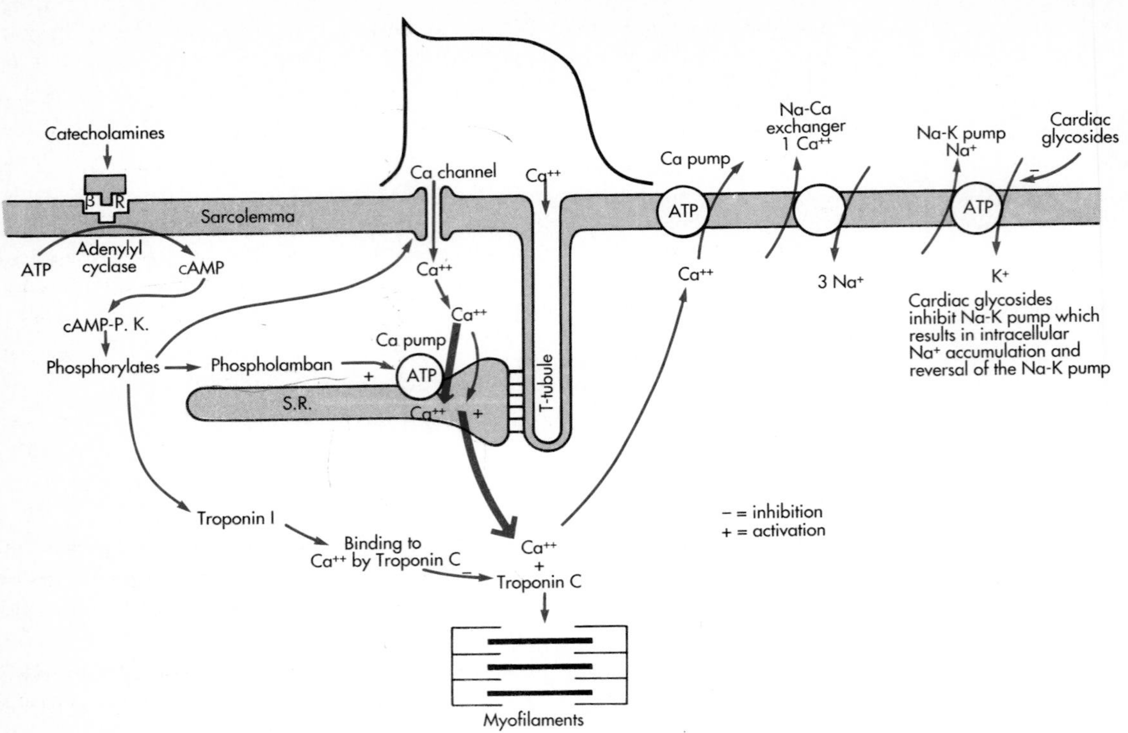

Fig. 3-5 ■ Schematic diagram of the movements of calcium in excitation-contraction coupling in cardiac muscle. The influx of Ca^{++} from the interstitial fluid during excitation triggers the release of Ca^{++} from the sarcoplasmic reticulum *(SR)*. The free cytosolic Ca^{++} activates contraction of the myofilaments (systole). Relaxation (diastole) occurs as a result of uptake of Ca^{++} by the sarcoplasmic reticulum, extrusion of intracellular Ca^{++} by $Na^{+}-Ca^{++}$ exchange and to a limited degree by the Ca pump. *βR,* beta-adrenergic receptor; *cAMP,* cyclic adenosine monophosphate; *cAMP-PK,* cyclic AMP-dependent protein kinase.

be caused by phosphorylation of the channel proteins by a cyclic AMP (cAMP)-dependent protein kinase. The primary source of extracellular Ca^{++} is the interstitial fluid (10^{-3}M of Ca^{++}). Some Ca^{++} also may be bound to the sarcolemma and to the **glycocalyx,** a mucopolysaccharide that covers the sarcolemma. The amount of calcium entering the cell interior from the extracellular space is not sufficient to induce contraction of the myofibrils, but it serves as a trigger **(trigger Ca^{++})** to release Ca^{++} from the intracellular Ca^{++} stores, the sarcoplasmic reticulum (Fig. 3-5). The cytosolic free Ca^{++} increases from a resting level of about 10^{-7}M to levels of 10^{-6} to 10^{-5}M during excitation, and the Ca^{++} binds to the protein troponin C. The Ca^{++}-troponin complex interacts with tropomyosin to unblock active sites between the actin and myosin filaments, which allows crossbridge cycling and hence contraction of the myofibrils (systole).

Mechanisms that raise cytosolic Ca^{++} increase the developed force and those that lower Ca^{++} decrease the developed force. For example, catecholamines increase the movement of Ca^{++} into the cell by phosphorylation of the Ca^{++} channels by a cAMP-dependent protein kinase. An increase in cytosolic Ca^{++} is also achieved by increasing extracellular Ca^{++} or decreasing the Na^{+} gradient across the sarcolemma.

The sodium gradient can be reduced by increasing intracellular Na^{+} or by decreasing extracellular Na^{+}. Cardiac glycosides increase intracellular Na^{+} by poisoning the Na-K pump, which results in an accumulation of Na^{+} in the cells. The elevated cytosolic Na^{+} reverses the Na-Ca exchanger so that less Ca^{++} is removed from the cell. A lowered extracellular Na^{+} results in a reduction in Na^{+} entry into the cell and hence less exchange of Na^{+} for Ca^{++} (see Fig. 3-5).

Developed tension is diminished by a reduction in extracellular Ca^{++}, an increase in the Na^{+} gradient across the sarcolemma, or by the administration of Ca^{++} blockers that prevent Ca^{++} from entering the myocardial cell (see Fig. 2-10).

At the end of systole the Ca^{++} influx ceases and the sarcoplasmic reticulum is no longer stimulated to release Ca^{++}. In fact, the sarcoplasmic reticulum avidly takes up Ca^{++} by means of an ATP-energized calcium pump that is stimulated by phospholamban after the phospholamban is phosphorylated by cAMP-dependent protein kinase. Phosphorylation of troponin I inhibits the Ca^{++} binding of troponin C, which permits tropomyosin to again block the sites for interaction between the actin and myosin filaments, and relaxation (diastole) occurs. Cardiac contraction and relaxation are both accelerated by catecholamines and adenylyl cyclase activation. The resulting increase in cAMP activates the cAMP-dependent protein kinase, which phosphorylates the Ca channel in the sarcolemma. This allows a greater influx of Ca^{++} into the cell, and thereby accelerates contraction. However, it also accelerates relaxation by phosphorylating phospholamban, which enhances Ca^{++} uptake by the sarcoplasmic reticulum, and by phosphorylating troponin I, which inhibits the Ca^{++} binding of troponin C. Thus the phosphorylations by cAMP-dependent protein kinase serve to increase both the speed of contraction *and* the speed of relaxation.

Mitochondria also take up and release Ca^{++}, but the process is too slow to be involved in excitation-contraction coupling. Only at very high intracellular Ca^{++} levels (pathological states) do the mitochondria take up a significant amount of Ca^{++}.

The Ca^{++} that enters the cell to initiate contraction must be removed during diastole. The removal is primarily accomplished by an electroneutral exchange of 3 Na^{+} for 1 Ca^{++} (see Fig. 3-5). Ca^{++} is also removed from the cell by an electrogenic pump that utilizes energy to transport Ca^{++} across the sarcolemma (see Fig. 3-5).

Myocardial Contractile Machinery and Contractility. Velocity and force of contraction are a function of the intracellular concentration of free Ca ions. *Force and velocity are inversely related, so that with no load, force is negligible and velocity is maximal. In an isometric contraction, where no external shortening occurs, force is maximal and velocity is zero.*

The sequence of events in a **preloaded** and **afterloaded** isotonic contraction of a papillary muscle is illustrated in Fig. 3-6. Point *A* represents the resting state in which the preload is responsible for the existing initial stretch. With stimulation the **contractile element** begins to shorten, and at point *B* the **elastic element** has been stretched, but the load has not yet been lifted because the overall length of the muscle has not changed; the muscle fibers have shortened at the expense of the elastic element.

This stretch of the elastic element (an expression of the muscle extensibility) consumes a certain amount of energy. To this energy is added the energy of shortening to obtain the

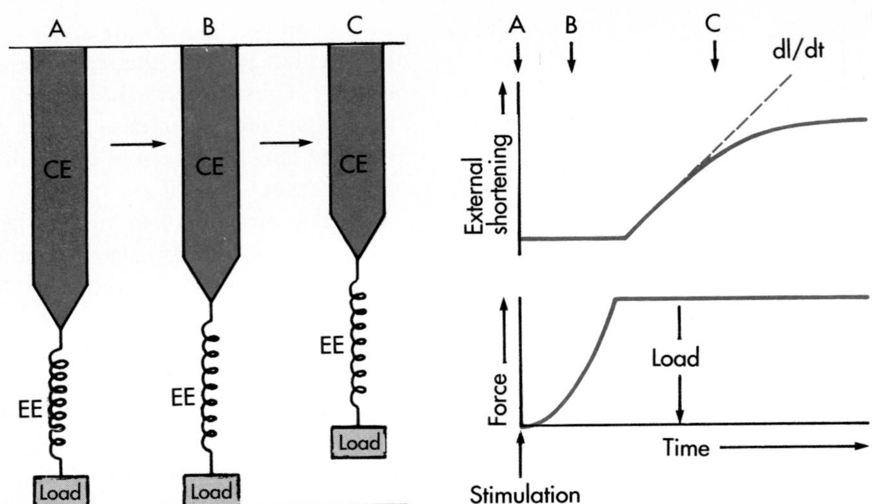

Fig. 3-6 ■ Model for a preloaded (isometric) and afterloaded (isotonic) contraction of papillary muscle. **A**, Muscle at rest. Preload is represented by partial stretch of the elastic element *(EE)*. **B**, Partial contraction of the contractile element *(CE)* with stretch of the *EE* elastic element and no external shortening (the isometric phase of the contraction). **C**, Further contraction of the contractile element with external shortening and lifting of the afterload. The tangent *(dl/dt)* to the initial slope of the shortening curve on the right is the velocity of initial shortening. (Redrawn from Sonnenblick, E.H.: The myocardial cell, Philadelphia, 1966, University of Pennsylvania Press.)

total energy expenditure of a single contraction. Stretch of the elastic element is represented in the diagram (see Fig. 3-6) as a progressive rise in force with no external shortening. At point *C* the force developed by the contractile element has equaled the load (the afterload), and the load has been raised without further stretch of the elastic element. This is represented in the diagram (see Fig. 3-6) as external shortening of the muscle without a further increase in force.

When these observations on papillary muscle are applied to the whole heart, the preload refers to the stretch of the left ventricle just before the onset of contraction (the so-called end-diastolic volume) and the afterload refers to the aortic pressure during the period when the aortic valve is open. The preload can be increased by greater filling of the left ventricle during diastole (see Fig. 3-1). At the lower end-diastolic volumes, increments in filling pressure during diastole elicit a greater systolic pressure during the subsequent contraction until a maximum systolic pressure is reached at the optimum preload. Further diastolic filling beyond this point results in no further increase in developed pressure; at very high filling pressures, peak pressure development in systole is reduced. At a constant preload, a higher systolic pressure can be reached during ventricular contractions by raising the afterload (e.g., increasing aortic pressure by preventing much of the runoff of blood to the periphery during diastole). Increments in afterload will produce progressively higher peak systolic pressures until the afterload is so great that the ventricle can no longer generate enough force to open the aortic valve. At this point ventricular systole is totally isometric; there is no ejection of blood, and hence no change in volume of the ventricle during systole. The maximal pressure developed by the left ventricle under these conditions is the maximal isometric force of which the ventricle is capable at a given preload. Of course, at preloads below the optimal filling volume an increase in preload can yield a greater maximal isometric force (see Fig. 3-1).

The preloads and afterloads depend on the characteristics of the vascular system and the behavior of the heart. With respect to the vasculature, the degree of venomotor tone and peripheral resistance influence preload and afterload. With respect to the heart, a change in rate or stroke volume can also alter preload and afterload. Hence, the cardiac and vascular factors are interactive in their effect on preload and afterload (see Chapter 9 for a full explanation).

If the initial velocity of shortening is plotted against the afterload, the force-velocity curves shown in Fig. 3-7 are obtained. The maximum velocity (V_0) may be estimated by extrapolation of the force-velocity curve back to zero load (as indicated by the dotted lines in Fig. 3-7) and represents the maximum rate of cycling of the crossbridges.

Contractility represents the performance of the heart at a given preload and afterload. It is the change in peak isometric force (isovolumic pressure) at a given initial fiber length (end-diastolic volume). Augmentation of contractility is observed with certain drugs, such as norepinephrine or digitalis, and with an increase in contraction frequency **(tachycardia).** The increase in contractility **(positive inotropic effect)** produced by any of these interventions is reflected by increments in developed force and V_0.

An increase in initial fiber length produces a more forceful contraction, as shown in Fig. 3-1. However, this greater force development is not associated with any change in contractility,

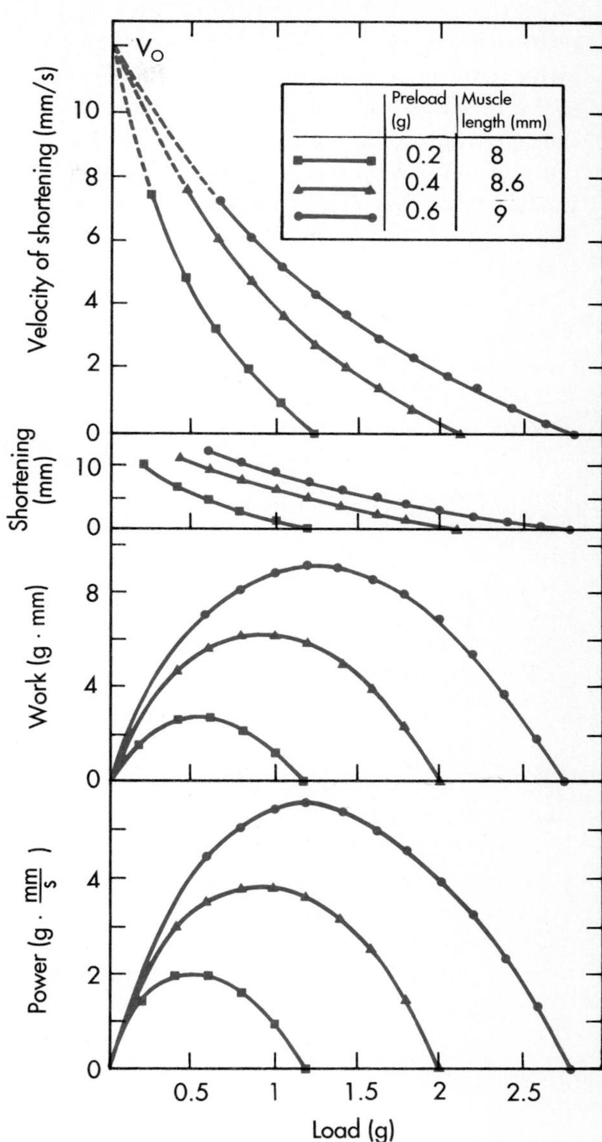

Fig. 3-7 ■ The effect of increasing initial length of a cat papillary muscle on the force-velocity relationship, degree of shortening, muscle work, and muscle power. (Redrawn and reproduced by permission from Am. J. Physiol. 202:931, 1962.)

as estimated by V_0 (see Fig. 3-7). Fig. 3-7 also illustrates that at any given preload, the degree of shortening, the work (load × shortening or force × distance), and the power (load × velocity or work/time) all increase with the initial length of the papillary muscle. It is apparent that with an increase in initial fiber length, greater force may be developed, but the estimated V_0 is the same for all three initial lengths. Hence changes in resting length may alter force development but not contractility. This conclusion is, of course, based on the assumption that the displayed extrapolation of the force-velocity curves back to the vertical axis provide the true value for V_0. This assumption has been challenged; some investigators have failed to obtain a hyperbolic force-velocity relationship and have observed changes in V_0 (inotropic state) with changes in initial length (that is, V_0 is **length-dependent**—activation of the contractile system is influenced by muscle length.). For this and several other reasons, estimates of V_0 are not a reliable index of contractility.

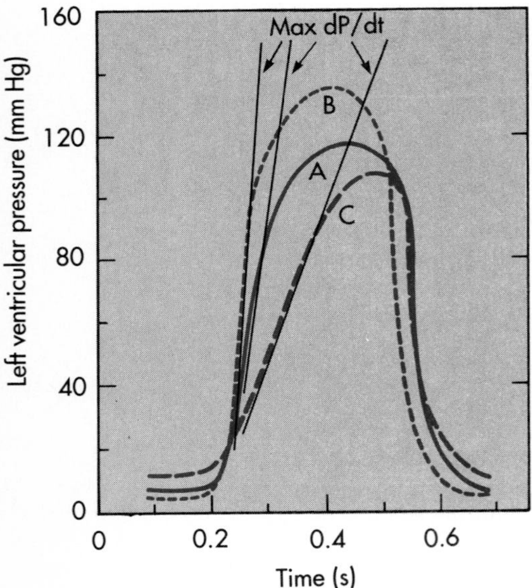

Fig. 3-8 ■ Left ventricular pressure curves with tangents drawn to the steepest portions of the ascending limbs to indicate maximum dP/dt values. *A,* Control; *B,* hyperdynamic heart, as with norepinephrine administration; *C,* hypodynamic heart, as in cardiac failure.

A reasonable index of myocardial contractility can be obtained from the contour of ventricular pressure curves (Fig. 3-8). A hypodynamic heart is characterized by an elevated end-diastolic pressure, a slowly rising ventricular pressure, and a somewhat reduced ejection phase (curve *C,* Fig. 3-8). A normal ventricle under adrenergic stimulation shows a reduced end-diastolic pressure, a fast-rising ventricular pressure, and a brief ejection phase (curve *B,* Fig. 3-8). The slope of the ascending limb of the ventricular pressure curve indicates the maximum rate of force development by the ventricle (maximum rate of change in pressure with time; maximum dP/dt, as illustrated by the tangents to the steepest portion of the ascending limbs of the ventricular pressure curves in Fig. 3-8). The slope is maximal during the isovolumic phase of systole (p. 71) and, at any given degree of ventricular filling, provides an index of the initial contraction velocity and hence of contractility. Similarly, one can obtain an indication of the contractile state of the myocardium from the initial velocity of blood flow in the ascending aorta (the initial slope of the aortic flow curve). The **ejection fraction,** which is the ratio of the volume of blood ejected from the left ventricle per beat **(stroke volume)** to the volume of blood in the left ventricle at the end of diastole is widely used clinically as an index of contractility. Other measurements or combinations of measurements that in general are concerned with the magnitude or velocity of the ventricular contraction also have been used to assess the contractile state of the cardiac muscle. There is no index that is entirely satisfactory at present, and this undoubtedly accounts for the several indices that are currently in use.

Cardiac Chambers

The atria are thin-walled, low-pressure chambers that function more as large reservoir conduits of blood for their respective ventricles than as important pumps for the forward propulsion of blood. The ventricles were once thought to be made up of bands of muscle. However, it now appears that they are formed by a continuum of muscle fibers that take origin from the fibrous skeleton at the base of the heart (chiefly around the aortic orifice). These fibers sweep toward the apex at the epicardial surface and also pass toward the endocardium as they gradually undergo a 180-degree change in direction to lie parallel to the epicardial fibers and form the endocardium and papillary muscles (Fig. 3-9). At the apex of the heart the fibers twist and turn inward to form papillary muscles, whereas at the base and around the valve orifices they form a thick powerful muscle that not only decreases ventricular circumference for ejection of blood but also narrows the AV valve orifices as an aid to valve closure. In addition to a reduction in circumference, ventricular ejection is accomplished by a decrease in the longitudinal axis with descent of the base of the heart. The earlier contraction of the apical part of the ventricles coupled with approximation of the ventricular walls propels the blood toward the outflow tracts. The right ventricle, which develops a mean pressure about one seventh that developed by the left ventricle, is considerably thinner than the left.

Cardiac Valves

The cardiac valves consist of thin flaps of flexible, tough endothelium-covered fibrous tissue firmly attached at the base to the fibrous valve rings. Movements of the valve leaflets are essentially passive, and the orientation of the cardiac valves is responsible for unidirectional flow of blood through the heart. There are two

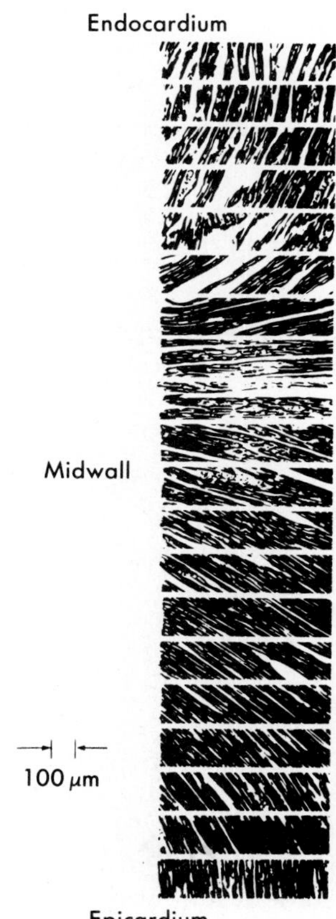

Fig. 3-9 ■ Sequence of photomicrographs showing fiber angles in successive sections taken from the middle of the free wall of the left ventricle from a heart in systole. The sections are parallel to the epicardial plane. Fiber angle is 90 degrees at the endocardium, running through 0 degrees at the midwall to −90 degrees at the epicardium. (From Streeter, D.D., Jr., Spotnitz, H.M., Patel, D.P., Ross, J., Jr., and Sonnenblick, E.H.: Circ. Res. 24:339, 1969. By permission of the American Heart Association, Inc.)

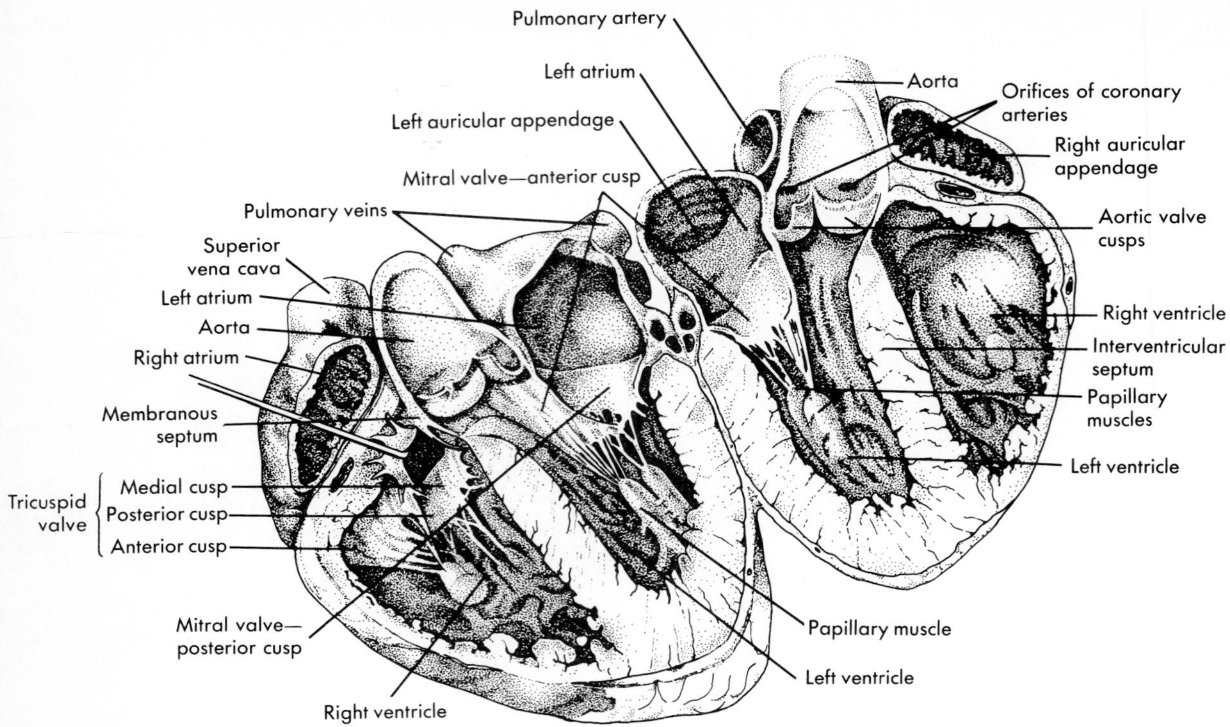

Fig. 3-10 ■ Drawing of a heart split perpendicular to the interventricular septum to illustrate the anatomical relationships of the leaflets of the AV and aortic valves.

types of valves in the heart—the **atrioventricular valves,** or **AV valves,** and the **semilunar valves** (Figs. 3-10 and 3-11).

Atrioventricular Valves. The valve between the right atrium and right ventricle is made up of three cusps **(tricuspid valve),** whereas that between the left atrium and left ventricle has two cusps **(mitral valve).** The total area of the cusps of each AV valve is approximately twice that of the respective AV orifice so that there is considerable overlap of the leaflets in the closed position (see Figs. 3-10 and 3-11). Attached to the free edges of these valves are fine, strong filaments **(chordae tendineae),** which arise from the powerful papillary muscles of the respective ventricles and prevent eversion of the valves during ventricular systole.

The mechanism of closure of the AV valves has been the subject of considerable investigation, and a number of factors are thought to play a role in approximating the valve leaflets. In the normal heart the valve leaflets are relatively close during ventricular filling and provide a funnel for the transfer of blood from atrium to ventricle. This partial approximation of the valve surfaces during diastole is believed to be caused by eddy currents behind the leaflets and possibly also by some tension on the free edges of the valves, exerted by the chordae tendineae and papillary muscles that are stretched by the filling ventricle. Movements

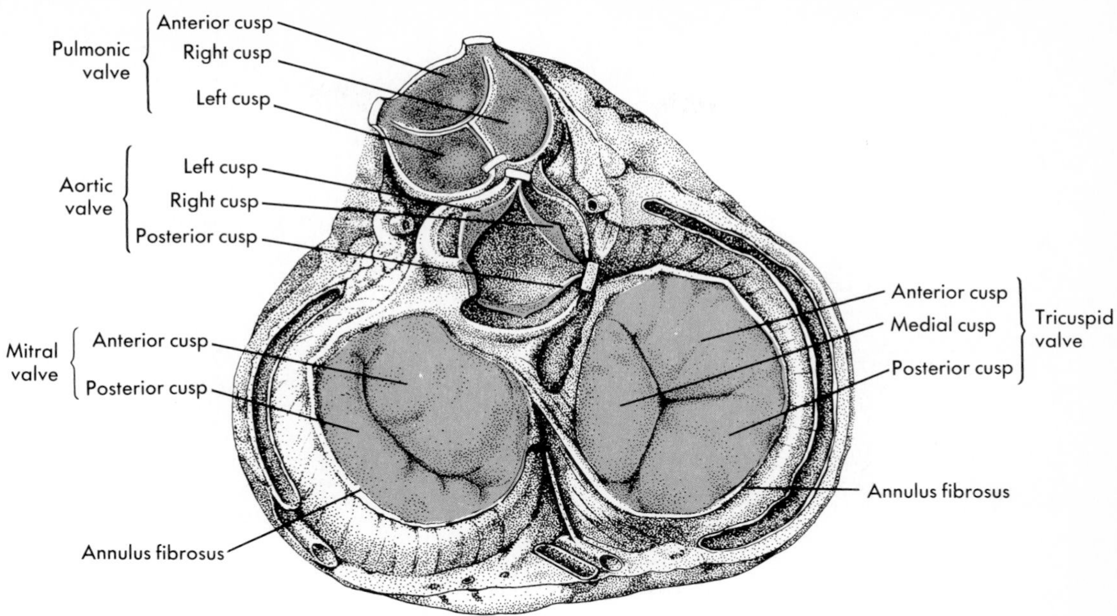

Fig. 3-11 ■ Four cardiac valves as viewed from the base of the heart. Note how the leaflets overlap in the closed valves.

of the mitral valve leaflets throughout the cardiac cycle are shown in an **echocardiogram** (Fig. 3-12). Echocardiography consists of sending short pulses of high-frequency sound waves (ultrasound) through the chest tissues and the heart and recording the echoes reflected from the various structures. The timing and the pattern of the reflected waves provide such information as the diameter of the heart, the ventricular wall thickness, and the magnitude and direction of the movements of various components of the heart.

In Fig. 3-12 the echocardiograph is positioned to depict movement of the anterior leaflet of the mitral valve. The posterior leaflet moves in a pattern that is a mirror image of the anterior leaflet, but in the projection shown in Fig. 3-12 the excursions appear much smaller. At point *D* the mitral valve opens, and during rapid filling (*D* to *E*) the anterior leaflet moves toward the ventricular septum. During the reduced filling phase (*E* to *F*) the valve leaflets float toward each other but the valve does not close. The ventricular filling contributed by atrial contraction (*F* to *A*) forces the leaflets apart, and a second approximation of the leaflets follows (*A* to *C*). At point *C* the valve is closed by ventricular contraction. The valve leaflets, which bulge toward the atrium, stay pressed together during ventricular systole (*C* to *D*).

Semilunar Valves. The valves between the right ventricle and the pulmonary artery and between the left ventricle and the aorta consist of three cuplike cusps attached to the valve rings (see Figs. 3-10 and 3-11). At the end of the reduced ejection phase of ventricular systole, there is a brief reversal of blood

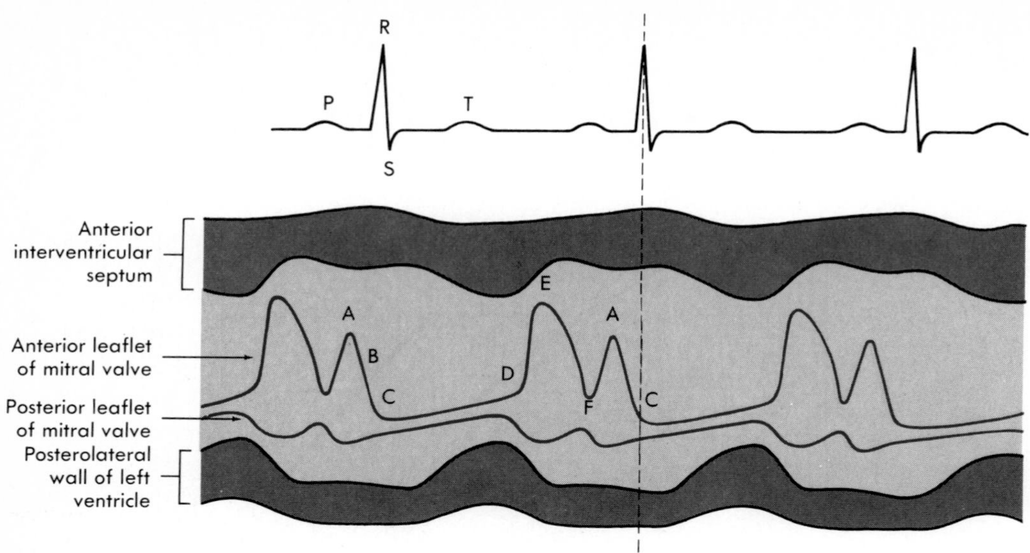

Fig. 3-12 ■ Drawing made from an echocardiogram showing movements of the mitral valve leaflets (particularly the anterior leaflet) and the changes in the diameter of the left ventricular cavity and the thickness of the left ventricular walls during cardiac cycles in a normal person. *D* to *C*, Ventricular diastole; *C* to *D*, ventricular systole; *D* to *E*, rapid filling; *E* to *F*, reduced filling (diastasis); *F* to *A*, atrial contraction. Mitral valve closes at *C* and opens at *D*. Simultaneously recorded electrocardiogram at top. (Original echocardiogram courtesy Dr. Sanjiv Kaul.)

flow toward the ventricles (shown as a negative flow in the phasic aortic flow curve in Fig. 3-13) that snaps the cusps together and prevents regurgitation of blood into the ventricles. During ventricular systole the cusps do not lie back against the walls of the pulmonary artery and aorta but float in the bloodstream approximately midway between the vessel walls and their closed position. Behind the semilunar valves are small outpocketings of the pulmonary artery and aorta **(sinuses of Valsalva),** where eddy currents develop that tend to keep the valve cusps away from the vessel walls. The orifices of the right and left coronary arteries are located behind the right and the left cusps, respectively, of the aortic valve. Were it not for the presence of the sinuses of Valsalva and the eddy currents developed therein, the coronary ostia could be blocked by the valve cusps.

The Pericardium

The pericardium is an epithelized fibrous sac. It closely invests the entire heart and the cardiac portion of the great vessels and is reflected onto the cardiac surface as the epicardium. The sac normally contains a small amount of fluid, which provides lubrication for the continuous movement of the enclosed heart. The distensibility of the pericardium is small, so that it strongly resists a large, rapid increase in cardiac size. Because of this characteristic, the pericardium plays a role in preventing sudden overdistension of the chambers of the heart. However, in congenital absence of the pericardium or after its surgical

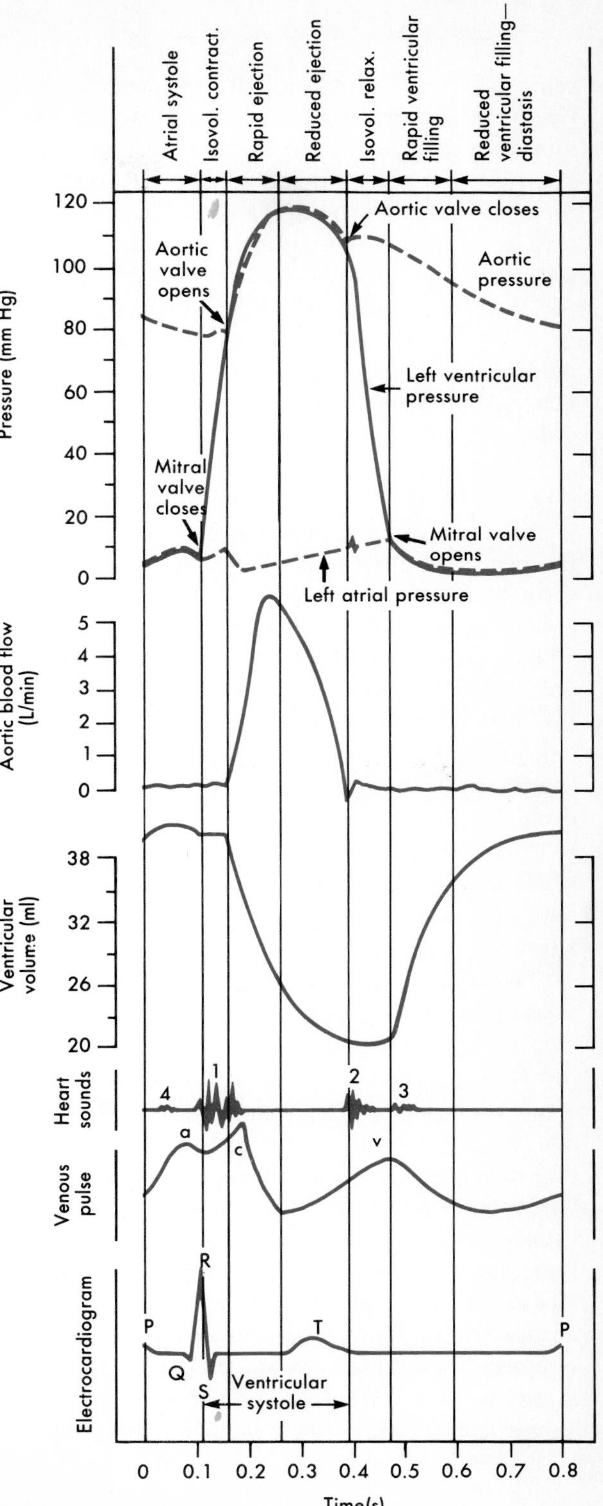

Fig. 3-13 ■ Left atrial, aortic, and left ventricular pressure pulses correlated in time with aortic flow, ventricular volume, heart sounds, venous pulse, and the electrocardiogram for a complete cardiac cycle in the dog.

removal, cardiac function is within physiological limits. Nevertheless, with the pericardium intact, an increase in diastolic pressure in one ventricle increases the pressure and decreases the compliance of the other ventricle. In contrast to an acute change in intracardiac pressure, progressive and sustained distension of the heart (as occurs in cardiac hypertrophy) or a slow progressive increase in pericardial fluid (as occurs in pericarditis with pericardial effusion) gradually stretches the intact pericardium.

Heart Sounds

There are usually four sounds produced by the heart, but only two are ordinarily audible through a stethoscope. With electronic amplification the less intense sounds can be detected and recorded graphically as a **phonocardiogram.** This means of registering heart sounds that may be inaudible to the human ear aids in delineating the precise timing of the heart sounds relative to other events in the cardiac cycle.

The first heart sound is initiated at the onset of ventricular systole (see Fig. 3-13) and consists of a series of vibrations of mixed, unrelated, low frequencies (a noise). It is the loudest and longest of the heart sounds, has a crescendo-decrescendo quality, and is heard best over the apical region of the heart. The tricuspid valve sounds are heard best in the fifth intercostal space just to the left of the sternum, and the mitral sounds are heard best in the fifth intercostal space at the cardiac apex.

The first heart sound is chiefly caused by the oscillation of blood in the ventricular chambers and vibration of the chamber walls. The vibrations are engendered in part by the abrupt rise of ventricular pressure with acceleration of blood back toward the atria, but primarily by sudden tension and recoil of the AV valves and adjacent structures with deceleration of the blood by closure of the AV valves. The vibrations of the ventricles and the contained blood are transmitted through surrounding tissues and reach the chest wall where they may be heard or recorded. The intensity of the first sound is a function of the force of ventricular contraction and of the distance between the valve leaflets. When the leaflets are farthest apart, either when the interval between atrial and ventricular systoles is prolonged and AV valve leaflets float apart or when ventricular systole immediately follows atrial systole, the first sound is loudest.

The second heart sound, which occurs with closure of the semilunar valves (see Fig. 3-13), is composed of higher frequency vibrations (higher pitch), is of shorter duration and lower intensity, and has a more snapping quality than the first heart sound. The second sound is caused by abrupt closure of the semilunar valves, which initiates oscillations of the columns of blood and the tensed vessel walls by the stretch and recoil of the closed valve. The second sound caused by closure of the pulmonic valve is heard best in the second thoracic interspace just to the left of the sternum, whereas that caused by closure of the aortic valve is heard best in the same intercostal space but to the right of the sternum. Conditions that bring about a more rapid closure of the semilunar valves, such as increases in pulmonary artery or aortic pressure (for example, pulmonary or systemic hypertension), will increase the intensity of the second heart sound. In the adult the aortic valve sound is usually louder than the pulmonic, but in cases of pulmonary hypertension the reverse is often true.

A normal phonocardiogram taken simultaneously with an electrocardiogram is illustrated in Fig. 3-14. Note that the first sound, which starts just beyond the peak of the R wave, is composed of irregular waves and is of greater intensity and duration than the second sound, which appears at the end of the T wave. A third and fourth heart sound do not appear on this record.

The third heart sound, which is sometimes heard in children with thin chest walls or in patients with left ventricular failure, consists of a few low-intensity, low-frequency vibrations heard best in the region of the apex. It occurs in early diastole and is believed to be the result of vibrations of the ventricular walls caused by abrupt cessation of ventricular distension and deceleration of blood entering the ventricles. This occurs in overloaded hearts when the ventricular volume is very large and the ventricular walls are stretched to the point where distensibility abruptly decreases. A third heart sound in patients with heart disease is usually a grave sign.

A fourth, or atrial, sound, consisting of a few low-frequency oscillations, is occasionally heard in normal individuals. It is caused by oscillation of blood and cardiac chambers created by atrial contraction (see Fig. 3-13).

Because the onset and termination of right and left ventricular systoles are not precisely synchronous, differences in the time of vibration of the two AV valves or two semilunar valves can sometimes be detected with the stethoscope. Such asynchrony of valve vibrations, which may sometimes indicate abnormal cardiac function, is manifest as a **split sound** over the apex of the heart for the AV valves and over the base for the semilunar valves. The heart sounds also may be altered by deformities of the valves; **murmurs** may be produced, and the character of the murmur serves as an important guide in the diagnosis of valvular disease. When the third and fourth (atrial) sounds are accentuated, as occurs in certain abnormal conditions, triplets of sounds may occur, resembling the sound of a galloping horse. These **gallop rhythms** are essentially of two types—**presystolic gallop** caused by accentuation of the atrial sound, and **protodiastolic gallop** caused by accentuation of the third heart sound.

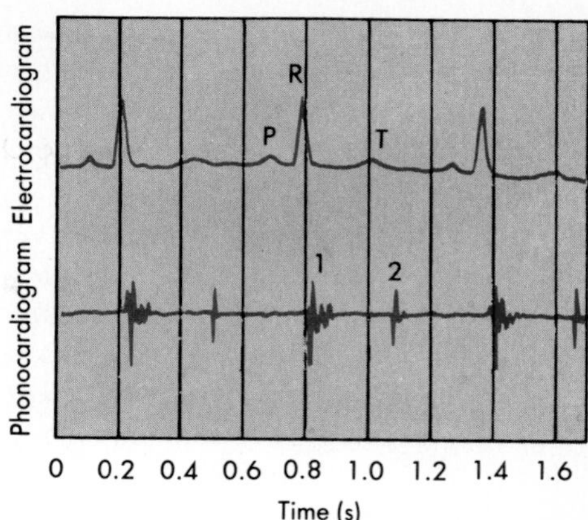

Fig. 3-14 ■ Phonocardiogram illustrating the first and second heart sounds and their relationship to the P, R, and T waves of the electrocardiogram. (Time lines = 0.04 s.)

■ CARDIAC CYCLE

Ventricular Systole

Isovolumic Contraction. The onset of ventricular contraction coincides with the peak of the R wave of the electrocardiogram and the initial vibration of the first heart sound. It is indicated on the ventricular pressure curve as the earliest rise in ventricular pressure after atrial contraction. The interval of time between the start of ventricular systole and the opening of the semilunar valves (when ventricular pressure rises abruptly) is termed **isovolumic contraction,** because ventricular volume is constant during this brief period (see Fig. 3-13).

The increment in ventricular pressure during isovolumic contraction is transmitted across the closed valves and is evident in Fig. 3-13 as a small oscillation on the aortic pressure curve. Isovolumic contraction also has been referred to as isometric contraction. However, some fibers shorten and others lengthen, as evidenced by changes in ventricular shape; it is therefore not a true isometric contraction.

Ejection. Opening of the semilunar valves marks the onset of the ejection phase, which may be subdivided into an earlier, shorter phase **(rapid ejection)** and a later, longer phase **(reduced ejection).** The rapid ejection phase is distinguished from the reduced ejection phase by (1) the sharp rise in ventricular and aortic pressures that terminates at the peak ventricular and aortic pressures, (2) a more abrupt decrease in ventricular volume, and (3) a greater aortic blood flow (see Fig. 3-13). The sharp decrease in the left atrial pressure curve at the onset of ejection results from the descent of the base of the heart and stretch of the atria. During the reduced ejection period, runoff of blood from the aorta to the periphery exceeds ventricular output and therefore aortic pressure declines. Throughout ventricular systole the blood returning to the atria produces a progressive increase in atrial pressure. Note that during approximately the first third of the ejection period left ventricular pressure slightly exceeds aortic pressure and flow accelerates (continues to increase), whereas during the last two thirds of ventricular ejection the reverse holds true. This reversal of the ventricular/aortic pressure gradient in the presence of continued flow of blood from the left ventricle to the aorta (caused by the momentum of the forward blood flow) is the result of the storage of potential energy in the stretched arterial walls, which produces a deceleration of blood flow into the aorta. The peak of the flow curve coincides in time with the point at which the left ventricular pressure curve intersects the aortic pressure curve during ejection. Thereafter, flow decelerates (continues to decrease) because the pressure gradient has been reversed.

With right ventricular ejection there is shortening of the free wall of the right ventricle (descent of the tricuspid valve ring) in addition to lateral compression of the chamber. However, with left ventricular ejection there is very little shortening of the base-to-apex axis, and ejection is accomplished chiefly by compression of the left ventricular chamber.

The effect of ventricular systole on left ventricular diameter is shown in an echocardiogram (see Fig. 3-12). During ventricular systole (see Fig. 3-12, *C* to *D*) the septum and the free wall of the left ventricle become thicker and move closer to each other.

The venous pulse curve shown in Fig. 3-13 has been taken from a jugular vein, and the *c* wave is caused by impact of the adjacent common carotid artery and to some extent by transmission of a pressure wave produced by the abrupt closure of the tricuspid valve in early ventricular systole. Note that except for the *c* wave, the venous pulse closely follows the atrial pressure curve.

At the end of ejection, a volume of blood approximately equal to that ejected during systole remains in the ventricular cavities. This **residual volume** is fairly constant in normal hearts but is smaller with increased heart rate or reduced outflow resistance and larger when the opposite conditions prevail. An increase in myocardial contractility may decrease residual volume and increase stroke volume and ejection fraction, especially in the depressed heart. With severely hypodynamic and dilated hearts, as in **heart failure,** the residual volume can become many times greater than the stroke volume. In addition to serving as a small adjustable blood reservoir, the residual volume to a limited degree can permit transient disparities between the outputs of the two ventricles.

Ventricular Diastole

Isovolumic Relaxation. Closure of the aortic valve produces the incisura on the descending limb of the aortic pressure curve and the second heart sound (with some vibrations evident on the atrial pressure curve) and marks the end of ventricular systole. The period between closure of the semilunar valves and opening of the AV valves is termed **isovolumic** (or **isometric**) relaxation and is characterized by a precipitous fall in ventricular pressure without a change in ventricular volume.

Rapid Filling Phase. The major part of the ventricular filling occurs immediately on opening of the AV valves when the blood that had returned to the atria during the previous ventricular systole is abruptly released into the relaxing ventricles. This period of ventricular filling is called the **rapid filling phase.** In Fig. 3-13 the onset of the rapid filling phase is indicated by the decrease in left ventricular pressure below left atrial pressure, resulting in the opening of the mitral valve. The rapid flow of blood from atria to relaxing ventricles produces a decrease in atrial and ventricular pressures and a sharp increase in ventricular volume.

The decrease in pressure from the peak of the *v* wave of the venous pulse is caused by transmission of the pressure decrease incident to the abrupt transfer of blood from the right atrium to the right ventricle with opening of the tricuspid valve. Elastic recoil of the previous ventricular contraction may aid in drawing blood into the relaxing ventricle when residual volume is small, especially when ventricular contractility is enhanced, as produced by catecholamines. However, this mechanism probably does not play a significant role in ventricular filling under most normal conditions.

Diastasis. The rapid filling phase is followed by a phase of slow filling, called **diastasis.** During diastasis, blood returning from the periphery flows into the right ventricle and blood from the lungs into the left ventricle. This small, slow addition to ventricular filling is indicated by a gradual rise in atrial, ventricular, and venous pressures and in ventricular volume (see Fig. 3-13).

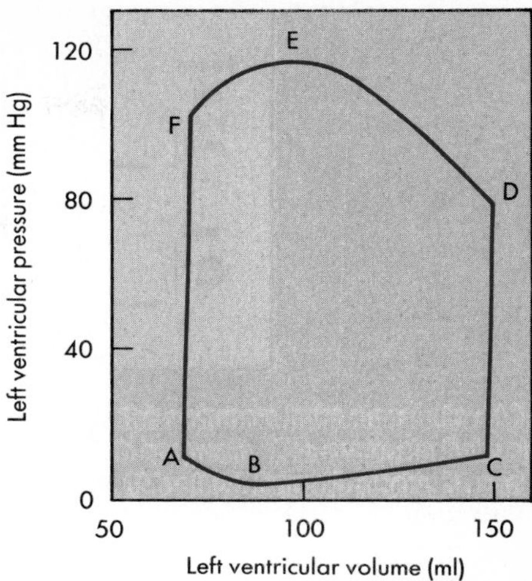

Fig. 3-15 ■ Pressure-volume loop of the left ventricle for a single cardiac cycle *(ABCDEF).*

Pressure-Volume Relationship. The changes in left ventricular pressure and volume throughout the cardiac cycle are summarized in Fig. 3-15. The element of time is not considered in this **pressure-volume loop.** Diastolic filling starts at *A* and terminates at *C*, when the mitral valve closes. The initial decrease in left ventricular pressure (*A* to *B*), despite the rapid inflow of blood from the atrium, is due to progressive ventricular relaxation and distensibility. During the remainder of diastole (*B* to *C*) the increase in ventricular pressure reflects ventricular filling and the passive elastic characteristics of the ventricle. Note that only a small increase in pressure occurs with the increase in ventricular volume during diastole (*B* to *C*). With isovolumic contraction (*C* to *D*) there is a steep rise in pressure and no change in ventricular volume. At *D* the aortic valve opens and during the first phase of ejection (rapid ejection, *D* to *E*), the large reduc-

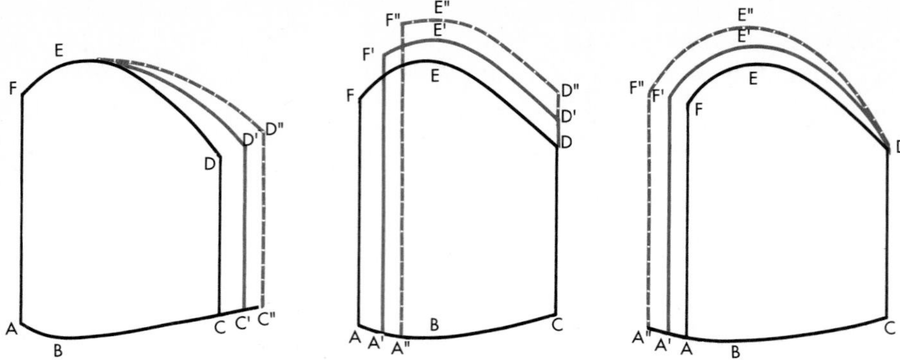

Fig. 3-16 ■ The effects of increases in preload **A**, afterload **B**, and contractility **C**, on the pressure-volume relationships of the left ventricle during a complete cardiac cycle.

tion in volume is associated with a continued but less steep increase in ventricular pressure than that which occurred during isovolumic contraction. This volume reduction is followed by reduced ejection (*E* to *F*) and a small decrease in ventricular pressure. The aortic valve closes at *F*, and this event is followed by isovolumic relaxation (*F* to *A*), which is characterized by a sharp drop in pressure and no change in volume. The mitral valve opens at *A* to complete one cardiac cycle.

With changes in preload, afterload, or myocardial contractility, the contours of the pressure volume loops are altered (Fig. 3-16). Increases in preload by greater filling of the ventricles are depicted in Fig. 3-16, *A* as an extension of the diastolic volume curve upward and to the right (C to C′ and to C″). This greater diastolic filling results in a larger stroke volume (D′ and D″ to F) but peak pressure (E) is unchanged because the afterload (aortic pressure) is unchanged. When the afterload is increased (higher aortic pressure) at a constant preload (Fig. 3-16, *B*), a greater ventricular pressure is reached (D, E, F to D′, E′, F′ and D″, E″, F″). However, less blood is ejected from the ventricle (A to A′ and to A″) (smaller stroke volume and hence a greater residual volume) because of the increased opposition to left ventricular outflow by the high aortic pressure. An increase in contractility without change in preload or afterload, as produced by cardiac sympathetic nerve stimulation or by administration of catecholamines (Fig. 3-16, *C*,) results in a greater pressure development and a greater emptying of the ventricle (larger stroke volume and smaller residual volume). This is shown in Fig. 3-16, *C* as a shift from D, E, F, A to D′, E′, F′, A′, and to D″, E″, F″, A″.

Atrial Systole. The onset of atrial systole occurs soon after the beginning of the P wave of the electrocardiogram (curve of atrial depolarization), and the transfer of blood from atrium to ventricle made by the peristalsis-like wave of atrial contraction completes the period of ventricular filling. Atrial systole is responsible for the small increases in atrial, ventricular, and venous (*a* wave) pressures, as well as in ventricular volume shown in Fig. 3-13. Throughout ventricular diastole, atrial pressure barely exceeds ventricular pressure, indicating a low-resistance pathway across the open AV valves during ventricular filling. A few small vibrations produced by atrial systole constitute the fourth, or atrial, heart sound.

Because there are no valves at the junctions of the venae cavae and right atrium or of the pulmonary veins and left atrium, atrial contraction can force blood in both directions. Actually, little blood is pumped back into the venous tributaries during the brief atrial contraction, mainly because of the inertia of the inflowing blood.

Atrial contraction is not essential for ventricular filling, as can be observed in atrial fibrillation or complete heart block. However, its contribution is governed to a great extent by the heart rate and the structure of the AV valves. At slow heart rates, filling practically ceases toward the end of diastasis, and atrial contraction contributes little additional filling. During tachycardia diastasis is abbreviated and the atrial contribution can become substantial, especially if it occurs immediately after the rapid filling phase when the AV pressure gradient is maximal. Should tachycardia become so great that the rapid filling phase is encroached on, atrial contraction assumes great importance in rapidly propelling blood into the ventricle during this brief period of the cardiac cycle. Of course, if the period of ventricular relaxation is so brief that filling is seriously impaired, even atrial contraction cannot prevent inadequate ventricular filling. The consequent reduction in cardiac output may result in syncope. Obviously, if atrial contraction occurs simultaneously with ventricular contraction, no atrial contribution to ventricular filling can occur. In certain disease states the AV valves may be markedly narrowed **(stenotic).** Under such conditions atrial contraction may play a much more important role in ventricular filling than it does in the normal heart.

Ventricular contraction has been shown to aid indirectly in right ventricular filling by its effect on the right atrium. Descent of the base of the heart stretches the right atrium downward, and pressure measurements indicate a sharp reduction in right atrial pressure associated with acceleration of blood flow in the venae cavae toward the heart. Enhancement of venous return by ventricular systole provides an additional supply of atrial blood for ventricular filling during the subsequent rapid filling phase of diastole. However, this mechanism is probably of little physiological importance, except possibly at rapid heart rates.

■ MEASUREMENT OF CARDIAC OUTPUT

Fick Principle

In 1870, the German physiologist, Adolph Fick, contrived the first method for measuring cardiac output in intact animals and people. The basis for this method, called the **Fick principle,** is simply an application of the law of conservation of mass. It is derived from the fact that the quantity of oxygen (O_2) delivered to the pulmonary capillaries via the pulmonary artery plus the quantity of O_2 that enters the pulmonary capillaries from the alveoli must equal the quantity of O_2 that is carried away by the pulmonary veins.

This is depicted schematically in Fig. 3-17. The rate, q_1, of O_2 delivery to the lungs equals the O_2 concentration in the pulmonary arterial blood, $[O_2]_{pa}$, times the pulmonary arterial blood flow, Q, which equals the cardiac output; that is,

$$q_1 = Q[O_2]_{pa} \quad (1)$$

Let q_2 be the net rate of O_2 uptake by the pulmonary capillaries from the alveoli. At equilibrium, q_2 equals the **O_2 consumption** of the body. The rate, q_3, at which O_2 is carried away by the pulmonary veins equals the O_2 concentration in the pulmonary venous blood, $[O_2]_{pv}$, times the total pulmonary venous flow, which is virtually equal to the pulmonary arterial blood flow, Q; that is,

$$q_3 = Q[O_2]_{pv} \quad (2)$$

From conservation of mass,

$$q_1 + q_2 = q_3 \quad (3)$$

Therefore,

$$Q[O_2]_{pa} + q_2 = Q[O_2]_{pv} \quad (4)$$

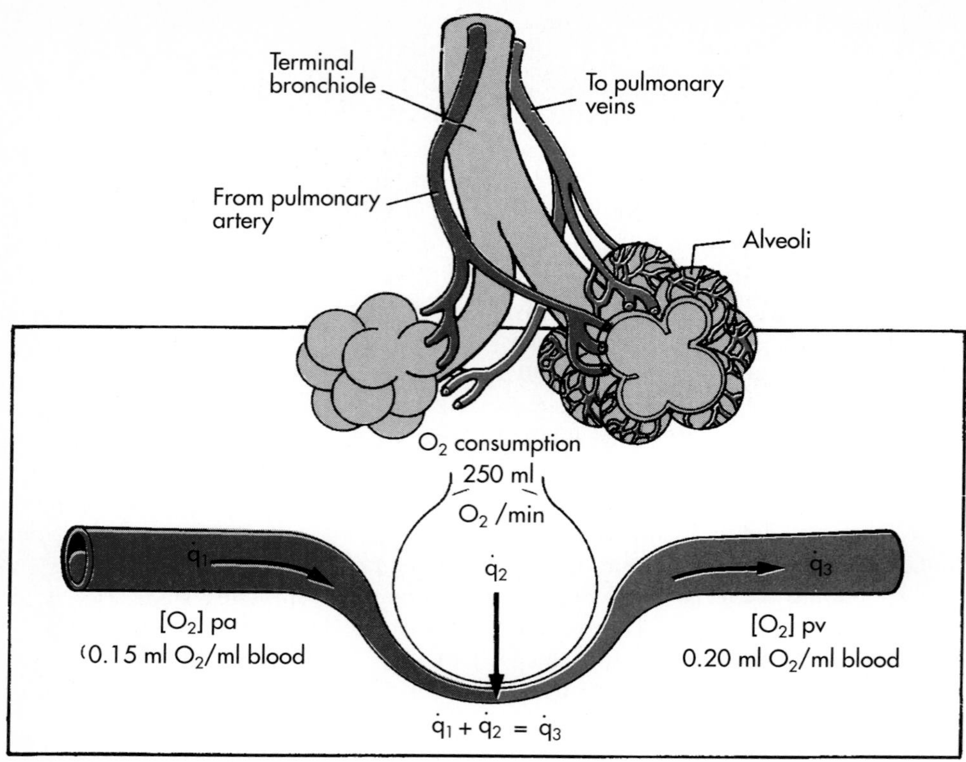

Fig. 3-17 ■ Schema illustrating the Fick principle for measuring cardiac output. The change in color from pulmonary artery to pulmonary vein represents the change in color of the blood as venous blood becomes fully oxygenated.

Solving for cardiac output,

$$Q = q_2/([O_2]_{pv} - [O_2]_{pa}) \qquad (5)$$

Equation 5 is the statement of the Fick principle.

In the clinical determination of cardiac output, O_2 consumption is computed from measurements of the volume and O_2 content of expired air over a given interval of time. Because the O_2 concentration of peripheral arterial blood is essentially identical to that in the pulmonary veins, $[O_2]_{pv}$ is determined on a sample of peripheral arterial blood withdrawn by needle puncture. Pulmonary arterial blood actually represents mixed systemic venous blood. Samples for O_2 analysis are obtained from the pulmonary artery or right ventricle through a catheter. In the past a stiff catheter was used, and it had to be introduced into the pulmonary artery under fluoroscopic guidance. Now, a very flexible catheter with a small balloon near the tip can be inserted into a peripheral vein. As the tube is advanced, it is carried by the flowing blood toward the heart. By following the pressure changes, the physician is able to advance the catheter tip into the pulmonary artery without the aid of fluoroscopy.

An example of the calculation of cardiac output in a normal, resting adult is illustrated in Fig. 3-17. With an O_2 consumption of 250

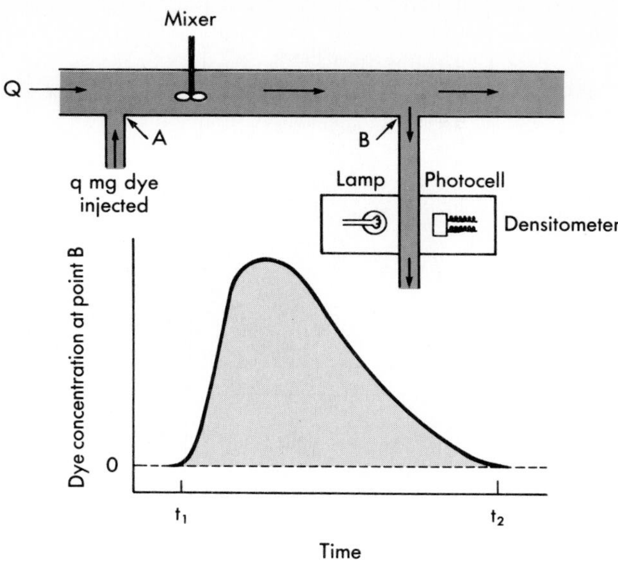

Fig. 3-18 ■ The indicator dilution technique for measuring cardiac output. In this model, in which there is no recirculation, q mg of dye are injected instantaneously at point *A* into a stream flowing at Q ml/min. A mixed sample of the fluid flowing past point *B* is withdrawn at a constant rate through a densitometer. The resulting dye concentration curve at point *B* has the configuration shown in the lower section of the figure.

ml/min, an arterial (pulmonary venous) O_2 content of 0.20 ml O_2/ml blood, and a mixed venous (pulmonary arterial) O_2 content of 0.15 ml O_2/ml blood, the cardiac output would equal 250 ÷ (0.20 − 0.15) = 5000 ml/min.

The Fick principle is also used for estimating the O_2 consumption of organs in situ, when blood flow and the O_2 contents of the arterial and venous blood can be determined. Algebraic rearrangement reveals that O_2 consumption equals the blood flow times the arteriovenous O_2 concentration difference. For example, if the blood flow through one kidney is 700 ml/min, arterial O_2 content is 0.20 ml O_2/ml blood, and renal venous O_2 content is 0.18 ml O_2/ml blood, then the rate of O_2 consumption by that kidney must be 700 (0.20 − 0.18) = 14 ml O_2/min.

Indicator Dilution Techniques

The indicator dilution technique for measuring cardiac output is also based on the law of conservation of mass and is illustrated by the model in Fig. 3-18. Let a liquid flow through a tube at a rate of Q ml/s, and let q mg of dye be injected as a slug into the stream at point *A*. Let mixing occur at some point downstream. If a small sample of liquid is continually withdrawn from point *B* farther downstream and passed through a densitometer, a curve of the dye concentration, c, may be recorded as a function of time, t, as shown in the lower half of the figure.

If no dye is lost between points *A* and *B*, the amount of dye, q, passing point *B* between times t_1 and t_2 will be

$$q = \bar{c}Q(t_2 - t_1) \quad (6)$$

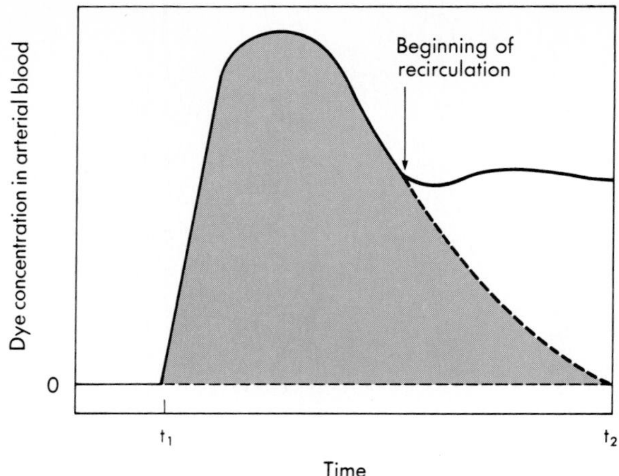

Fig. 3-19 ■ Typical dye concentration curve recorded from a human. Because of recirculation of the dye, the concentration does not return to 0, as in the model in Fig. 3-18. The dashed line on the descending limb represents the semilogarithmic extrapolation of the upper portion of the descending limb, before the beginning of recirculation.

where $\bar{c}$ is the mean concentration of dye. The value of $\bar{c}$ may be computed by dividing the area of the dye concentration by the duration $(t_2 - t_1)$ of that curve; that is

$$\bar{c} = \int_{t1}^{t2} c\, dt/(t_2 - t_1) \quad (7)$$

Substituting this value of $\bar{c}$ into equation 6, and solving for Q yields

$$Q = \frac{q}{\int_{t1}^{t2} c\, dt} \quad (8)$$

Thus, flow may be measured by dividing the amount of indicator injected upstream by the area under the downstream concentration curve.

This technique has been widely used to estimate cardiac output in humans. A measured quantity of some indicator (a dye or isotope that remains within the circulation) is injected rapidly into a large central vein or into the right side of the heart through a catheter. Arterial blood is continuously drawn through a detector (densitometer or isotope rate counter), and a curve of indicator concentration is recorded as a function of time.

Because some of the indicator recirculates and reappears at the site of arterial withdrawal before the entire curve is inscribed, the concentration curve is not as simple as that shown in Fig. 3-18. Instead, on the downstroke of the curve a secondary increase in concentration (Fig. 3-19) appears as the recirculated dye becomes mixed with the last portions of dye still undergoing its primary passage past the site of withdrawal. To compute the area under the concentration curve, the downslope of the curve beyond the beginning of recirculation is extrapolated to zero concentration (dashed line, Fig. 3-19). The extrapolation, of course, introduces some error into the estimation of cardiac output.

Presently the most popular indicator dilution technique is **thermodilution.** The indicator is cold saline. The temperature and volume of the saline are measured accurately before injection. A flexible catheter is introduced into a peripheral vein and advanced so that the tip lies in the pulmonary artery. A small thermistor at the catheter tip records the changes in temperature. The opening in the catheter lies a few inches proximal to the tip. When the tip is in the pulmonary artery, the opening lies in or near the right atrium. The cold saline is injected rapidly into the right atrium through the catheter. The resultant change in temperature downstream is recorded by the thermistor in the pulmonary artery.

The thermodilution technique has the following advantages: (1) an arterial puncture is not necessary; (2) the small volumes of saline used in each determination are innocuous, allowing repeated determinations to be made; and (3) recirculation is negligible. Temperature equilibration takes place as the cooled blood flows through the pulmonary and systemic capillary beds, before it flows by the thermistor in the pulmonary artery the second time. Therefore, the curve of temperature change resembles that shown in Fig. 3-18, and the extrapolation errors are averted.

■ SUMMARY

1. An increase in myocardial fiber length, as occurs with an augmented ventricular filling during diastole (preload), produces a more forceful ventricular contraction. This relation between fiber length and strength of contraction is known as Starling's law of the heart.
2. Although the myocardium is made up of individual cells with discrete membrane boundaries, the cardiac myocytes that comprise the ventricles contract almost in unison, as do those of the atria. The myocardium functions as a syncytium with an all-or-none response to excitation. Cell to cell conduction occurs through gap junctions that connect the cytosol of adjacent cells.
3. On excitation, voltage gated calcium channels open to admit extracellular Ca^{++} into the cell. The influx of Ca^{++} triggers the release of Ca^{++} from the sarcoplasmic reticulum. The elevated intracellular Ca^{++} produces contraction of the myofilaments. Relaxation is accomplished by restoration of the resting cytosolic Ca^{++} level by pumping it back into the sarcoplasmic reticulum and exchanging it for extracellular Na^{+} across the sarcolemma.
4. Velocity and force of contraction are functions of the intracellular concentration of free Ca ions. Force and velocity are inversely related, so that with no load, force is negligible and velocity is maximal. In an isometric contraction, where no external shortening occurs, force is maximal and velocity is zero.
5. In ventricular contraction the preload is the stretch of the fiber by the blood during ventricular filling and the afterload is the aortic pressure against which the left ventricle ejects the blood.
6. Contractility is an expression of cardiac performance at a given preload and afterload. Contractility is increased by stimulation of cardiac sympathetic nerves and decreased by stimulation of the cardiac branches of the vagus nerves.
7. Simultaneous recording of the left atrial, left ventricular and aortic pressures, ventricular volume, heart sounds, and electrocardiogram graphically portray the sequential and related electrical and cardiodynamic events throughout a cardiac cycle.
8. As illustrated by pressure-volume loops of the left ventricle, an increment in preload increases stroke volume, an increase in afterload results in an increase in peak pressure, but a decrease in stroke volume and an increase in contractility produces a greater peak pressure and a greater stroke volume.
9. Cardiac output can be determined, according to the Fick principle, by measuring the oxygen consumption of the body (MVO_2) and the oxygen content of arterial $[O_2]_{pa}$ and mixed venous $[O_2]_{pv}$ blood − cardiac output $= MVO_2/([O_2]_{pv} - [O_2]_{pa})$. It can

also be measured by dye dilution or thermodilution techniques. The greater the cardiac output the greater the dilution of the injected dye or cold saline by the arterial blood.

■ BIBLIOGRAPHY

Journal Articles

Alpert, N.R., Hamrell, B.B., and Mulieri, L.A.: Heart muscle mechanics, Ann. Rev. Physiol. 41:521, 1979.

Bers, D.M., Lederer, W.J., and Berlin, J.R.: Intracellular Ca transients in rat cardiac myocytes: role of Na-Ca exchange in excitation-contraction coupling, Am. J. Physiol. 258:C944, 1990.

Blaustein, M.P.: Sodium/calcium exchange and the control of contractility in cardiac muscle and vascular smooth muscle, J. Cardiovas. Pharmacol. 12:S56, 1988.

Brutsaert, D.L., and Sys, S.U.: Relaxation and diastole of the heart, Physiol. Rev. 69:1228, 1989.

Carafoli, E.: The homeostasis of calcium in heart cells, J. Mol. Cell. Cardiol., 17:203, 1985.

Chapman, R.A.: Control of cardiac contractility at the cellular level, Am. J. Physiol. 245:H535, 1983.

Fabiato, A., and Fabiato, F.: Calcium and cardiac excitation-contraction coupling, Ann. Rev. Physiol. 41:473, 1979.

Gilbert, J.C., and Glantz, S.A.: Determinants of left ventricular filling and of the diastolic pressure-volume relation, Circ. Res. 64:827, 1989.

Jewell, B.R.: A reexamination of the influence of muscle length on myocardial performance, Circ. Res. 40:221, 1977.

Katz, A.M.: Interplay between inotropic and lusitropic effects of cyclic adenosine monophosphate on the myocardial cell, Circ. 82:I-7, 1990.

Katz, A.M.: Cyclic adenosine monophosphate effects on the myocardium: A man who blows hot and cold with one breath, J. Am. Coll. Cardiol., 2:143, 1983.

Sagawa, K.: The ventricular pressure-volume diagram revisited, Circ. Res. 43:677, 1978.

Sonnenblick, E.: Force-velocity relations in mammalian heart muscle, Am. J. Physiol. 202:931, 1962.

Streeter, D.D., Jr., Spotnitz, H.M., Patel, D.P., et al: Fiber orientation in the canine left ventricle during diastole and systole, Circ. Res. 24:339, 1969.

Books and Monographs

Brady, A.J.: Mechanical properties of cardiac fibers. In Handbook of physiology, section 2: The cardiovascular system—the heart, vol. I, Bethesda, Md., 1979, American Physiological Society.

Braunwald, E., Ross, J., Jr., and Sonnenblick, E.H.: Mechanisms of contraction of the normal and failing heart, ed. 2, Boston, 1976, Little, Brown & Co.

Katz, A.M.: Role of calcium in contraction of cardiac muscle. In Stone, P.H., and Antman, E.M., editors: Calcium channel blocking agents in the treatment of cardiovascular disorders, Mt. Kisco, N.Y., 1983, Futura Publishing Co., Inc.

Katz, A.M., Takenaka, H., and Watras, J.: The sarcoplasmic reticulum. In Fozzard, H.A. et al, editor: The heart and cardiovascular system, New York, 1986, Raven Press.

Parmley, W.W., and Talbot, L.: Heart as a pump. In Handbook of physiology; section 2: The cardiovascular system—the heart, vol. I, Bethesda, Md., 1979, American Physiological Society.

Ruegg, J.C.: Calcium in muscle activation, Springer-Verlag, Heidelberg, 1988.

Sheu, S.S., and Blaustein, M.P.: Sodium/calcium exchange and control of cell calcium and contractility in cardiac muscle and vascular smooth muscle. In Fozzard H.A. et al, editor: The heart and cardiovascular system, New York, 1991, Raven Press.

Sommer, J.R., and Johnson, E.A.: Ultrastructure of cardiac muscle. In Handbook of physiology, section 2: The cardiovascular system—the heart, vol. I, Bethesda, Md., 1979, American Physiological Society.

4 Regulation of the Heartbeat

The quantity of blood pumped by the heart each minute (i.e., the **cardiac output,** CO) may be varied by changing the frequency of its beats (i.e., the **heart rate**, HR) or the volume ejected per stroke (i.e., the **stroke volume,** SV). Cardiac output is the product of heart rate and stroke volume; i.e.,

$$CO = HR \times SV$$

A discussion of the control of cardiac activity may therefore be subdivided into a consideration of the regulation of pacemaker activity and the regulation of myocardial performance. However, in the intact organism, a change in the behavior of one of these features of cardiac activity almost invariably alters the other.

Certain local factors, such as temperature changes and tissue stretch, can affect the discharge frequency of the SA node. However, the principal control of heart rate is relegated to the autonomic nervous system, and the discussion will be restricted to this aspect of heart rate control. Relative to myocardial performance, intrinsic and extrinsic factors will be considered.

■ NERVOUS CONTROL OF HEART RATE

In normal adults the average heart rate at rest is approximately 70 beats per minute, but it is significantly greater in children. During sleep the heart rate diminishes by 10 to 20 beats per minute, but during emotional excitement or muscular activity it may accelerate to rates considerably above 100. In well-trained athletes at rest the rate is usually only about 50 beats per minute.

The SA node is usually under the tonic influence of both divisions of the autonomic nervous system. The sympathetic system enhances automaticity, whereas the parasympathetic system inhibits it. Changes in heart rate usually involve a reciprocal action of the two divisions of the autonomic nervous system. Thus an increased heart rate is produced by a diminution of parasympathetic activity and concomitant increase in sympathetic activity; deceleration is usually achieved by the opposite mechanisms. Under certain conditions the heart rate may change by selective action of just one division of the autonomic nervous system, rather than by reciprocal changes in both divisions.

Ordinarily, in healthy, resting individuals parasympathetic tone predominates. Abolition of parasympathetic influences by the administration of atropine usually increases heart rate substantially, whereas abrogation of sympathetic effects by the administration of propranolol usually decreases heart rate only slightly (Fig. 4-1). When both divisions of the autonomic nervous system are blocked, the heart

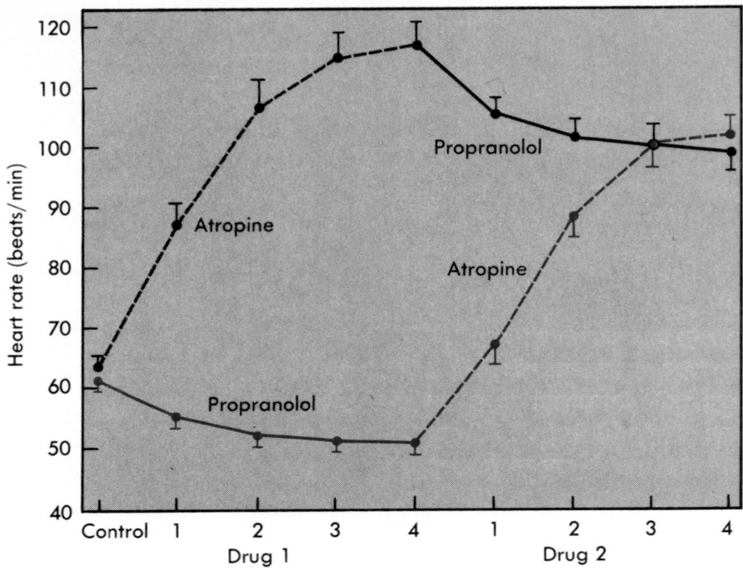

Fig. 4-1 ■ The effects of four equal doses of atropine (0.04 mg/kg total) and of propranolol (0.2 mg/kg total) on the heart rate of 10 healthy young men (mean age, 21.9 years). In half of the trials, atropine was given first *(top curve)*; in the other half, propranolol was given first *(bottom curve)*. (Redrawn from Katona, P.G., McLean, M., Dighton, D.H., and Guz, A.: J. Appl. Physiol. 52:1652, 1982.)

rate of young adults averages about 100 beats per minute. The rate that prevails after complete autonomic blockade is called the **intrinsic heart rate.**

Parasympathetic Pathways

The cardiac parasympathetic fibers originate in the medulla oblongata, in cells that lie in the **dorsal motor nucleus** of **the vagus** or in the **nucleus ambiguus.** The precise location varies from species to species. Centrifugal vagal fibers pass inferiorly through the neck close to the common carotid arteries and then through the mediastinum to synapse with postganglionic cells located on the epicardial surface or within the walls of the heart itself. Most of the cardiac ganglion cells are located near the SA node and AV conduction tissue.

The right and left vagi are distributed differentially to the various cardiac structures. The right vagus nerve affects the SA node predominantly. Stimulation slows SA nodal firing or may even stop it for several seconds. The left vagus nerve mainly inhibits AV conduction tissue, to produce various degrees of AV block. However, the efferent vagal fibers overlap, such that left vagal stimulation also depresses the SA node and right vagal stimulation impedes AV conduction.

The SA and AV nodes are rich in **cholinesterase.** Hence the effects of any given vagal impulse are ephemeral because the acetylcholine released at the nerve terminals is rapidly hydrolyzed. Furthermore, the effects of vagal activity on SA and AV nodal function have a very short latency (about 50 to 100 ms), because the released acetylcholine activates special K^+ channels in the cardiac cells. Opening

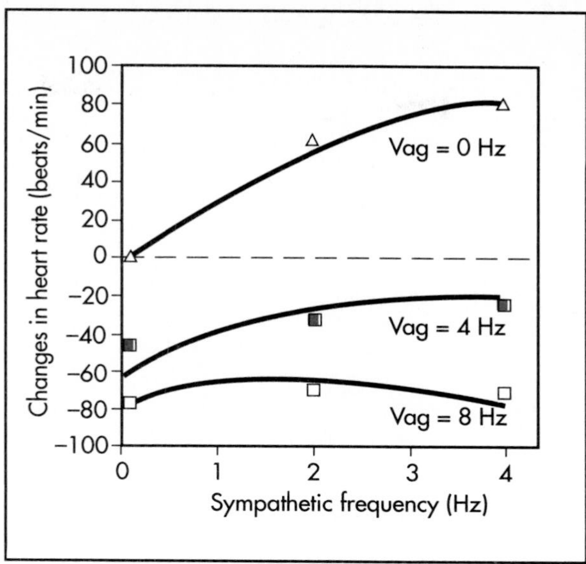

Fig. 4-2 ■ The changes in heart rate in an anesthetized dog when the vagus and cardiac sympathetic nerves were stimulated simultaneously. The sympathetic nerves were stimulated at 0, 2, and 4 Hz; the vagus nerves at 0, 4, and 8 Hz. The symbols represent the observed changes in heart rate; the curves were derived from the computed regression equation. (Modified from Levy, M.N., and Zieske, H.: J. Appl. Physiol. 27:465, 1969.)

of these channels is so prompt because it does not require the operation of a second messenger system, such as the adenylyl cyclase system. The combination of the brief latency and the rapid decay of the response (because of the abundance of cholinesterase) provides the potential for the vagus nerves to exert a beat by beat control of SA and AV nodal function.

Parasympathetic influences preponderate over sympathetic effects at the SA node, as shown in Fig. 4-2. As the frequency of sympathetic stimulation in an anesthetized dog was increased from 0 to 4 Hz, the heart rate increased by about 80 beats per minute in the absence of vagal stimulation (Vag = 0 Hz). However, when the vagi were stimulated at 8 Hz, increasing the sympathetic stimulation frequency from 0 to 4 Hz had a negligible influence on heart rate.

Sympathetic Pathways

The cardiac sympathetic fibers originate in the intermediolateral columns of the upper five or six thoracic and lower one or two cervical segments of the spinal cord. They emerge from the spinal column through the white communicating branches and enter the paravertebral chains of ganglia. The anatomical details of the sympathetic innervation of the heart vary among mammalian species; the innervation has been elaborated in detail in the dog (Fig. 4-3). The synapses between the preganglionic and postganglionic neurons synapse mainly in the stellate or caudal cervical ganglia, depending on the species. The caudal (or middle) cervical ganglia lie close to the vagus nerves in the superior portion of the mediastinum. Sympathetic and parasympathetic fibers then join to form a complex plexus of

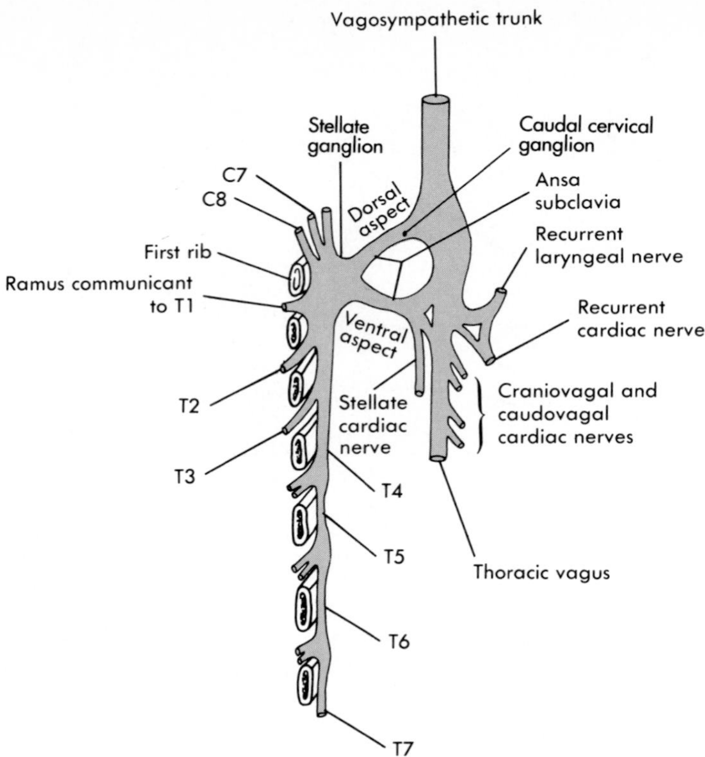

Fig. 4-3 ■ Upper thoracic sympathetic chain and the cardiac autonomic nerves on the right side in the dog. (Modified from Mizeres, N.J.: Anat. Rec. 132:261, 1958.)

mixed efferent nerves to the heart (see Fig. 4-3).

The postganglionic cardiac sympathetic fibers approach the base of the heart along the adventitial surface of the great vessels. On reaching the base of the heart, these fibers are distributed to the various chambers as an extensive epicardial plexus. They then penetrate the myocardium, usually accompanying the coronary vessels. The adrenergic receptors in the nodal regions and in the myocardium are predominantly of the beta type; that is, they are responsive to beta-adrenergic agonists, such as isoproterenol, and are inhibited by beta-adrenergic blocking agents, such as propranolol.

As with the vagus nerves, there is a differential distribution of the left and right sympathetic fibers. In the dog, for example, the fibers on the left side have more pronounced effects on myocardial contractility than do fibers on the right side, whereas the fibers on the left side have much less effect on heart rate than do the fibers on the right side (Fig. 4-4). In some dogs left cardiac sympathetic nerve stimulation may not affect heart rate at all. This bilateral asymmetry probably also exists in humans. In a group of patients right stellate ganglion blockade caused a mean reduction in heart rate of 14 beats per minute, whereas left-sided blockade decreased heart rate by only 2 beats per minute.

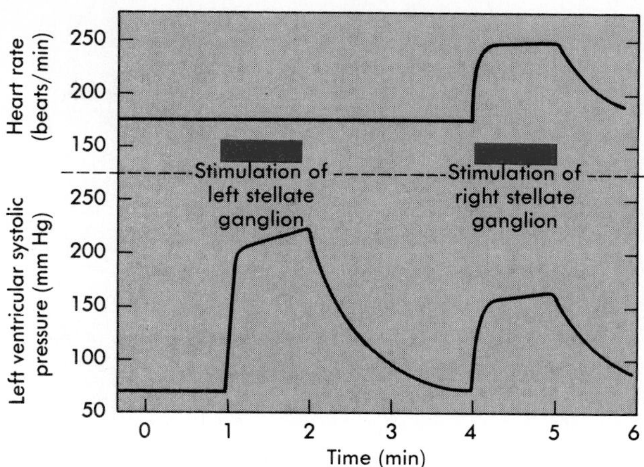

Fig. 4-4 ■ In the dog, stimulation of the left stellate ganglion has a greater effect on ventricular contractility than does right-sided stimulation, but it has a lesser effect on heart rate. In this example, traced from an original record, left stellate ganglion stimulation had no detectable effect at all on heart rate but had a considerable effect on ventricular performance in an isovolumic left ventricle preparation. (From Levy, M.N.: unpublished tracing.)

It is evident from Fig. 4-4 that the effects of sympathetic stimulation decay very gradually after the cessation of stimulation, in contrast to the abrupt termination of the response after vagal activity (not shown). Most of the norepinephrine released during sympathetic stimulation is taken up again by the nerve terminals, and much of the remainder is carried away by the bloodstream. These processes are relatively slow. Furthermore, at the beginning of sympathetic stimulation, the facilitatory effects on the heart attain steady state values much more slowly than do the inhibitory effects of vagal stimulation. Recent studies suggest that some of the ionic channels (e.g., the Ca^{++} channels) that regulate cardiac activity may be coupled to the beta-adrenergic receptors **directly** through G proteins, as well as **indirectly** through second messenger systems (mainly the adenylyl cyclase system). Even though the direct coupling may afford a more rapid cardiac response than does the slower second messenger system, sympathetic activity alters heart rate and AV conduction much more slowly than does vagal activity. Therefore, vagal activity can exert beat by beat control of cardiac function, whereas sympathetic activity cannot.

Control by Higher Centers

Dramatic alterations in cardiac rate, rhythm, and contractility have been induced experimentally by stimulation of various regions of the brain. In the cerebral cortex the centers regulating cardiac function are located mostly in the anterior half of the brain, principally in the frontal lobe, the orbital cortex, the motor and premotor cortex, the anterior part of the temporal lobe, the insula, and the cingulate gyrus. In the thalamus, tachycardia may be induced by stimulation of the midline, ventral, and medial groups of nuclei. Variations in heart rate also may be evoked by stimulating the posterior and posterolateral regions of the hypothalamus. Stimuli applied to the H_2 fields of Forel in the diencephalon elicit a variety of cardiovascular responses, including tachycardia; such changes simulate closely those ob-

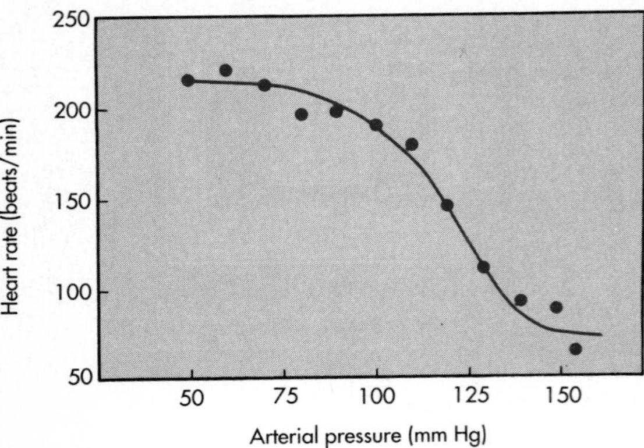

Fig. 4-5 ■ Heart rate as a function of mean arterial pressure in a group of five conscious, chronically instrumented monkeys. The mean control arterial pressure was 114 mm Hg. Pressure was increased above the control value by infusing phenylephrine and was decreased below the control value by infusing nitroprusside. (Adapted from Cornish, K.G., et al.: Am. J. Physiol. 257:R595, 1989.)

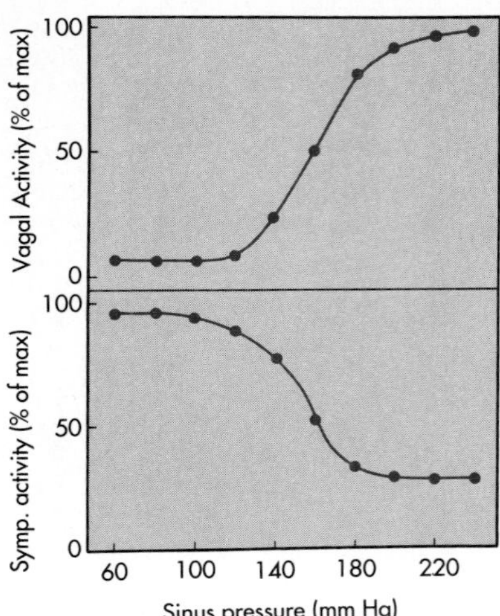

Fig. 4-6 ■ The changes in neural activity in cardiac vagal and sympathetic nerve fibers induced by changes in pressure in the isolated carotid sinuses in an anesthetized dog. Over the pressure range of about 100 to 200 mm Hg, pressure increments increased vagal activity and decreased sympathetic activity. At pressures below about 100 mm Hg, sympathetic activity was maximal (100%), and vagal activity was minimal. At pressures above about 200 mm Hg, vagal activity was maximal (100%) and sympathetic activity remained at a low constant level (about 25% of the maximum value). (Adapted from Kollai, M., and Koizumi, K.: Pflügers Arch. Ges. Physiol. 413:365, 1989.)

served during muscular exercise. Undoubtedly the cortical and diencephalic centers are responsible for initiating the cardiac reactions that occur during excitement, anxiety, and other emotional states. The hypothalamic centers are also involved in the cardiac response to alterations in environmental temperature. Recent studies have shown that localized temperature changes in the preoptic anterior hypothalamus alter heart rate and peripheral resistance.

Stimulation of the parahypoglossal area of the medulla produces a reciprocal activation of cardiac sympathetic and inhibition of cardiac parasympathetic pathways. In certain dorsal regions of the medulla, distinct cardiac accelerator and augmentor sites have been detected in animals with transected vagi. Stimulation of accelerator sites increases heart rate, whereas stimulation of augmentor sites increases cardiac contractility. The accelerator regions were found to be more abundant on the right and the augmentor sites more prevalent on the left. A similar distribution also exists in the hypothalamus. It appears, therefore, that for the most part the sympathetic fibers descend the brainstem ipsilaterally.

Baroreceptor Reflex

Acute changes in arterial blood pressure reflexly elicit inverse changes in heart rate (Fig. 4-5) via the baroreceptors located in the aortic arch and carotid sinuses (p. 184). The inverse relation between heart rate and arterial blood pressure is usually most pronounced over an intermediate range of arterial blood pressures.

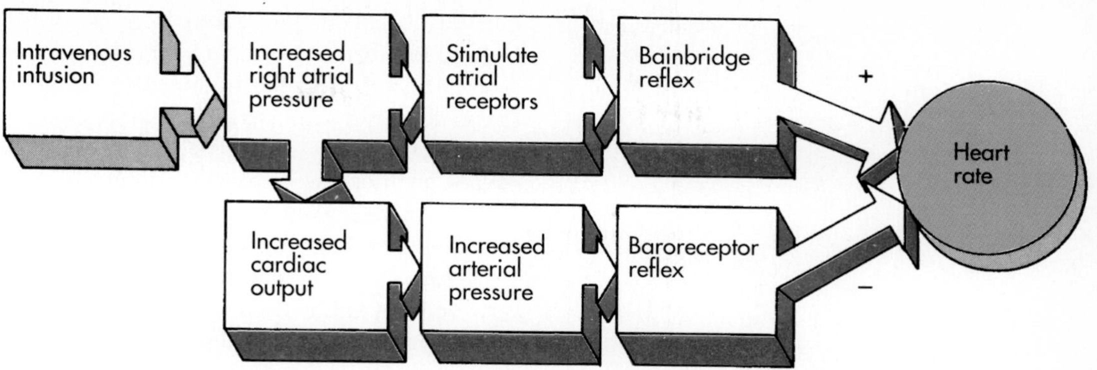

Fig. 4-7 ■ Intravenous infusions of blood or electrolyte solutions tend to increase heart rate via the Bainbridge reflex and to decrease heart rate via the baroreceptor reflex. The actual change in heart rate induced by such infusions is the result of these two opposing effects.

In an experiment conducted on a conscious, chronically instrumented monkey (see Fig. 4-5), this range varied between about 70 and 160 mm Hg. Below the intermediate range of pressures, the heart rate maintains a constant, high value, whereas above this pressure range, the heart rate maintains a constant, low value.

The effects of changes in carotid sinus pressure on the activity in the cardiac autonomic nerves of an anesthetized dog are shown in Fig. 4-6. Over an intermediate range of arterial pressures, the alterations in heart rate are achieved by reciprocal changes in vagal and sympathetic neural activity. Below this range of arterial blood pressures, the high heart rate is achieved by intense sympathetic activity and the virtual absence of vagal activity. Conversely, above the intermediate range of arterial blood pressures, the low heart rate is achieved by intense vagal activity and a constant low level of sympathetic activity.

Bainbridge Reflex and Atrial Receptors

In 1915 Bainbridge reported that infusions of blood or saline accelerated the heart rate in dogs. This increase in heart rate occurred whether arterial blood pressure did or did not rise. Acceleration was observed whenever central venous pressure rose sufficiently to distend the right side of the heart, and the effect was abolished by bilateral transection of the vagi.

Numerous investigators have confirmed Bainbridge's observations. However, the magnitude and direction of the response depends on the prevailing heart rate. When the heart rate is slow, intravenous infusions usually accelerate the heart. At more rapid heart rates, however, infusions will ordinarily slow the heart. Increases in blood volume not only evoke the Bainbridge reflex, but they also activate other reflexes (notably the baroreceptor reflex) that tend to change the heart rate in the opposite direction. The actual change in heart rate evoked by an alteration of blood volume is therefore the resultant of these antagonistic reflex effects (Fig. 4-7).

In unanesthetized dogs, volume loading with blood increased heart rate and cardiac output proportionately (Fig. 4-8). Consequently, stroke volume remained virtually constant. Conversely, reductions in blood volume diminished the cardiac output but increased heart

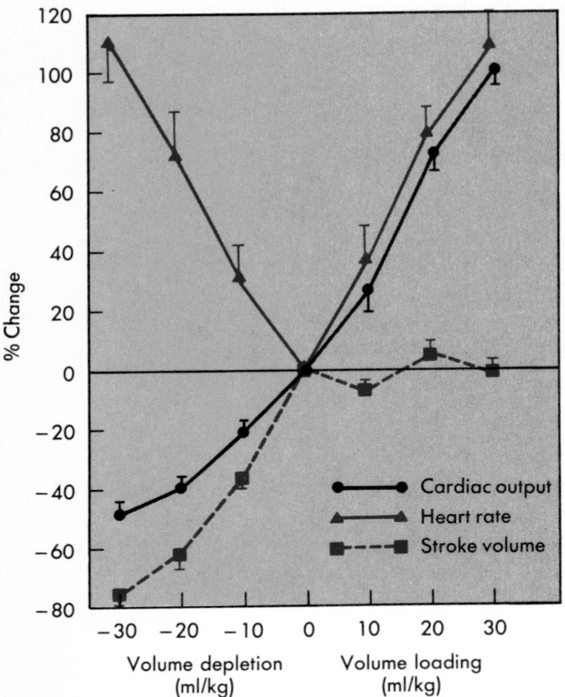

Fig. 4-8 ■ Effects of blood transfusion and of bleeding on cardiac output, heart rate, and stroke volume in unanesthetized dogs. (From Vatner, S.F., and Boettcher, D.H.: Circ. Res. 42:557, 1978. By permission of the American Heart Association, Inc.)

rate. Undoubtedly, the Bainbridge reflex was prepotent over the baroreceptor reflex when the blood volume was raised, but the baroreceptor reflex prevailed over the Bainbridge reflex when the blood volume was diminished.

Receptors that influence heart rate exist in both atria. They are located principally in the venoatrial junctions—in the right atrium at its junctions with the venae cavae and in the left atrium at its junctions with the pulmonary veins. Distension of these atrial receptors sends impulses centripetally in the vagi. The efferent impulses are carried by fibers from both autonomic divisions to the SA node. The cardiac response is highly selective. Even when the reflex increase in heart rate is large, changes in ventricular contractility have been negligible. Furthermore, the increase in heart rate is unattended by an increase of sympathetic activity to the peripheral arterioles.

Stimulation of the atrial receptors also causes an increase in urine volume. Reduced activity in the renal sympathetic nerve fibers might be partially responsible for this diuresis. However, the principal mechanism appears to be a neurally mediated reduction in the secretion of vasopressin (antidiuretic hormone) by the posterior pituitary gland.

A peptide, called **atrial natriuretic factor** (ANF), is released from atrial tissue in response to increases in blood volume, presumably because of the resultant stretch of the atrial walls. ANF consists of 28 amino acids, and it has potent diuretic and natriuretic effects on the kidneys and vasodilator effects on the resistance and capacitance blood vessels. Thus, ANF plays an important role in the regulation of blood volume and blood pressure.

Respiratory Cardiac Arrhythmia

Rhythmic variations in heart rate, occurring at the frequency of respiration, are detectable in most individuals and tend to be more pronounced in children. Typically the cardiac rate accelerates during inspiration and decelerates during expiration (Fig. 4-9).

Recordings from the autonomic nerves to the heart reveal that the neural activity increases in the sympathetic fibers during inspiration, whereas the neural activity in the vagal fibers increases during expiration (Fig. 4-10). The acetylcholine released at the vagal endings is removed so rapidly that the rhythmic changes in activity are able to elicit rhythmic variations in heart rate. Conversely, the norepinephrine released at the sympathetic endings is removed more slowly, thus damping out the effects of rhythmic variations in norepinephrine release on heart rate. Hence, rhythmic changes in heart rate are ascribable almost en-

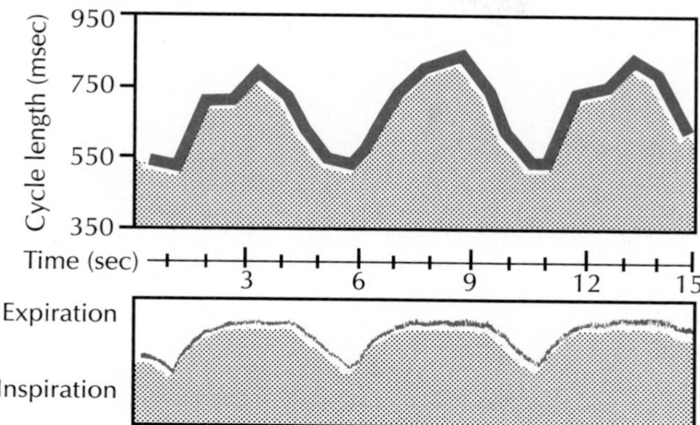

Fig. 4-9 ■ Respiratory sinus arrhythmia in a resting, unanesthetized dog. Note that the cardiac cycle length increases during expiration and decreases during inspiration. (Modified from Warner, M.R. et al.: Am. J. Physiol. 251:H1134, 1986.)

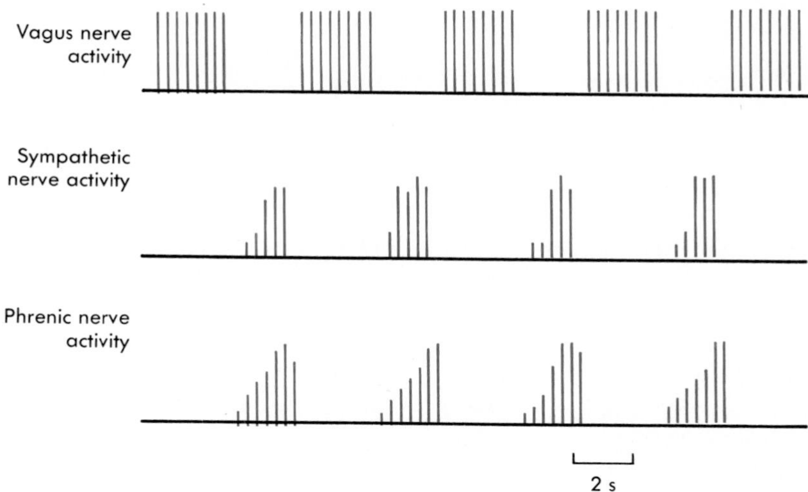

Fig. 4-10 ■ The respiratory fluctuations in efferent neural activity in the cardiac nerves of an anesthetized dog. Note that the sympathetic nerve activity occurs synchronously with the phrenic nerve discharges (which initiate diaphragmatic contraction), whereas the vagus nerve activity occurs between the phrenic nerve discharges. (From Kollai, M., and Koizumi, K.: J. Auton. Nerv. Syst. 1:33, 1979.)

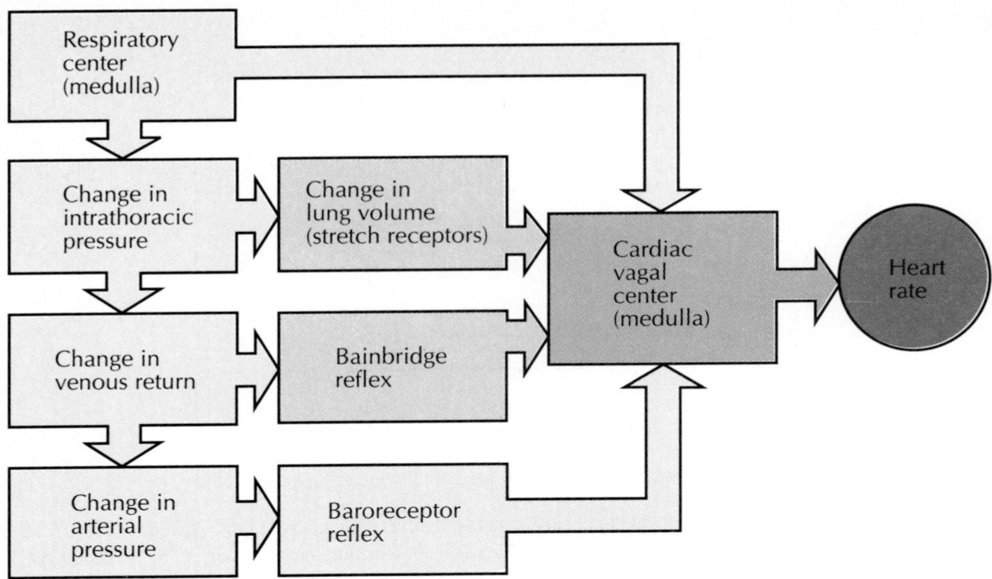

Fig. 4-11 ■ Respiratory sinus arrhythmia is generated by a direct interaction between the respiratory and cardiac centers in the medulla, as well as by reflexes originating from stretch receptors in the lungs, stretch receptors in the right atrium (Bainbridge reflex), and baroreceptors in the carotid sinuses and aortic arch.

tirely to the oscillations in vagal activity. Respiratory sinus arrhythmia is exaggerated when vagal tone is enhanced.

Both reflex and central factors contribute to the genesis of the respiratory cardiac arrhythmia (Fig. 4-11). During inspiration the intrathoracic pressure decreases and therefore venous return to the right side of the heart is accelerated (see p. 215), which elicits the Bainbridge reflex (see Fig. 4-11). After the time delay required for the increased venous return to reach the left side of the heart, left ventricular output increases and raises arterial blood pressure. This in turn reduces heart rate reflexly through baroreceptor stimulation (see Fig. 4-11).

Fluctuations in sympathetic activity to the arterioles cause peripheral resistance to vary at the respiratory frequency. Consequently, arterial blood pressure fluctuates rhythmically, which affects heart rate via the baroreceptor reflex. Stretch receptors in the lungs may also affect heart rate (see Fig. 4-11). Moderate pulmonary inflation may increase heart rate reflexly. The afferent and efferent limbs of this reflex are located in the vagus nerves.

Central factors are also responsible for respiratory cardiac arrhythmia (see Fig. 4-11). The respiratory center in the medulla influences the cardiac autonomic centers. In heart-lung bypass experiments conducted on animals, the chest is open, the lungs are collapsed, venous return is diverted to a pump-oxygenator, and arterial blood pressure is maintained at a constant level. In such experiments, rhythmic movements of the rib cage attest to the activity of the medullary respiratory centers, and the movements of the rib cage are often accompanied by rhythmic changes in heart rate at the respiratory frequency. This respira-

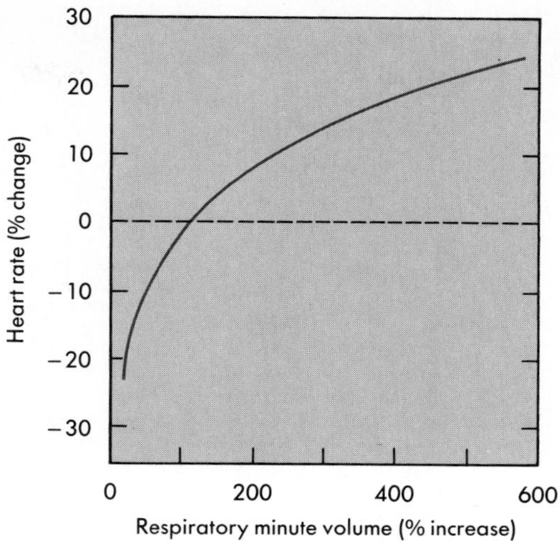

Fig. 4-12 ■ Relationship between the change in heart rate and the change in respiratory minute volume during carotid chemoreceptor stimulation in spontaneously breathing cats and dogs. When respiratory stimulation was relatively slight, heart rate usually diminished; when respiratory stimulation was more pronounced, heart rate usually increased. (Modified from Daly, M.deB., and Scott, M.J.: J. Physiol. 144:148, 1958.)

tory cardiac arrhythmia is almost certainly induced by an interaction between the respiratory and cardiac centers in the medulla (see Fig. 4-11).

Chemoreceptor Reflex

The cardiac response to peripheral chemoreceptor stimulation merits special consideration because it illustrates the complexity that may be introduced when one stimulus excites two organ systems simultaneously. In intact animals, stimulation of the carotid chemoreceptors consistently increases ventilatory rate and depth but ordinarily changes heart rate only slightly.

The directional change in heart rate is related to the enhancement of pulmonary ventilation, as shown in Fig. 4-12. When respiratory stimulation is mild, heart rate usually diminishes; when the increase in pulmonary ventilation is more pronounced, heart rate usually accelerates.

The cardiac response to peripheral chemoreceptor stimulation is the resultant of primary and secondary reflex mechanisms (Fig. 4-13). The primary reflex effect of carotid chemoreceptor excitation is mainly to facilitate the medullary vagal center and thereby to decrease heart rate. Secondary effects are mediated by the respiratory system. The respiratory stimulation by the arterial chemoreceptors tend to inhibit the medullary vagal center. This inhibitory effect varies with the concomitant stimulation of respiration.

An example of the primary inhibitory influence is displayed in Fig. 4-14. In this experiment on an anesthetized dog, the lungs were completely collapsed and blood oxygenation was accomplished by an artificial oxygenator. When the carotid chemoreceptors were stimulated, an intense bradycardia and some degree of AV block ensued. Such effects are mediated primarily by efferent vagal fibers.

The identical primary inhibitory effect also

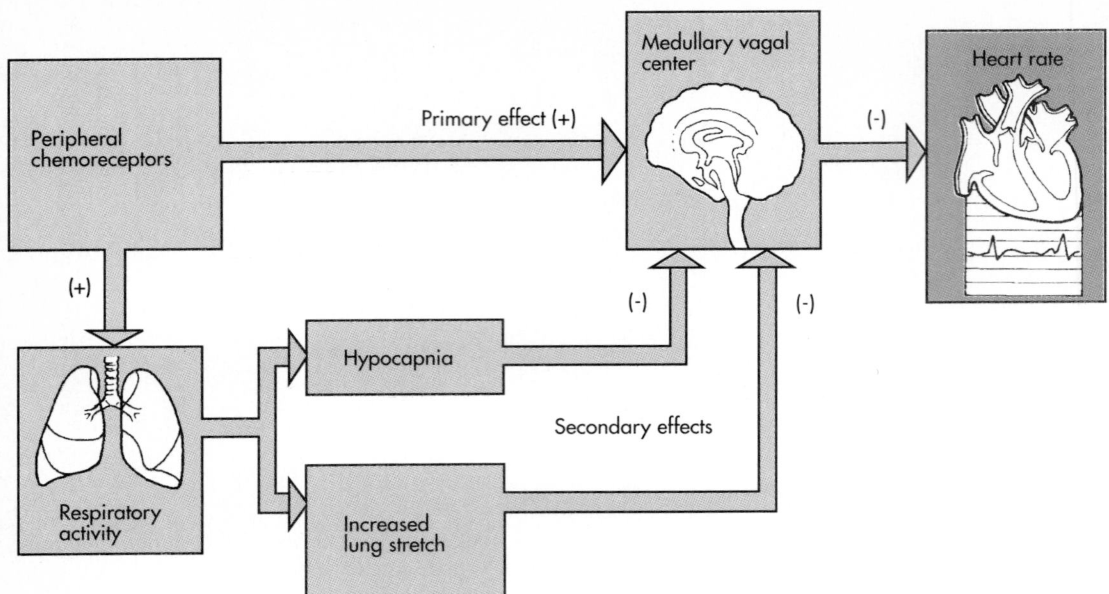

Fig. 4-13 ■ The primary effect of stimulation of the peripheral chemoreceptors on heart rate is to excite the cardiac vagal center in the medulla and thus to decrease heart rate. Peripheral chemoreceptor stimulation also excites the respiratory center in the medulla. This effect produces hypocapnia and increases lung inflation, both of which secondarily inhibit the medullary vagal center. Thus these secondary influences attenuate the primary reflex effect of peripheral chemoreceptor stimulation on heart rate.

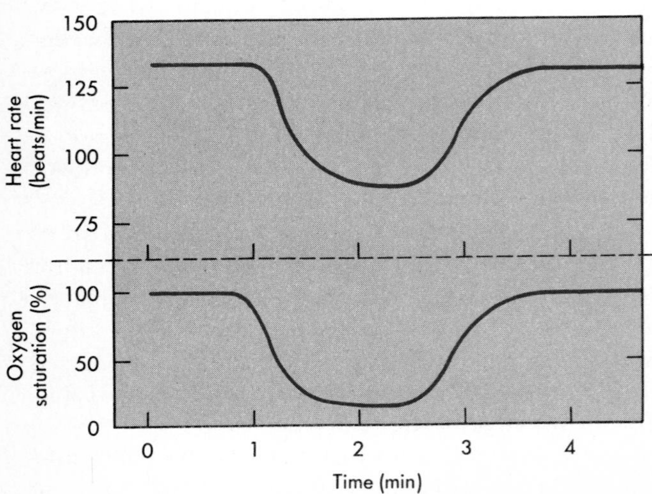

Fig. 4-14 ■ Changes in heart rate during carotid chemoreceptor stimulation in an anesthetized dog on total heart bypass. The lungs remain deflated and respiratory gas exchange is accomplished by an artificial oxygenator. The lower tracing represents the oxygen saturation of the blood perfusing the carotid chemoreceptors. The blood perfusing the remainder of the animal, including the myocardium, was fully saturated with oxygen throughout the experiment. (Modified from Levy, M.N., DeGeest, H., and Zieske, H.: Circ. Res. 18:67, 1966.)

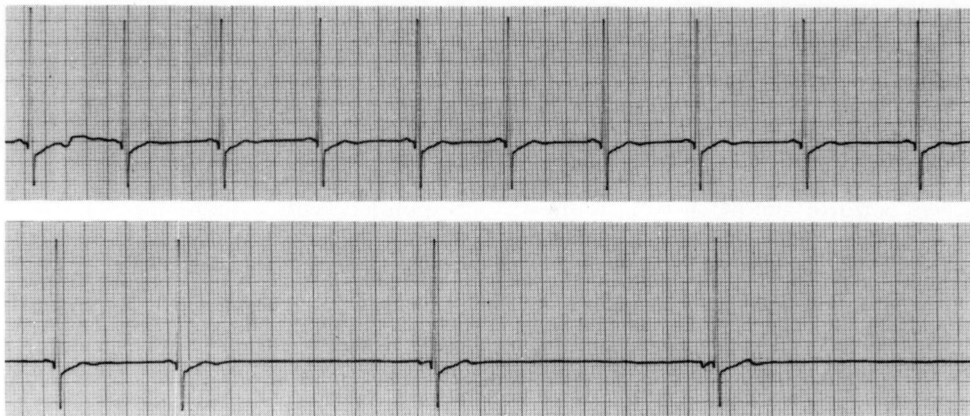

Fig. 4-15 ■ Electrocardiogram of a 30-year-old quadriplegic man who could not breathe spontaneously and required tracheal intubation and artificial respiration. The two strips are continuous. The tracheal catheter was temporarily disconnected from the respirator at the beginning of the top strip, at which time his heart rate was 65 beats per minute. In less than 10 s, his heart rate decreased to about 20 beats per minute. (Modified from Berk, J.L., and Levy, M.N.: Eur. Surg. Res. 9:75, 1977.)

operates in humans. The electrocardiogram in Fig. 4-15 was recorded from a quadriplegic patient who could not breathe spontaneously, but required tracheal intubation and artificial respiration. When the tracheal catheter was briefly disconnected to permit nursing care, the patient quickly developed a profound bradycardia. His heart rate was 65 beats per minute just before the tracheal catheter was disconnected. In less than 10 s after cessation of artificial respiration, his heart rate dropped to about 20 beats per minute. This bradycardia could be prevented by blocking the effects of efferent vagal activity with atropine, and its onset could be delayed considerably by hyperventilating the patient before disconnecting the tracheal catheter.

The pulmonary hyperventilation that is ordinarily evoked by carotid chemoreceptor stimulation influences heart rate secondarily, both by initiating more pronounced pulmonary inflation reflexes and by producing hypocapnia (see Fig. 4-13). Each of these influences tends to depress the primary cardiac response to chemoreceptor stimulation and thereby to accelerate the heart. Hence when pulmonary hyperventilation is not prevented, the primary and secondary effects tend to neutralize each other, and carotid chemoreceptor stimulation affects heart rate only minimally.

Ventricular Receptor Reflexes

Sensory receptors located near the endocardial surfaces of the ventricular walls initiate reflex effects similar to those elicited by the arterial baroreceptors. Excitation of these endocardial receptors diminishes the heart rate and peripheral resistance. Other sensory receptors have been identified in the epicardial regions of the ventricles. Ventricular receptors are excited by a variety of mechanical and chemical stimuli, but their physiological functions are not clear.

■ INTRINSIC REGULATION OF MYOCARDIAL PERFORMANCE

Just as the heart can initiate its own beat in the absence of any nervous or hormonal control, so also can the myocardium adapt to changing hemodynamic conditions by mechanisms that are intrinsic to cardiac muscle itself. Experiments on denervated hearts reveal that this organ adjusts remarkably well to stress. For example, racing greyhounds with denervated hearts perform almost as well as those with intact innervation. Their maximal running speed was found to be only 5% less after complete cardiac denervation. In these dogs, the threefold to fourfold increase in cardiac output was achieved principally by an increase in stroke volume. In normal dogs the increase of cardiac output with exercise is accompanied by a proportionate increase of heart rate; stroke volume does not change much (see Chapter 12). It is unlikely that the cardiac adaptation in the denervated animals is achieved entirely by intrinsic mechanisms; circulating catecholamines undoubtedly contribute. If the beta-adrenergic receptors are blocked in greyhounds with denervated hearts, their racing performance is severely impaired.

The heart is partially or completely denervated in a variety of clinical situations: (1) the surgically transplanted heart is totally decentralized, although the intrinsic, postganglionic parasympathetic fibers persist; (2) atropine blocks vagal effects on the heart, and propranolol blocks sympathetic beta-adrenergic influences; (3) certain drugs, such as reserpine, deplete cardiac norepinephrine stores and thereby restrict or abolish sympathetic control; and (4) in chronic congestive heart failure, cardiac norepinephrine stores are often severely diminished, thereby attenuating any sympathetic influences.

The intrinsic cardiac adaptation that has received the greatest attention involves changes in the resting length of the myocardial fibers. This adaptation is designated **Starling's law of the heart** or the **Frank-Starling mechanism.** The mechanical, ultrastructural, and physiological bases for this mechanism have been explained in Chapter 3.

Frank-Starling Mechanism

Isolated Hearts. In 1895 Frank described the response of the isolated heart of the frog to alterations in the load on the myocardial fibers just before contraction—the **preload.** He observed that as the preload increased, the heart responded with a more forceful contraction. Frank recognized that cardiac muscle behavior was similar to that of skeletal muscle when it is stretched to progressively greater initial lengths before contraction.

In 1914 Starling described the intrinsic response of the heart to changes in right atrial and aortic pressure in the canine heart-lung preparation, which is depicted in Fig. 4-16. In this preparation the right atrium is filled with blood from an elevated reservoir. Right atrial pressure is varied either by altering the height of the reservoir or by adjusting a screw clamp on the connecting tube. From the right atrium, blood enters the right ventricle, which then pumps it through the pulmonary vessels to the left atrium. The trachea is cannulated and the lungs are artificially ventilated.

The aorta is ligated distal to the arch, and a cannula is inserted into the brachiocephalic artery. Blood is pumped by the left ventricle through this cannula and through rubber tubing that ultimately conducts the blood back through a heating coil to the right atrial reservoir. A pressure limiting system, known as a **Starling resistance,** is installed in the rubber tubing to permit changes in peripheral resistance. The volume of both ventricles is recorded by a special device. Cardiac output is determined by measuring the flow from the rubber tubing back into the venous reservoir connected to the right atrium.

The response of the isolated heart to a sudden augmentation of right atrial pressure (increased preload) is shown in Fig. 4-17. Aortic pressure was permitted to increase only slightly. In the top tracing, an increase of ventricular volume is registered as a downward deflection. Hence the upper border of the trac-

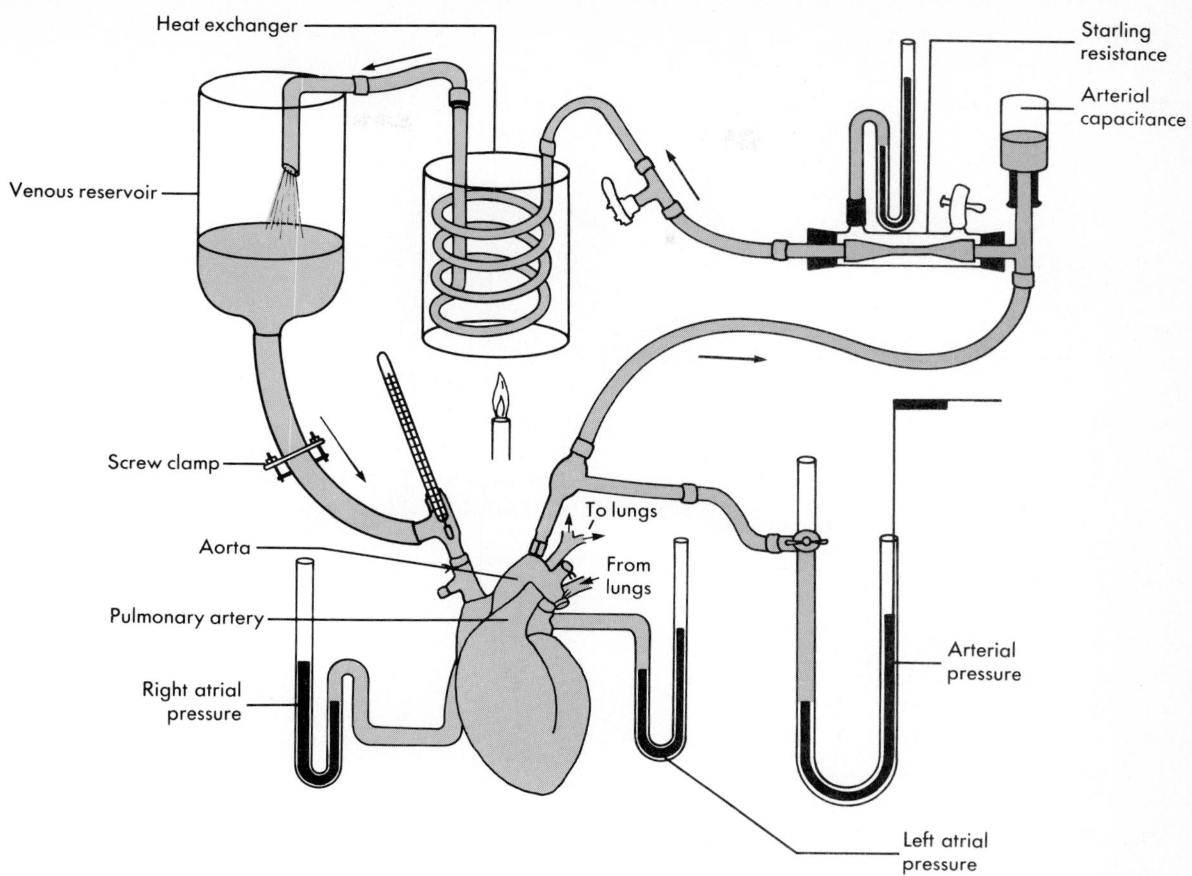

Fig. 4-16 ■ Heart-lung preparation. (Redrawn from Patterson, S.W., and Starling, E.H.: J. Physiol. 48:357, 1914.)

ing represents the systolic volume, the lower border indicates the diastolic volume, and the amplitude of the deflections reflects the stroke volume.

For several beats after the rise in right atrial pressure, the ventricular volume progressively increased. This indicates that during these few beats a disparity must have existed between ventricular inflow during diastole and ventricular output during systole. Thus, during this transient period before equilibrium was attained, the stroke volume must have been less than the filling volume. The consequent accumulation of blood dilated the ventricles and lengthened the individual myocardial fibers that comprised the walls of the ventricles.

The increased diastolic fiber length somehow facilitates ventricular contraction and enables the ventricles to pump a greater stroke volume, so that at equilibrium cardiac output exactly matches the augmented venous return. Increased fiber length alters cardiac performance mainly by changing the number of myofilament crossbridges that can interact and by changing the calcium sensitivity of the myofilaments (see Chapter 3). An optimum fiber

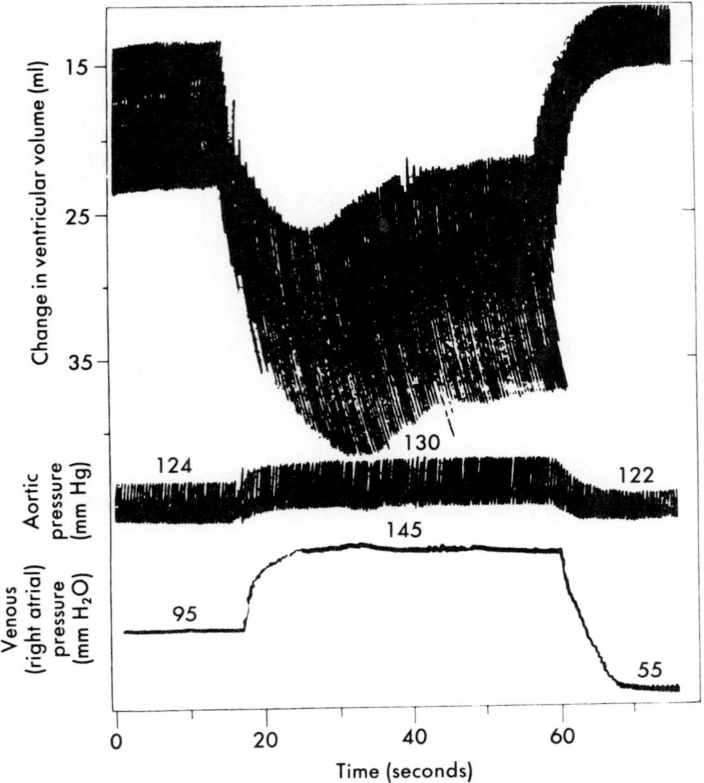

Fig. 4-17 ■ Changes in ventricular volume in a heart-lung preparation when the venous reservoir was suddenly raised (right atrial pressure increased from 95 to 145 mm H_2O) and subsequently lowered (right atrial pressure decreased from 145 to 55 mm H_2O). Note that an increase in ventricular volume is registered as a downward shift in the volume tracing. (Redrawn from Patterson, S.W., Piper, H., and Starling, E.H.: J. Physiol. 48:465, 1914.)

length apparently exists, beyond which contraction is actually impaired. Therefore, excessively high filling pressures may depress rather than enhance the pumping capacity of the ventricles by overstretching the myocardial fibers.

Changes in diastolic fiber length also permit the isolated heart to compensate for an increase of peripheral resistance. In the experiment depicted in Fig. 4-18 the arterial resistance was abruptly raised in three steps, whereas venous inflow was held constant. Each rise in resistance increased the arterial pressure and ventricular volume. With each abrupt elevation of arterial pressure (increased afterload), the left ventricle was at first unable to pump a normal stroke volume. Because venous return was held constant, the diminution of stroke volume was attended by a rise in ventricular diastolic volume and therefore in the length of the myocardial fibers. This change in end-diastolic fiber length finally enabled the ventricle to pump a given stroke volume against a greater peripheral resistance.

The external work performed per stroke by

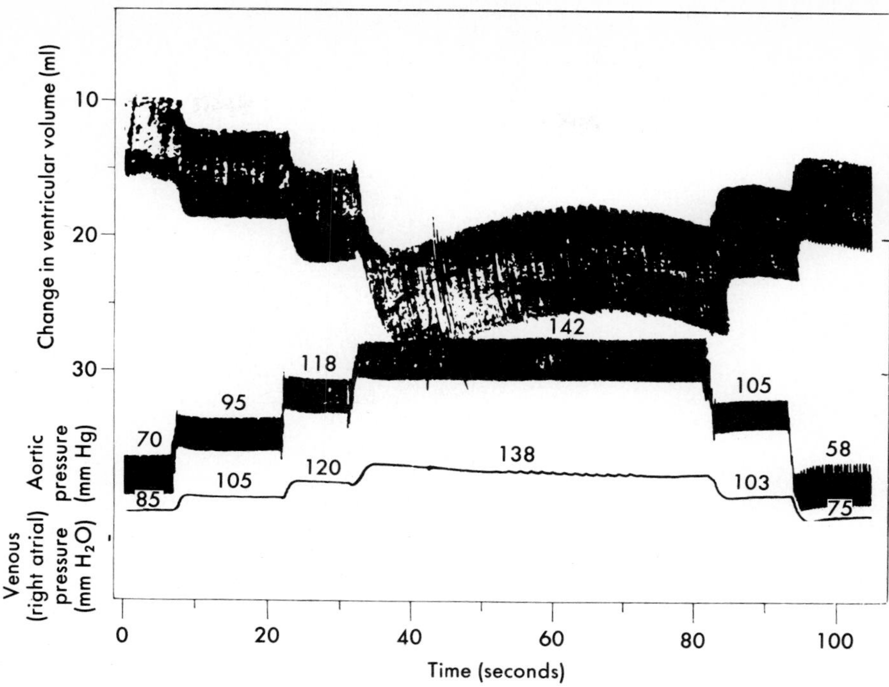

Fig. 4-18 ■ Changes in ventricular volume, aortic pressure, and right atrial pressure in a heart-lung preparation when peripheral resistance was raised and subsequently lowered in several steps. Note that an increase in ventricular volume is registered as a downward shift in the volume tracing. (Redrawn from Patterson, S.W., Piper, H., and Starling, E.H.: J. Physiol. 48:465, 1914.)

the left ventricle is approximately equal to the product of the mean arterial pressure and stroke volume (p. 138). Therefore, the increased diastolic length of the cardiac muscle fiber increases the work production by the left ventricle. However, at an excessively high peripheral resistance, further augmentation of resistance will reduce stroke volume and stroke work.

Changes in ventricular volume are also involved in the cardiac adaptation to alterations in heart rate. During bradycardia, for example, the increased duration of diastole permits greater ventricular filling. The consequent augmentation of myocardial fiber length increases stroke volume. Therefore, the reduction in heart rate may be fully compensated by the increase in stroke volume, such that cardiac output may remain constant (see Fig. 9-14).

When cardiac compensation involves ventricular dilation, the force required by each myocardial fiber to generate a given intraventricular systolic pressure must be appreciably greater than that developed by the fibers in a ventricle of normal size. The relationship between wall tension and cavity pressure resembles that for cylindrical tubes (p. 154) in that for a constant internal pressure, wall tension varies directly with the radius. As a consequence, the dilated heart requires considerably more oxygen to perform a given amount of external work than does the normal heart.

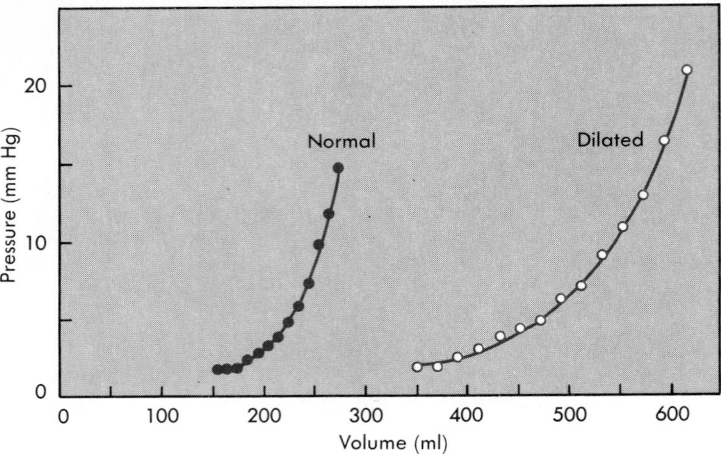

Fig. 4-19 ■ Pericardial pressure-volume relations in a normal dog and in a dog with experimentally induced chronic cardiac hypertrophy. (Modified from Freeman, G.L., and Le Winter, M.M.: Circ. Res. 54:294, 1984. By permission of the American Heart Association, Inc.)

In the intact animal, the heart is enclosed in the pericardial sac. The relatively rigid pericardium determines the pressure-volume relationship at high levels of pressure and volume. The pericardium exerts this limitation of volume even under normal conditions, when an individual is at rest and the heart rate is slow. In the cardiac dilation and hypertrophy that accompanies chronic heart failure, the pericardium is stretched considerably (Fig. 4-19). The pericardial limitation of cardiac filling is exerted at pressures and volumes that are entirely different from those in normal individuals.

Intact Preparations. The major problem of assessing the role of the Frank-Starling mechanism in intact animals and humans is the difficulty of measuring end-diastolic myocardial fiber length. The Frank-Starling mechanism has been represented graphically by plotting some index of ventricular performance along the ordinate and some index of fiber length along the abscissa. The most commonly used indices of ventricular performance are cardiac output, stroke volume, and stroke work. The indices of fiber length include ventricular end-diastolic volume, ventricular end-diastolic pressure, ventricular circumference, and mean atrial pressure.

The Frank-Starling mechanism is better represented by a family of so-called ventricular function curves, rather than by a single curve. To construct a given ventricular function curve, blood volume is altered over a wide range of values, and stroke work and end-diastolic pressure are measured at each step. Similar observations are then made during the desired experimental intervention. For example, the ventricular function curve obtained during a norepinephrine infusion lies above and to the left of a control ventricular function curve (Fig. 4-20). It is evident that, for a given level of left ventricular end-diastolic pressure, the left ventricle performs more work during a norepinephrine infusion than during control conditions. Hence a shift of the ventricular

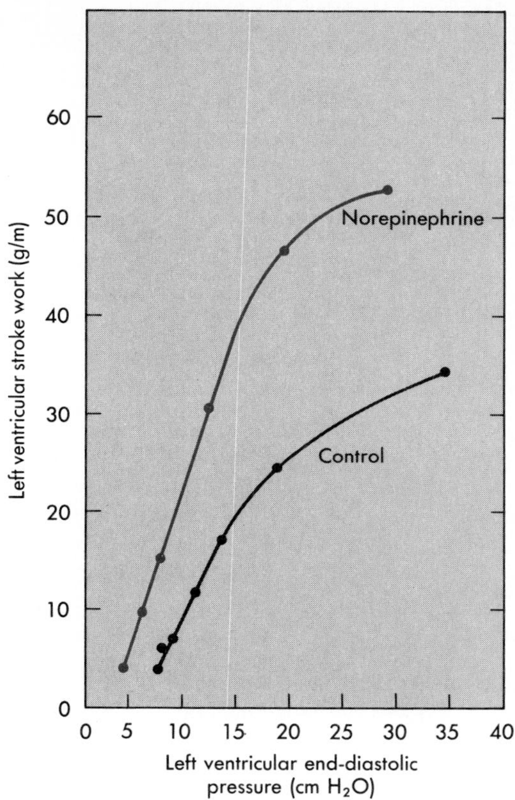

Fig. 4-20 ■ A constant infusion of norepinephrine in a dog shifts the ventricular function curve to the left. This shift signifies an enhancement of ventricular contractility. (Redrawn from Sarnoff, S.J., Brockman, S.K., Gilmore, J.P., Linden, R.J., and Mitchell, J.H.: Circ. Res. 8:1108, 1960.)

function curve to the left usually signifies an improvement of ventricular contractility (p. 206); a shift to the right usually indicates an impairment of contractility and a consequent tendency toward **cardiac failure.**

A shift in a ventricular function curve does not uniformly indicate a change in contractility, however. **Contractility** is a measure of cardiac performance at a given level of preload and afterload. The end-diastolic pressure is ordinarily a good index of preload, whereas the aortic systolic pressure is a good index of afterload. In assessing myocardial contractility, the cardiac afterload must be held constant as the end-diastolic pressure is varied over a range of values.

The Frank-Starling mechanism is ideally suited for matching the cardiac output to the venous return. Any sudden, excessive output by one ventricle soon increases the venous return to the other ventricle. The consequent increase in diastolic fiber length augments the output of the second ventricle to correspond with that of its mate. Therefore, it is the Frank-Starling mechanism that maintains a precise balance between the outputs of the right and left ventricles. Because the two ventricles are arranged in series in a closed circuit, even a small, but maintained, imbalance in the outputs of the two ventricles would otherwise be catastrophic.

The curves relating cardiac output to mean atrial pressure for the two ventricles are not coincident; the curve for the left ventricle usually lies below that for the right, as shown in Fig. 4-21. At equal right and left atrial pressures (points *A* and *B*) right ventricular output would exceed left ventricular output. Hence venous return to the left ventricle (a function of right ventricular output) would exceed left ventricular output, and left ventricular diastolic volume and pressure would rise. By the Frank-Starling mechanism, left ventricular output would therefore increase (from *B* toward *C*). Only when the outputs of both ventricles are identical (points *A* and *C*) would the equilibrium be stable. Under such conditions, however, left atrial pressure *(C)* would exceed right atrial pressure *(A),* and this is precisely the relationship that ordinarily prevails. This difference in atrial pressures accounts for the observation that in **congenital atrial septal defects,** where the two atria communicate,

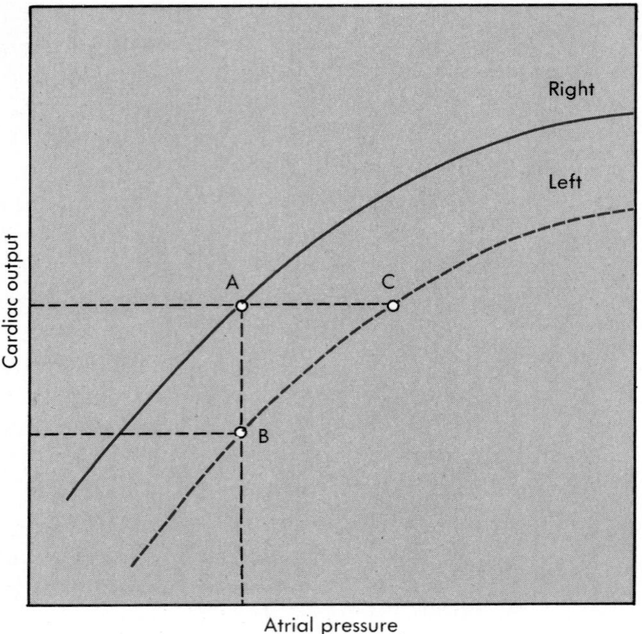

Fig. 4-21 ■ Curves relating the outputs of right and left ventricles to mean right and left atrial pressure, respectively. At a given level of cardiac output, mean left atrial pressure (for example, point *C*) exceeds mean right atrial pressure (point *A*).

the direction of the shunt flow is usually from left to right.

Rate-Induced Regulation

The effects of a sustained frequency of contraction on the force developed in an isometrically contracting cat papillary muscle are shown in Fig. 4-22, *B*. Initially, the strip of cardiac muscle was stimulated to contract only once every 20 s. When the muscle was suddenly made to contract once every 0.63 s, the developed force increased progressively over the next several beats. This progressive increase in developed force induced by a change in contraction frequency is known as the **staircase**, or **Treppe, phenomenon.**

At the new steady state, the developed force was more than five times as great as it was at the larger contraction interval. A return to the larger interval (20 s) had the opposite influence on developed force.

The effect of the interval between contractions on the steady-state level of developed force is shown in panel *A* (see Fig. 4-22) for a wide range of intervals. As the interval is diminished from 300 s down to about 20 s, there is little change in developed force. As the interval is reduced further, to a value of about 0.5 s, force increases sharply. Further reduction of the interval to 0.2 s has little additional effect on developed force.

The initial progressive rise in developed force when the interval between beats is suddenly decreased (e.g., from 20 to 0.63 s in panel B) (Fig. 4-22) is ascribable to a gradual increase in intracellular Ca^{++} content. Two

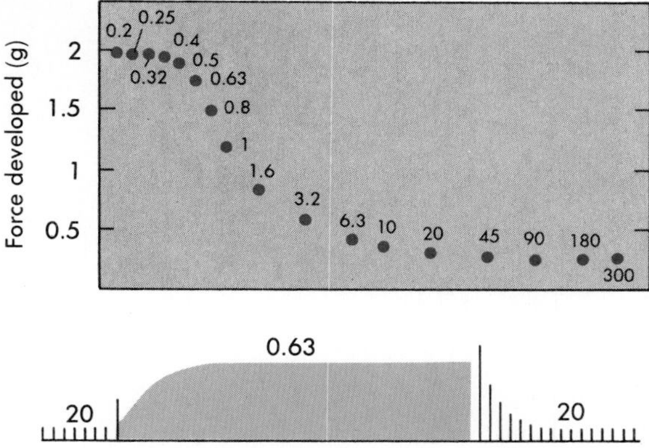

Fig. 4-22 ■ Changes in force development in an isolated papillary muscle from a cat as the interval between contractions is varied. The numbers in both sections of the record denote the interval (in seconds) between beats. In section **A** the points represent the steady-state forces developed at the intervals indicated. (Redrawn from Koch-Weser, J., and Blinks, J.R.: Pharmacol. Rev. 15:601, 1963.)

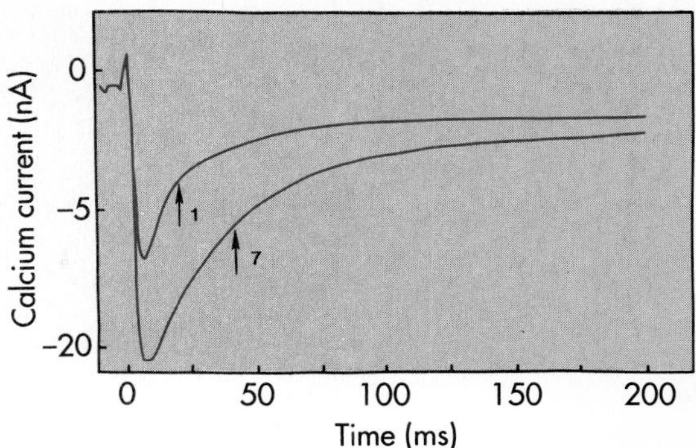

Fig. 4-23 ■ The calcium currents induced in a guinea pig myocyte during the first and seventh depolarizations in a sequence of depolarizations. The arrows indicate the half-times of inactivation. Note that during the seventh depolarization, the maximum inward Ca^{++} current and the halftime of inactivation were greater than the respective values for the first depolarization. (Modified from Lee, K.S.: Proc. Natl. Acad. Sci. 84:3941, 1987.)

mechanisms contribute to the rise in Ca^{++} content: (1) an increase in the number of depolarizations per minute, and (2) an increase in the inward Ca^{++} current per depolarization.

With respect to the first mechanism, Ca^{++} enters the myocardial cell during each action potential plateau (see Fig. 2-9). As the interval between beats is diminished, the number of plateaus per minute increases. Even though the duration of each action potential (and of each plateau) decreases as the interval between beats is reduced (see Fig. 2-19), the overriding effect of the increased number of plateaus per minute on the influx of Ca^{++} would prevail, and the intracellular content of Ca^{++} would increase.

With respect to the second mechanism, as the interval between beats is suddenly diminished, the inward Ca^{++} current (i_{Ca}) progressively increases with each successive beat until a new steady state is attained at the new basic cycle length. Figure 4-23 shows that in an isolated ventricular myocyte that was subjected to repetitive depolarizations, the influx of Ca^{++} into the myocyte increased on successive beats. For example, the maximum i_{Ca} was considerably greater during the seventh depolarization than it was during the first depolarization. Furthermore, the decay of that current (i.e., its inactivation) was substantially slower during the seventh depolarization than during the first depolarization. Both of these characteristics of the i_{Ca} would result in a greater influx of Ca^{++} into the myocyte during the seventh depolarization than during the first depolarization. The greater influx of Ca^{++} would, of course, strengthen the contraction.

Transient changes in the intervals between beats also profoundly affect the strength of contraction. When a premature ventricular systole (Fig. 4-24, beat *A*) occurs, the premature contraction (extrasystole) itself is feeble, whereas the beat after the compensatory pause is very strong. This response is partly ascrib-

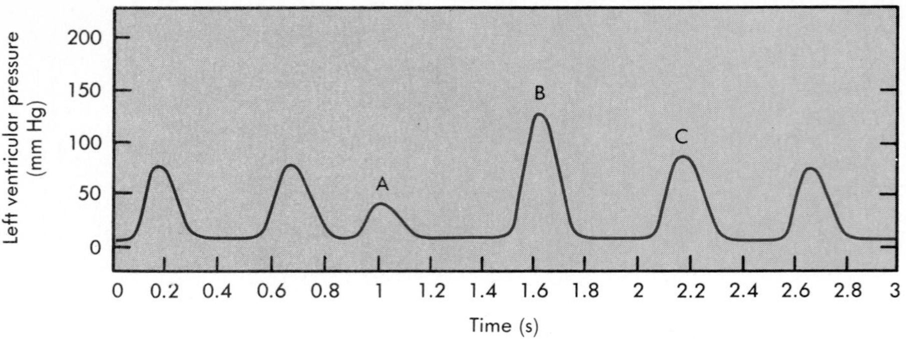

Fig. 4-24 ■ In an isovolumic canine left ventricle preparation a premature ventricular systole (beat *A*) is typically feeble, whereas the postextrasystolic contraction (beat *B*) is characteristically strong, and the enhanced contractility may persist to a diminishing degree over a few beats (for example, contraction *C*). (From Levy, M.N.: unpublished tracing.)

able to the Frank-Starling mechanism. Inadequate ventricular filling just before the premature beat accounts partly for the weak premature contraction. Subsequently, the exaggerated degree of filling associated with the compensatory pause explains in part the vigorous postextrasystolic contraction.

Although the Frank-Starling mechanism is certainly involved in the usual ventricular adaptation to a premature beat, it is not the exclusive mechanism. For example, in the ventricular pressure curves recorded from an isovolumic left ventricle preparation (see Fig. 4-24), in which neither filling nor ejection takes place during the cardiac cycle, the premature beat *(A)* is feeble and the succeeding contraction *(B)* is supernormal. Such enhanced contractility in contraction B is an example of **postextrasystolic potentiation,** and it may persist for one or more additional beats (for example, contraction *C*).

The weakness of the premature beat is directly related to the degree of prematurity. Conversely, as the time **(coupling interval)** between the premature beat and the preceding beat is increased, the more nearly normal will be the premature beat. The curve that relates the strength of contraction of a premature beat to the coupling interval is called a **mechanical restitution curve.** Fig. 4-25 shows the restitution curve obtained by varying the coupling intervals of test beats in an isolated ventricular muscle preparation from a guinea pig.

The restitution of contractile strength probably depends on the time course of the intracellular circulation of Ca^{++} during the contraction and relaxation process (see Fig. 3-5). During relaxation, the Ca^{++} that dissociates from the contractile proteins is taken up by the sarcoplasmic reticulum for subsequent release. However, about 500 to 800 ms are required before the Ca^{++} that had been taken up becomes available for release in response to the next depolarization.

The premature beat itself (see Fig. 4-24, beat *A*) is feeble probably because not enough time has elapsed to allow much of the Ca^{++} taken up by the sarcoplasmic reticulum during the preceding relaxation to become available for release in response to the premature depolarization. The postextrasystolic beat (see Fig. 4-24, beat *B*), conversely, is considerably

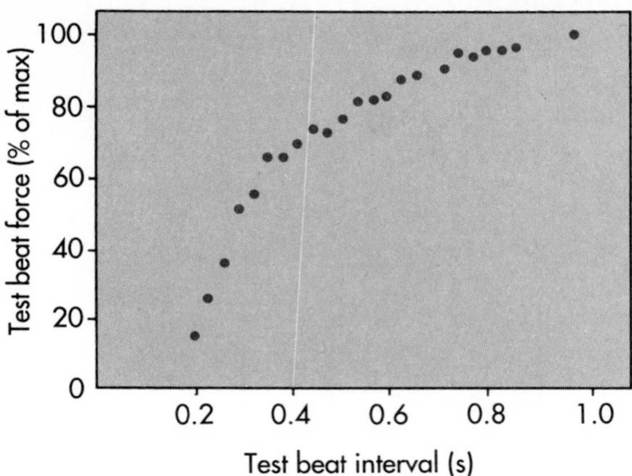

Fig. 4-25 ■ The force generated during premature contractions in a guinea pig isolated ventricular muscle preparation. The muscle was driven to contract once per second. Periodically, the muscle was stimulated to contract prematurely. The scale along the X-axis denotes the time between the driven and premature beat. The Y-axis scale denotes the ratio of the contractile force of the premature beat to that of the driven beat. (Modified from Seed, W.A., and Walker, J.M.: Cardiovasc. Res. 22:303, 1988.)

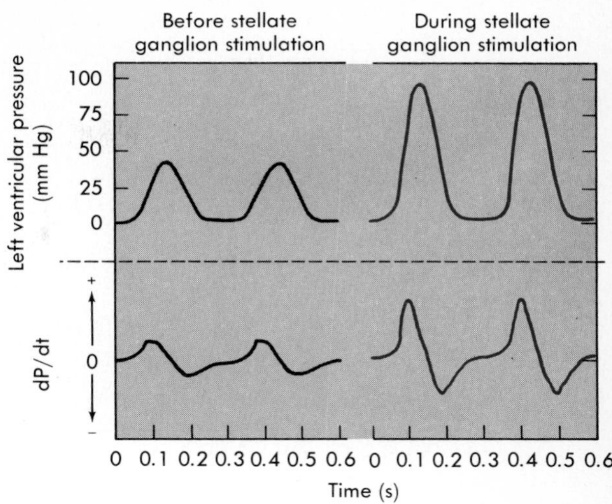

Fig. 4-26 ■ In an isovolumic left ventricle preparation, stimulation of cardiac sympathetic nerves evokes a substantial rise in peak left ventricular pressure and in the maximum rates of intraventricular pressure rise and fall *(dP/dt)*. (From Levy, M.N.: unpublished tracing.)

stronger than normal. A plausible reason is that after the compensatory pause (p. 47) between beats A and B, the sarcoplasmic reticulum will have available for release the Ca^{++} that had been taken up during two heartbeats: the extrasystole (beat *A*) and the normal beat that had preceded it.

■ EXTRINSIC REGULATION OF MYOCARDIAL PERFORMANCE

Although the completely isolated heart can adapt well to changes in preload and afterload, various extrinsic factors also influence the heart in the intact animal. Under many natural conditions these extrinsic regulatory mechanisms may overwhelm the intrinsic mechanisms. These extrinsic regulatory factors may be subdivided into nervous and chemical components.

Nervous Control

Sympathetic Influences. Sympathetic nervous activity enhances atrial and ventricular contractility. Effects of increased cardiac sympathetic activity on the ventricular myocardium are asymmetrical. The cardiac sympathetic nerves on the left side of the body usually have a much greater effect on ventricular contraction than do those on the right side (see Fig. 4-4).

The alterations in ventricular contraction evoked by electrical stimulation of the left stellate ganglion in a canine isovolumic left ventricle preparation are shown in Fig. 4-26. The peak pressure and the maximum rate of pressure rise (dP/dt) during systole are markedly increased. Also, the duration of systole is reduced and the rate of ventricular relaxation is increased during the early phases of diastole. The shortening of systole and more rapid ven-

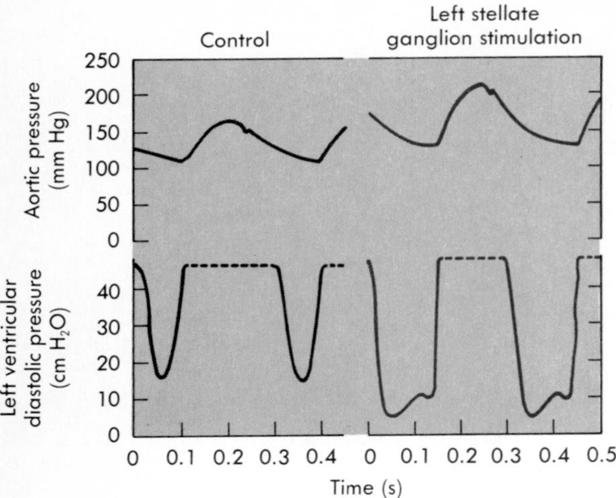

Fig. 4-27 ■ Stimulation of the left stellate ganglion of a dog increases arterial pressure, stroke volume, and stroke work despite a concomitant reduction in ventricular end-diastolic pressure. Note also the abridgment of systole, thereby allowing more time for ventricular filling; the heart was paced at a constant rate. In the ventricular pressure tracings the pen excursion is limited at 45 mm Hg; actual ventricular pressures during systole can be estimated from the aortic pressure tracings. (Redrawn from Mitchell, J.H., Linden, R.J., and Sarnoff, S.J.: Circ. Res. 8:1100, 1960.)

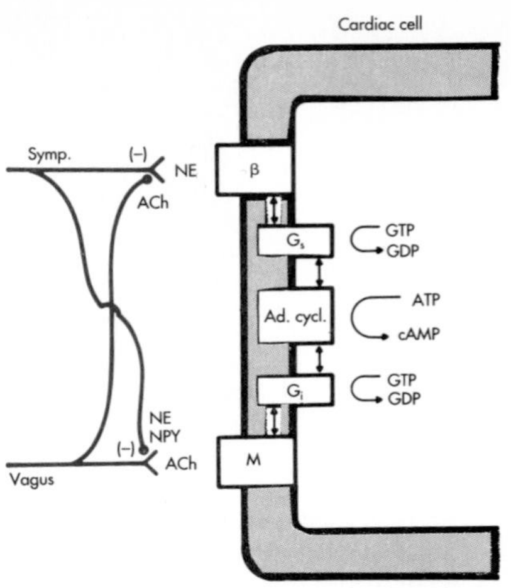

Fig. 4-28 ■ The interneuronal and intracellular mechanisms responsible for the interactions between the sympathetic and parasympathetic systems in the neural control of cardiac function. (From Levy, M.N.: Neurocardiology. In Kulbertus, H.E., and Franck, G., editors: Mt. Kisco, N.Y. 1988, Futura Publishing Co.)

tricular relaxation assist ventricular filling. For a given cardiac cycle length, the abbreviation of systole allows more time for diastole and hence for ventricular filling. In the experiment shown in Fig. 4-27, for example, the animal's heart was paced at a constant rapid rate. Sympathetic stimulation (right panel) shortened systole, which allowed substantially more time for ventricular filling.

Sympathetic nervous activity enhances myocardial performance. Neurally released norepinephrine or circulating catecholamines interact with beta-adrenergic receptors on the cardiac cell membranes (Fig. 4-28). This reaction activates adenylyl cyclase, which raises the intracellular levels of cyclic AMP (cAMP). As a consequence, protein kinases are activated that promote the phosphorylation of various proteins within the myocardial cells. Phosphorylation of specific sarcolemmal proteins activates the calcium channels in the myocardial cell membranes.

Activation of the calcium channels increases the influx of Ca^{++} during the action potential plateau, and more Ca^{++} is released from the sarcoplasmic reticulum in response to each cardiac excitation. The contractile strength of the heart is thereby increased. Fig. 4-29 shows the correlation between the contractile force developed by a thin strip of ventricular muscle and the Ca^{++} concentration (as reflected by the aequorin light signal) in the myocytes as the concentration of isoproterenol (a beta-adrenergic agonist) was increased in the tissue bath.

The overall effect of increased cardiac sympathetic activity in intact animals can best be appreciated in terms of families of ventricular function curves. When stepwise increases in

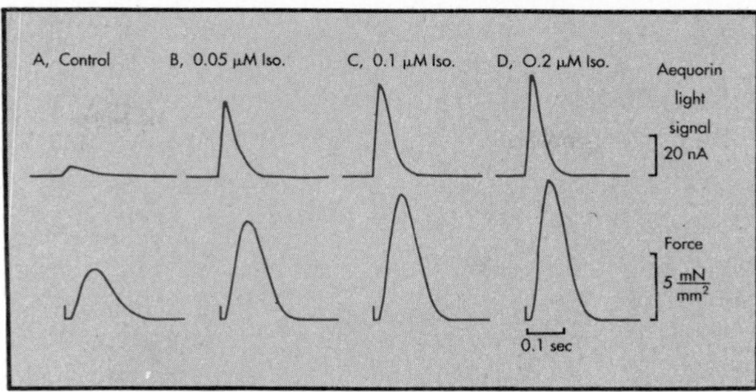

Fig. 4-29 ■ Effects of various concentrations of isoproterenol (Iso) on the aequorin light signal (in nA) and contractile force (in mN/mm^2) in a rat ventricular muscle injected with aequorin. The aequorin light signal reflects the instantaneous changes in intracellular Ca^{++} concentration. (Modified from Kurihara, S., and Konishi, M.: Effects of β-adrenoreceptor stimulation on intracellular Ca transients and tension in rat ventricular muscle, Pflügers Arch., 409:427, 1987.)

the frequency of electrical stimulation are applied to the left stellate ganglion, the ventricular function curves shift progressively to the left. The changes parallel those produced by catecholamine infusions (see Fig. 4-20). Hence, for any given left ventricular end-diastolic pressure, the ventricle is capable of performing more work as the level of sympathetic nervous activity is raised.

During cardiac sympathetic stimulation the increase in work is usually accompanied by a reduction in left ventricular end-diastolic pressure. An example of the response to stellate ganglion stimulation in a heart paced at a constant frequency is shown in Fig. 4-27. In this experiment, stroke work increased by about 50%, despite a reduction in the left ventricular end-diastolic pressure. Note also the pronounced shortening of ventricular systole, with the consequent lengthening of the filling period. The reason for the reduction in ventricular end-diastolic pressure is explained on p. 207.

Parasympathetic Influences. The vagus nerves inhibit the cardiac pacemaker, atrial myocardium, and AV conduction tissue. The vagus nerves also depress the ventricular myocardium, but the effects are less pronounced.

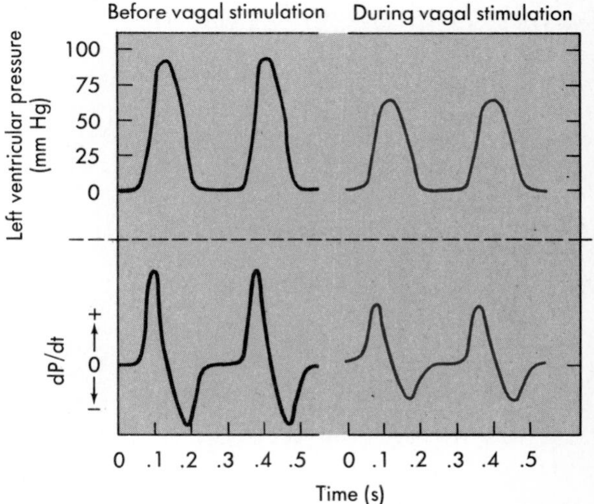

Fig. 4-30 ■ In an isovolumic left ventricle preparation, when the ventricle is paced at a constant frequency, vagal stimulation decreases the peak left ventricular pressure and diminishes the maximum rates of pressure rise and fall *(dP/dt)*. (From Levy, M.N.: unpublished tracing.)

In the isovolumic left ventricle preparation, vagal stimulation decreases the peak left ventricular pressure, maximum rate of pressure development (dP/dt), and maximum rate of pressure decline during diastole (Fig. 4-30). In pumping heart preparations the ventricular function curve shifts to the right during vagal stimulation.

The vagal effects on the ventricular myocardium are achieved by at least two mechanisms, as shown in Fig. 4-28. The acetylcholine (ACh) released from the vagal endings can interact with muscarinic (M) receptors in the cardiac cell membrane. This interaction leads to the inhibition of adenylyl cyclase. The consequent diminution in the intracellular concentration of cyclic AMP leads to a reduction in Ca^{++} conductance of the cell membrane, and hence a decrease in myocardial contractility.

The ACh released from the vagal endings can also inhibit the release of norepinephrine from neighboring sympathetic nerve endings (see Fig. 4-28). The experiment illustrated in Fig. 4-31 demonstrates that stimulation of the cardiac sympathetic nerves *(S)* results in the overflow of substantial amounts of norepinephrine into the coronary sinus blood. Concomitant vagal stimulation (S + V) reduces the overflow of norepinephrine by about 30%. The amount of norepinephrine overflowing into the coronary sinus blood probably parallels the amount released at the sympathetic terminals. Thus, vagal activity can decrease ventricular contractility partly by antagonizing the facilitatory effects of any concomitant sympathetic activity to enhance ventricular contractility. Similarly, sympathetic nerves release norepinephrine and certain neuropeptides, including neuropeptide Y *(NPY);* norepinephrine and NPY both inhibit the release of acetylcholine

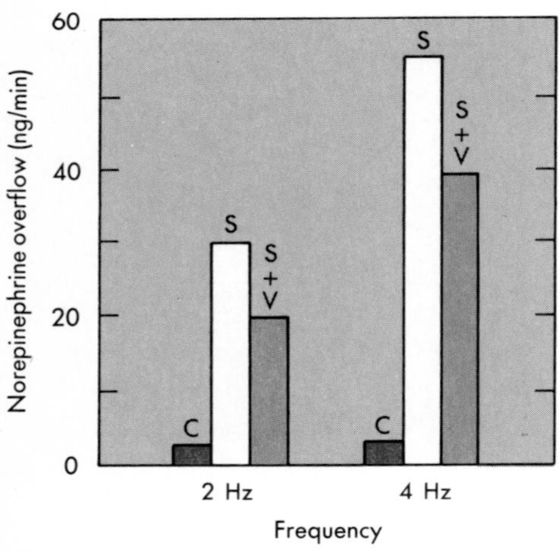

Fig. 4-31 ■ The mean rates of overflow of norepinephrine into the coronary sinus blood in a group of seven dogs under control conditions *(C),* during cardiac sympathetic stimulation *(S)* at 2 or 4 Hz and during combined sympathetic and vagal stimulation (*S* + *V*). The combined stimulus consisted of sympathetic stimulation at 2 or 4 Hz, and vagal stimulation at 15 Hz. (Redrawn from Levy, M.N., and Blattberg, B.: Circ. Res. 38:81, 1976. By permission of the American Heart Association, Inc.)

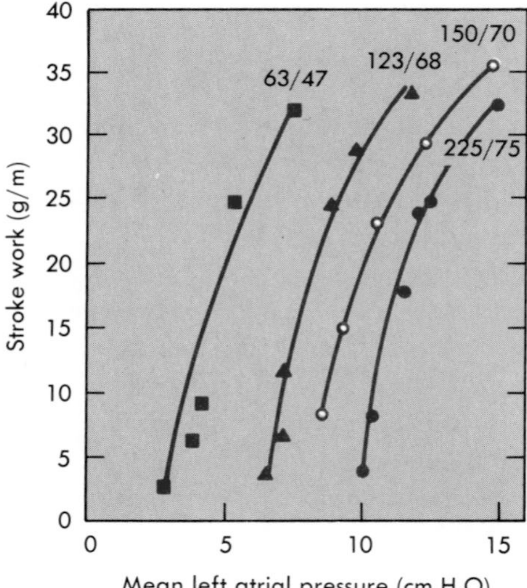

Fig. 4-32 ■ As the pressure in the isolated carotid sinus is progressively raised, the ventricular function curves shift to the right. The numbers at the tops of each curve represent the systolic/diastolic perfusion pressures (in millimeters of mercury) in the carotid sinus regions of the dog. (Redrawn from Sarnoff, S.J., Gilmore, J.P., Brockman, S.K., Mitchell, J.H., and Linden, R.J.: Circ. Res. 8:1123, 1960.)

from neighboring vagal fibers (see Fig. 4-28).

Baroreceptor Reflex. Just as stimulation of the carotid sinus and aortic arch baroreceptors may change heart rate (p. 86), so also may it alter myocardial performance. Evidence of reflex alterations of ventricular contractility is presented in Fig. 4-32. Ventricular function curves were obtained at four levels of carotid sinus pressure. With each successive rise in pressure, the ventricular function curves were displaced farther and farther to the right, denoting a progressively greater reflex depression of ventricular performance.

In normal, resting individuals and animals the tonic level of sympathetic activity is usually very low. Under such conditions, moderate changes in baroreceptor activity may have little reflex influence on myocardial contractility. In states of augmented sympathetic neural activity, however, the effects of the baroreceptor reflex on contractility may be substantial. In the adaptation to blood loss, for example, a reflex change in myocardial contractility may constitute an important compensation.

Chemical Control

Hormones

Adrenomedullary Hormones. The adrenal medulla is essentially a component of the autonomic nervous system. The principal hormone secreted by the adrenal medulla is epinephrine, although some norepinephrine is also released. The rate of secretion of catecholamines by the adrenal medulla is largely regulated by the same mechanisms that control the activity of the sympathetic nervous system. The concentrations of catecholamines in the blood rise under the same conditions that activate the sympathoadrenal system. However, the cardiovascular effects of circulating catecholamines are probably minimal under normal conditions. Instead, the cardiac effects of increased sympathoadrenal activity are mainly ascribable to the norepinephrine released at the sympathetic nerve endings in the heart.

The changes in myocardial contractility induced by norepinephrine infusions have been tested in resting, unanesthetized dogs. The maximum rate of rise of left ventricular pressure (dP/dt), an index of myocardial contractility, was found to be proportional to the norepinephrine concentration in the blood (Fig. 4-33). In these same animals, moderate exercise increased the maximum dP/dt by almost 100%, but it raised the circulating catecholamines by only 0.5 ng/ml. Such a rise in blood norepinephrine concentration, by itself, would have had only a negligible effect on left ventricular dP/dt

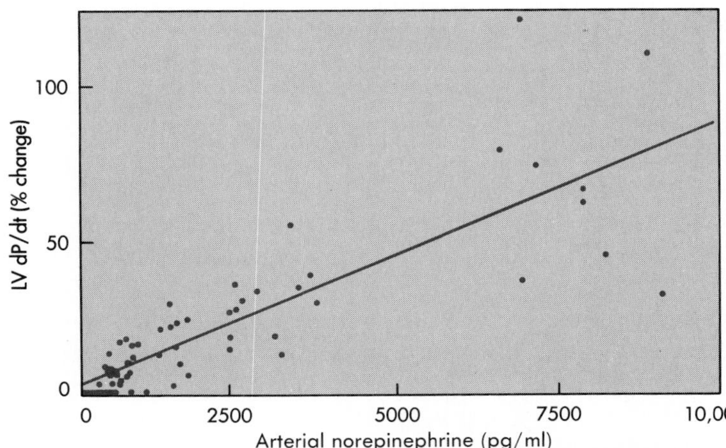

Fig. 4-33 ■ The effect of norepinephrine infusions on ventricular contractility in a group of resting, unanesthetized dogs. The plasma concentrations of norepinephrine *(pg/ml)* plotted along the abscissa are the increments above the control values. The maximum rate of rise of left ventricular pressure *(LV dP/dt)* is plotted along the ordinate as percent change from the control value; it is an index of contractility. (Redrawn from Young, M.A., Hintze, T.H., and Vatner, S.F.: Am. J. Physiol. 248:H82, 1985.)

(see Fig. 4-33). Hence, the pronounced change in dP/dt observed during exercise must have been ascribable mainly to the norepinephrine released from the cardiac sympathetic nerve fibers rather than to the catecholamines released from the adrenal medulla.

Adrenocortical Hormones. Cardiovascular problems are common in adrenocortical insufficiency **(Addison's disease).** The blood volume tends to fall, which may lead to severe hypotension and cardiovascular collapse, the so-called addisonian crisis.

The influence of adrenocortical steroids on the myocardium is controversial. Cardiac muscle removed from adrenalectomized animals and placed in a tissue bath is more likely to fatigue than that obtained from normal animals. In some species the adrenocortical hormones enhance contractility. Furthermore, hydrocortisone potentiates the cardiotonic effects of the catecholamines. This potentiation may be mediated in part by an inhibition of the uptake mechanisms for the catecholamines by the adrenocortical steroids.

Thyroid Hormones. Cardiac activity is sluggish in patients with inadequate thyroid function **(hypothyroidism);** that is, the heart rate is slow and cardiac output is diminished. The converse is true in patients with overactive thyroid glands **(hyperthyroidism).** Characteristically, hyperthyroid patients exhibit tachycardia, high cardiac output, palpitations, and arrhythmias (such as atrial fibrillation). In experimental animals the cardiovascular manifestations of hyperthyroidism may be simulated by the administration of thyroxine.

Numerous studies on intact animals and humans have demonstrated that thyroid hormones enhance myocardial contractility. The rates of Ca^{++} uptake and of ATP hydrolysis by the sarcoplasmic reticulum are increased in experimental hyperthyroidism, and the opposite effects occur in hypothyroidism. Thyroid hormones increase protein synthesis in the heart, which leads to cardiac hypertrophy. These hormones also affect the composition of myosin isoenzymes in cardiac muscle. They increase principally those isoenzymes with the greatest ATPase activity, which thereby enhances myocardial contractility.

The cardiovascular changes in thyroid dysfunction also depend on indirect mechanisms. Thyroid hyperactivity increases the body's metabolic rate, and this in turn results in arteriolar vasodilation. The consequent reduction in the total peripheral resistance increases cardiac output, as explained on p. 209. Substantial evidence indicates that with hyperthyroidism either sympathetic neural activity is increased or the sensitivity of the heart to such activity is enhanced. However, other evidence contradicts these conclusions. Studies do agree, however, that thyroid hormone increases the density of beta-adrenergic receptors in cardiac tissue.

Insulin. Insulin has a prominent, direct, positive inotropic effect on the heart. The effect of insulin is evident even when hypoglycemia is prevented by glucose infusions and when the beta-adrenergic receptors are blocked. In fact, the positive inotropic effect of insulin is potentiated by beta-adrenergic receptor blockade. The enhancement of contractility cannot be explained satisfactorily by the concomitant augmentation of glucose transport into the myocardial cells.

Glucagon. Glucagon has potent positive inotropic and chronotropic effects on the heart. The endogenous hormone probably plays no significant role in the normal regulation of the cardiovascular system, but it has been used to treat a variety of cardiac conditions. The effects of glucagon on the heart closely resemble those of the catecholamines, and certain metabolic effects are similar. Both glucagon and catecholamines activate adenylyl cyclase to increase the myocardial tissue levels of cAMP. The catecholamines activate adenylyl cyclase by interacting with beta-adrenergic receptors, but glucagon activates this enzyme through a different mechanism. Nevertheless, the consequent rise in cAMP increases Ca^{++} influx through the Ca^{++} channels in the sarcolemma and facilitates Ca^{++} release and reuptake by the sarcoplasmic reticulum, just as do the catecholamines.

Anterior Pituitary Hormones. The cardiovascular derangements in hypopituitarism are related principally to the associated deficiencies in adrenocortical and thyroid function. Growth hormone does affect the myocardium, at least in combination with thyroxine. In hypophysectomized animals growth hormone alone has little effect on the depressed heart, whereas thyroxine by itself restores adequate cardiac performance under basal conditions. However, when blood volume or peripheral resistance is increased, thyroxine alone does not restore adequate cardiac function, but the combination of growth hormone and thyroxine does reestablish normal cardiac performance.

Blood Gases

Oxygen. Changes in oxygen tension (Pa_{O_2}) of the blood perfusing the brain and the peripheral chemoreceptors affect the heart through nervous mechanisms, as described earlier in this chapter. These indirect effects of hypoxia are usually prepotent. Moderate degrees of hypoxia characteristically increase heart rate, cardiac output, and myocardial contractility. These changes are largely abolished by beta-adrenergic receptor blockade.

The Pa_{O_2} of the blood perfusing the myocardium also influences myocardial performance directly. The effect of hypoxia is biphasic; moderate degrees are stimulatory and more severe degrees are depressant. As shown in Fig. 4-34, when the O_2 saturation is reduced to levels below 50% in isolated hearts, the peak left ventricular pressures are less than the control levels. However, with less severe degrees of hypoxia (O_2 saturation $>$ 50%), the peak pressures exceed the control level.

Carbon Dioxide and Acidosis. Changes in Pa_{CO_2} may also affect the myocardium directly

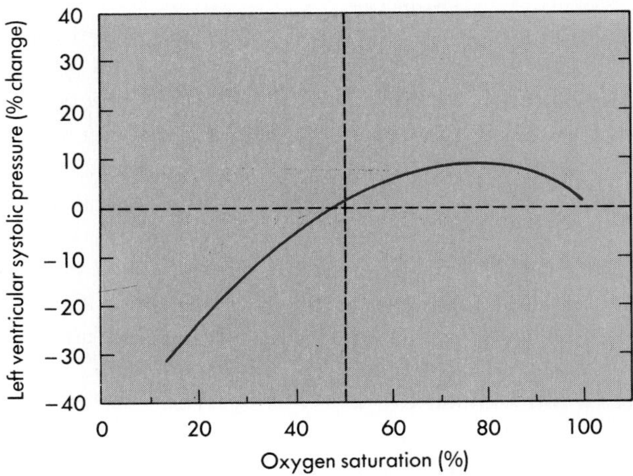

Fig. 4-34 ■ In the isovolumic left ventricle preparation, a reduction in the O_2 saturation of coronary arterial blood to between 45% and 100% stimulates ventricular contractility, whereas an O_2 saturation below 45% depresses ventricular contractility. (Redrawn from Ng, M.L., Levy, M.N., DeGeest, H., and Zieske, H.: Am. J. Physiol. 211:43, 1966.)

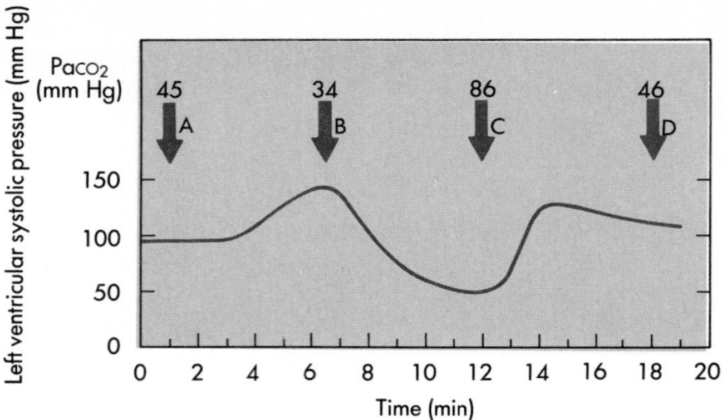

Fig. 4-35 ■ Decrease in $Paco_2$ increases left ventricular systolic pressure (arrow *B*) in an isovolumic left ventricle preparation; a rise in $Paco_2$ (arrow *C*) has the reverse effect. When the $Paco_2$ is returned to the control level (arrow *D*), left ventricular systolic pressure returns to its original value (arrow *A*). (Levy, M.N.: unpublished tracing.)

and indirectly. The indirect, neurally mediated effects produced by increased $Paco_2$ are similar to those evoked by a decrease in Pao_2.

With respect to the direct effects on the heart, alterations in myocardial performance elicited by changes of $Paco_2$ in the coronary arterial blood are illustrated in Fig. 4-35. In this experiment on an isolated left ventricle preparation, the control $Paco_2$ was 45 mm Hg (arrow *A*). Decreasing the $Paco_2$ to 34 mm Hg (arrow *B*) was stimulatory, whereas increasing $Paco_2$ to 86 mm (arrow *C*) was depressant. In intact animals, systemic hypercapnia activates the sympathoadrenal system, which tends to compensate for the direct depressant effect of the increased $Paco_2$ on the heart.

Neither the $Paco_2$ nor the blood pH are primary determinants of myocardial behavior. The resultant change in intracellular pH is the critical factor. The reduced intracellular pH diminishes the amount of Ca^{++} released from the sarcoplasmic reticulum in response to excitation. The diminished pH also decreases the sensitivity of the myofilaments to Ca^{++}. When they are exposed to a given concentration of Ca^{++}, the lower the prevailing pH, the less force the myofibrils develop.

■ SUMMARY

1. Cardiac function is regulated by a number of intrinsic and extrinsic mechanisms.
2. Heart rate is regulated mainly by the autonomic nervous system. Sympathetic nervous activity increases heart rate, whereas parasympathetic (vagal) activity decreases heart rate. When both systems are active, the vagal effects usually dominate.
3. The following reflexes regulate heart rate: baroreceptor, chemoreceptor, pulmonary inflation, atrial receptor (Bainbridge), and ventricular receptor reflexes.
4. The principal intrinsic mechanisms that regulate myocardial contraction are the Frank-Starling mechanism and rate induced regulation.
   a. Frank-Starling mechanism: a change in the resting length of the muscle influences the subsequent contraction by altering the number of interacting cross-bridges between the thick and thin filaments and by altering the affinity of the myofilaments for calcium.
   b. Rate induced regulation: a sustained

change in contraction frequency affects the strength of contraction by altering the influx of Ca^{++} into the cell per minute, whereas a transient change in contraction frequency alters contractile strength because an appreciable delay exists between the time that Ca^{++} is taken up by the sarcoplasmic reticulum and the time that it becomes available again for release.

5. The autonomic nervous system regulates myocardial performance mainly by varying the Ca^{++} conductance of the cell membrane via the adenylyl cyclase system.
6. Various hormones, including epinephrine, adrenocortical steroids, thyroid hormones, insulin, glucagon, and anterior pituitary hormones regulate myocardial performance.
7. Changes in the blood concentrations of O_2, CO_2, and H^+ alter cardiac function directly and, via the chemoreceptors, reflexly.

■ BIBLIOGRAPHY

Journal articles

Bouchard, R.A., and Bose, D.: Analysis of the interval-force relationship in rat and canine ventricular myocardium, Am. J. Physiol. 257:H2036, 1989.

Cantin, M., and Genest, J.: The heart as an endocrine gland, Hypertension 10(Suppl. I):I-118-I-121, 1987.

Chernow, B., Reed, L., Geelhoed, G.W., Anderson, M., Teich, S., Meyerhoff, J., Beardsley, D., Lake, C.R., and Holaday, J.W.: Glucagon: Endocrine effects and calcium involvement in cardiovascular actions in dogs, Circ. Shock 19:393, 1986.

Dampney, R.A.L.: Functional organization of central cardiovascular pathways, Clin. Exp. Pharmacol. Physiol. 8:241, 1981.

Endoh, M., and Blinks, J.R.: Actions of sympathomimetic amines on the Ca^{2+} transients and contractions of rabbit myocardium: Reciprocal changes in myofibrillar responsiveness to Ca^{2+} mediated through α- and β-adrenoceptors, Circ. Res. 62:247, 1988.

Farah, A.E.: Glucagon and the circulation, Pharmacol. Rev. 35:181, 1983.

Farah, A.E., and Alousi, A.A.: The actions of insulin on cardiac contractility, Life Sci. 29:975, 1981.

Hakumäki, M.O.K.: Seventy years of the Bainbridge reflex, Acta Physiol. Scand. 130:177, 1987.

Hathaway, D.R., and March, K.L.: Molecular cardiology: New avenues for the diagnosis and treatment of cardiovascular disease, J. Am. Coll. Cardiol. 13:265, 1989.

Josephson R.A., Spurgeon, H.A., and Lakatta, E.G.: The hyperthyroid heart. An analysis of systolic and diastolic properties in single rat ventricular myocytes, Circ. Res. 66:773, 1990.

Katona, P.G., McLean, M., Dighton, D.H., and Guz, A.: Sympathetic and parasympathetic cardiac control in athletes and nonathletes at rest, J. Appl. Physiol. 52:1652, 1982.

Klein, I., and Levey, G.S.: New perspectives on thyroid hormone, catecholamines, and the heart, Am. J. Med. 76:167, 1984.

Kohmoto, O., Spitzer, K.W., Movsesian, M.A., and Barry, W.H.: Effects of intracellular acidosis on $(Ca^{2+})_i$ transients, transsarcolemmal Ca^{2+} fluxes, and contraction in ventricular myocytes, Circ. Res. 66:622, 1990.

Kollai, M., and Koizumi, K.: Cardiac vagal and sympathetic nerve responses to baroreceptor stimulation in the dog, Pflügers Arch. 413:365, 1989.

Kuhn, H.J., Bletz, C., and Rüegg, J.C.: Stretch-induced increase in the Ca^{2+} sensitivity of myofibrillar ATPase activity in skinned fibres from pig ventricles, Pflügers Arch. 415:741, 1990.

Kurihara, S., and Konishi, M.: Effects of β-adrenoceptor stimulation on intracellular Ca transients and tension in rat ventricular muscle, Pflügers Arch. 409:427, 1987.

Lakatta, E.G.: Starling's law of the heart is explained by an intimate interaction of muscle length and myofilament calcium activation, J. Am. Coll. Cardiol. 10:1157, 1987.

Levy, M.N.: Autonomic interactions in cardiac control, Ann. N.Y. Acad. of Sci. 601:209, 1990.

Löffelholz, K., and Pappano, A.J.: The parasympathetic neuroeffector junction of the heart, Pharmacol. Rev. 37:1, 1985.

Morkin, E., Flink, I.L., and Goldman, S.: Biochemical and physiologic effects of thyroid hormone on cardiac performance, Prog. Cardiovasc. Dis. 25:435, 1983.

Reiter, M.: Calcium mobilization and cardiac inotropic mechanisms, Pharmacol. Rev. 40:189, 1988.

Seed, W.A., and Walker, J.M.: Relation between beat interval and force of the heartbeat and its clinical implications, Cardiovasc. Res. 22:303, 1988.

Spyer, K.M.: Neural organisation and control of the baroreceptor reflex, Rev. Physiol. Biochem. Pharmacol. 88:23, 1981.

Vanhoutte, P.M., and Levy, M.N.: Prejunctional cholinergic modulation of adrenergic neurotransmission in the cardiovascular system, Am. J. Physiol. 238:H275, 1980.

Watanabe, A.M., Jones, L.R., Manalan, A.S., and Besch, H.R., Jr.: Cardiac autonomic receptors, Circ. Res. 50:161, 1982.

Winegrad, S.: Regulation of cardiac contractile proteins, Circ. Res. 55:565, 1984.

Young, M.A., Hintze, T.H., and Vatner, S.F.: Correlation between cardiac performance and plasma catecholamine levels in conscious dogs, Am. J. Physiol. 248:H82, 1985.

Books and monographs

Bishop, V.S., Malliani, A., and Thorén, P.: Cardiac mechanoreceptors. In Handbook of physiology; Section 2: The cardiovascular system—peripheral circulation and organ blood flow, vol. III, Bethesda, Md., 1983, American Physiological Society.

Downing, S.E.: Baroreceptor regulation of the heart. In Handbook of physiology; Section 2: Cardiovascular system—the heart, vol. I, Washington, D.C., 1979, American Physiologic Society.

Fowler, N.O.: Pericardium in health and disease, Mount Kisco, N.Y., 1985, Futura Publishing Co., Inc.

Levine, H.J., and Gaasch, W.H., editors: The ventricle: basic and clinical aspects, Hingham, Mass., 1985, Martinus Nijhoff Publishers.

Levy, M.N., and Martin, P.J.: Neural control of the heart. In Handbook of physiology; Section 2: Cardiovascular system—the heart, vol. I, Washington, D.C., 1979, American Physiological Society.

Opie, L., editor: The heart, Orlando, Fla., 1984, Grune & Stratton, Inc.

Randall, W.C., editor: Nervous control of cardiovascular function, New York, 1984, Oxford University Press.

Sagawa, K., Maughan, L., Suga, H., and Sunagawa, K.: Cardiac contraction and the pressure-volume relationship, New York, 1988, Oxford University Press.

Sperelakis, N., editor: Physiology and pathophysiology of the heart, ed. 2, Boston, 1989, Kluwer Academic Publishers.

Zucker, I.H., and Gilmore, J.P.: Reflex control of the circulation, Boca Raton, 1990, CRC Press, Inc.

5 Hemodynamics

The problem of treating the pulsatile flow of blood through the cardiovascular system in precise mathematical terms is insuperable. The heart is a complicated pump, and its behavior is affected by a variety of physical and chemical factors. The blood vessels are multibranched, elastic conduits of continuously varying dimensions. The blood itself is not a simple, homogeneous solution, but instead is a complex suspension of red and white corpuscles, platelets, and lipid globules dispersed in a colloidal solution of proteins.

Despite these complicating factors, considerable insight may be gained from understanding the elementary principles of fluid mechanics as they pertain to simple physical systems. Such principles will be expounded in this chapter to explain the interrelationships among velocity of blood flow, blood pressure, and the dimensions of the various components of the systemic circulation.

■ VELOCITY OF THE BLOODSTREAM

In describing the variations in blood flow in different vessels it is first essential to distinguish between the terms **velocity** and **flow**. The former term, sometimes designated as **linear** velocity, refers to the rate of displacement with respect to time and has the dimensions of distance per unit time, for example, cm/s. The latter term is frequently designated as **volume** flow and has the dimensions of volume per unit time, for example, cm^3/s. In a conduit of varying cross-sectional dimensions, velocity, v, flow, Q, and cross-sectional area, A, are related by the equation:

$$v = Q/A \qquad (1)$$

The interrelationships among velocity, flow, and area are portrayed in Fig. 5-1. The flow of an incompressible fluid past successive cross sections of a rigid tube must be constant. For a given constant flow the velocity varies inversely as the cross-sectional area (see Fig. 1-2). Thus for the same volume of fluid per second passing from section *a* into section *b*, where the cross-sectional area is five times greater, the velocity diminishes to one fifth of its previous value. Conversely, when the fluid proceeds from section *b* to section *c*, where the cross-sectional area is one tenth as great, the velocity of each particle of fluid must increase tenfold.

The velocity at any point in the system depends not only on area, but also on the flow, Q. This, in turn, depends on the pressure gradient, properties of the fluid, and dimensions of the entire hydraulic system, as discussed in

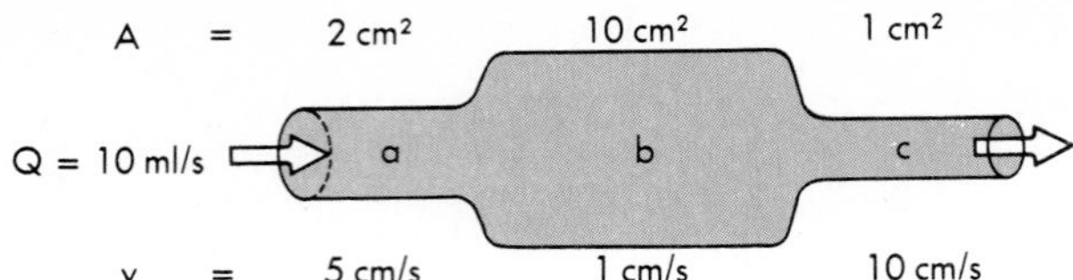

Fig. 5-1 ■ As fluid flows through a tube of variable cross-sectional area, *A*, the linear velocity, *v*, varies inversely as the cross-sectional area.

the following section. For any given flow, however, the ratio of the velocity past one cross section relative to that past a second cross section depends only on the inverse ratio of the respective areas; that is,

$$v_1/v_2 = A_2/A_1 \qquad (2)$$

This rule pertains regardless of whether a given cross-sectional area applies to a system that consists of a single large tube or to a system comprised of several smaller tubes in parallel.

As shown in Fig. 1-2, velocity decreases progressively as the blood traverses the aorta, its larger primary branches, the smaller secondary branches, and the arterioles. Finally, a minimum value is reached in the capillaries. As the blood then passes through the venules and continues centrally toward the venae cavae, the velocity progressively increases again. The relative velocities in the various components of the circulatory system are related only to the cross-sectional area. Thus each point on the cross-sectional area curve is inversely proportional to the corresponding point on the velocity curve (Fig. 1-2).

■ RELATIONSHIP BETWEEN VELOCITY AND PRESSURE

In that portion of a hydraulic system in which the total energy remains virtually constant, changes in velocity may be accompanied by appreciable alterations in the measured pressure. Consider three sections (**A, B,** and **C**) of such a hydraulic system, as depicted in Fig. 5-2. Six pressure probes, or **pitot tubes**, have been inserted. The opening of three of these (**2, 4,** and **6**) are tangential to the direction of flow and hence measure the **lateral**, or **static**, pressure within the tube. The openings of the remaining three pitot tubes (**1, 3,** and **5**) face upstream. Therefore, they detect the **total pressure**, which is the lateral pressure plus a dynamic pressure component ascribable to the kinetic energy of the flowing fluid. This dynamic component, P_d, of the total pressure may be calculated from the following equation:

$$P_d = \tfrac{1}{2}\rho v^2 \qquad (3)$$

where ρ is the density of the fluid, and v is the velocity. If the midpoints of segments *A, B,* and *C* are at the same hydrostatic level, then the corresponding total pressure, P_1, P_3, and P_5, will be equal, provided that the energy loss from viscosity in these segments is negligible. However, because of the changes in cross-sectional area, the concomitant velocity changes alter the dynamic component.

In sections *A* and *C*, let $\rho = 1\ g/cm^3$, and $v = 100$ cm/s. From equation 3

$$P_d = 5000\ dynes/cm^2$$
$$= 3.8\ mm\ Hg$$

since 1330 dynes/cm^2 = 1 mm Hg. In the narrow section, *B*, let the velocity be twice as great as in sections *A* and *C*. Therefore,

$$P_d = 20{,}000\ dynes/cm^2$$
$$= 15\ mm\ Hg$$

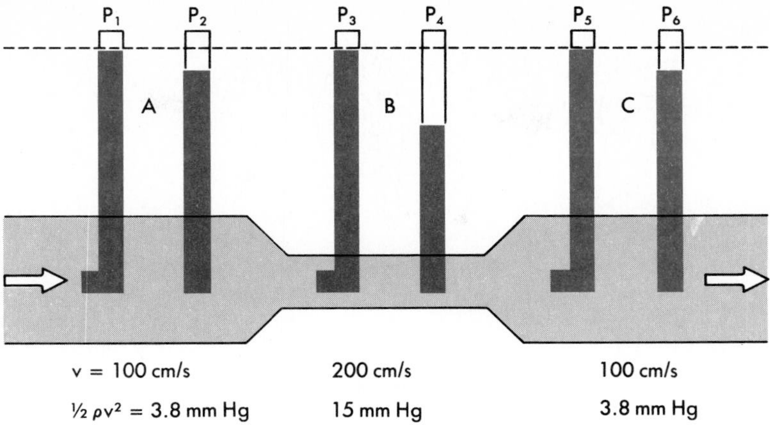

Fig. 5-2 ▪ In a narrow section, *B*, of a tube, the linear velocity, *v*, and hence the dynamic component of pressure, $\frac{1}{2}\rho v^2$, are greater than in the wide sections, *A* and *C*, of the same tube. If the total energy is virtually constant throughout the tube (that is, if the energy loss because of viscosity is negligible), the total pressures (P_1, P_3 and P_5) will not be detectably different, but the lateral pressure, P_4, in the narrow section will be less than the lateral pressures (P_2 and P_6) in the wide sections of the tube.

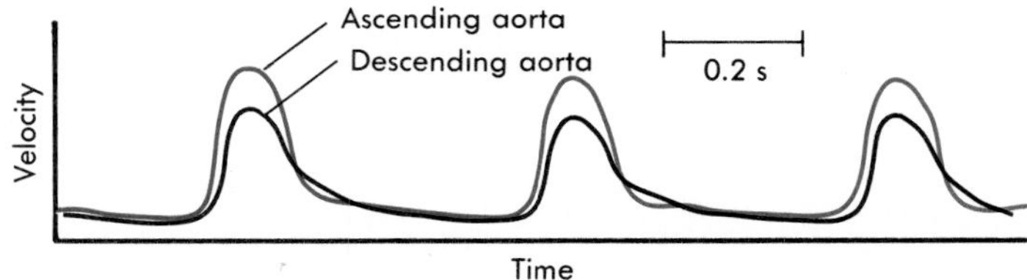

Fig. 5-3 ▪ Velocity of the blood in the ascending and descending aorta of a dog. (Redrawn from Falsetti, H.L., Kiser, K.M., Francis, G.P., and Belmore, E.R.: Circ. Res. 31:328, 1972. By permission of the American Heart Association, Inc.)

Hence, in the wide sections of the conduit, the lateral pressures (P_2 and P_6) will be only 3.8 mm Hg less than the respective total pressures (P_1 and P_5), whereas in the narrow section, the lateral pressure (P_4) is 15 mm Hg less than the total pressure (P_3).

The peak velocity of flow in the ascending aorta of normal dogs is about 150 cm/s. Therefore, the measured pressure may vary significantly, depending on the orientation of the pressure probe. In the descending thoracic aorta the peak velocity is substantially less than that in the ascending aorta (Fig. 5-3), and lesser velocities have been recorded in still more distal arterial sites. In most arterial locations the dynamic component will be a negligible fraction of the total pressure, and the orientation of the pressure probe will not materially influence the pressure recorded. At the site of a constriction, however, the dynamic pressure component may attain substantial values. In **aortic stenosis**, for example, the entire output of the left ventricle is ejected through a narrow valve orifice. The high flow velocity is

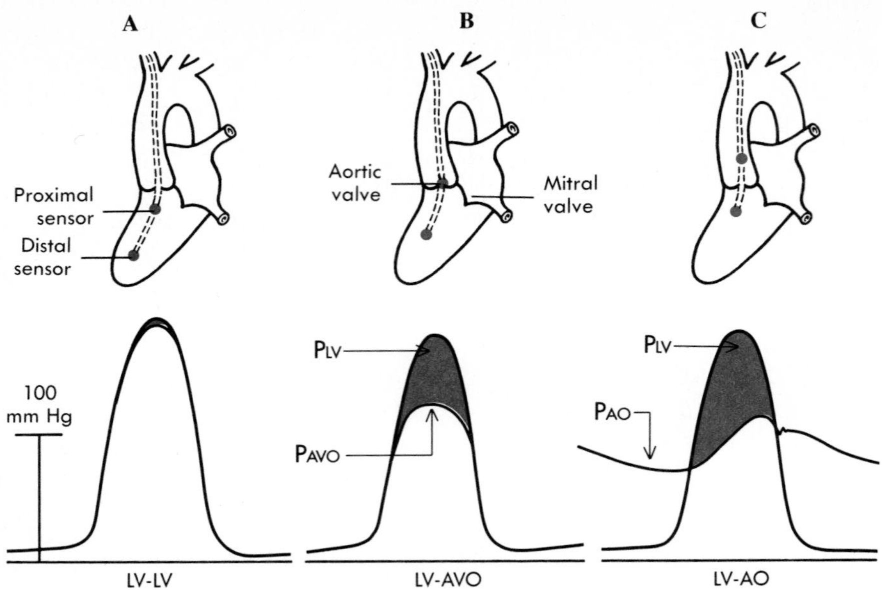

Fig. 5-4 ■ Pressures (P) recorded by two transducers in a patient with aortic stenosis. **A,** Both transducers were in the left ventricle (*LV-LV*). **B,** One transducer was in the left ventricle, and the other was in the aortic valve orifice (*LV-AVO*). **C,** One transducer was in the left ventricle, and the other was in the ascending aorta (*LV-AO*). (Redrawn from Pasipoularides, A., Murgo, J.P., Bird, J.J., and Craig, W.E.: Am. J. Physiol. 246:H542, 1984.)

associated with a large kinetic energy, and therefore the lateral pressure is correspondingly reduced.

The pressure tracings shown in Fig. 5-4 were obtained from two pressure transducers inserted into the left ventricle of a patient with aortic stenosis. The transducers were located on the same catheter and were 5 cm apart. When both transducers were well within the left ventricular cavity (Fig. 5-4, *A*), they both recorded the same pressures. However, when the proximal transducer was positioned in the aortic valve orifice (Fig. 5-4, *B*), the lateral pressure recorded during ejection was much less than that recorded by the transducer in the ventricular cavity. This pressure difference was ascribable almost entirely to the much greater velocity of flow in the narrowed valve orifice than in the ventricular cavity. The pressure difference reflects mainly the conversion of some potential energy to kinetic energy. When the catheter was withdrawn still farther, so that the proximal transducer was in the aorta (Fig. 5-4, *C*), the pressure difference was even more pronounced, because substantial energy was lost through friction (viscosity) as blood flowed rapidly through the narrow orifice.

The reduction of lateral pressure in the region of the stenotic valve orifice influences the coronary blood flow in patients with aortic stenosis. The orifices of the right and left coronary arteries are located in the sinuses of Valsalva, just behind the valve leaflets. Hence the initial segments of these vessels are oriented at right angles to the direction of blood flow through the aortic valves. Therefore, the lateral pressure is that component of the total pressure that propels the blood through the two major coronary arteries. During the ejection phase of the cardiac cycle, the lateral pressure is diminished by the conversion of potential energy to kinetic energy. This process is grossly exaggerated in aortic stenosis, because of the high flow velocities. Angiographic studies in patients with aortic stenosis have revealed that the direction of flow often reverses in the large coronary arteries toward the end of the ejection phase of systole; that is, blood flows toward the aorta rather than toward the myocardial capillaries. The decreased lateral pressure in the aorta in aortic stenosis is undoubtedly an important factor in causing this reversal of coronary blood flow.

An important aggravating feature in this condition is that the demands of the heart muscle for oxygen are greatly increased. Therefore, the pronounced drop in lateral pressure during cardiac ejection may contribute to the tendency for patients with severe aortic stenosis to experience **angina pectoris** (anterior chest pain associated with inadequate blood supply to the heart muscle) and to die suddenly.

■ RELATIONSHIP BETWEEN PRESSURE AND FLOW

The most fundamental law governing the flow of fluids through cylindrical tubes was derived empirically by Poiseuille. He was primarily interested in the physical determinants of blood flow, but substituted simpler liquids for blood in his measurements of flow through glass capillary tubes. His work was so precise and important that his observations have been designated **Poiseuille's law**. Subsequently, this same law has been derived theoretically.

Poiseuille's law is applicable to the flow of fluids through cylindrical tubes only under special conditions. It applies to the case of steady, laminar flow of newtonian fluids. The term **steady flow** signifies the absence of variations of flow in time, that is, a nonpulsatile flow. **Laminar flow** is the type of motion in which the fluid moves as a series of individual layers, with each stratum moving at a different velocity from its neighboring layers (see Fig. 5-12). In the case of flow through a tube, the fluid consists of a series of infinitesimally thin concentric tubes sliding past one another. Laminar flow will be described in greater detail below, where it will be distinguished from turbulent flow. Also a **newtonian fluid** will be defined more precisely. For the present discussion it may be considered to be a homogeneous fluid, such as water, in contradistinction to a suspension, such as blood.

Pressure is one of the principal determinants of the rate of flow. The pressure, P, in dynes/cm^2, at a distance h centimeters below the surface of a liquid is

$$P = h\rho g \tag{4}$$

where ρ is the density of the liquid in g/cm^3 and g is the acceleration of gravity in cm/s^2. For convenience, however, pressure is frequently expressed simply in terms of height, h, of the column of liquid above some arbitrary reference point.

Consider the tube connecting reservoirs R_1 and R_2 in Fig. 5-5, *A*. Let reservoir R_1 be filled with liquid to height h_1, and let reservoir R_2 be empty, as in section *1* of Fig. 5-5. The outflow pressure, P_o, is therefore equal to the atmospheric pressure, which shall be designated as the zero, or reference, level. The inflow pressure, P_i, is then equal to the same reference level plus the height, h_1, of the column of liquid in reservoir R_1. Under these conditions let the flow, Q, through the tube be 5 ml/s.

If reservoir R_1 is filled to height h_2, which is twice h_1, and reservoir R_2 is again empty (as in panel *B)*, the flow will be twice as great, that is, 10 ml/s. Thus with reservoir R_2 empty, the flow will be directly proportional to the inflow pressure, P_i.

If reservoir R_2 is now allowed to fill to height h_1, and the fluid level in R_1 is main-

A

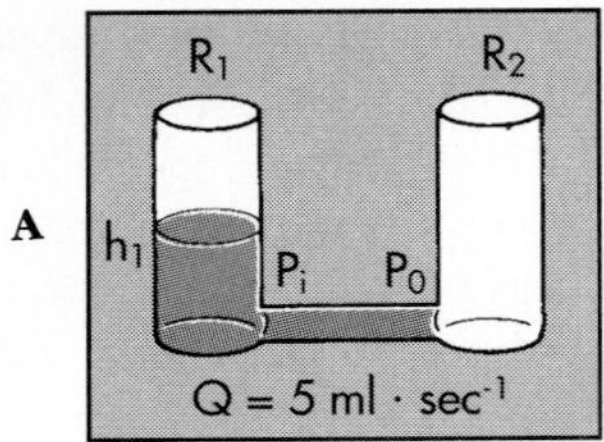

A, When R_2 is empty, fluid flows from R_1 to R_2 at a rate proportional to the pressure in R_1.

B

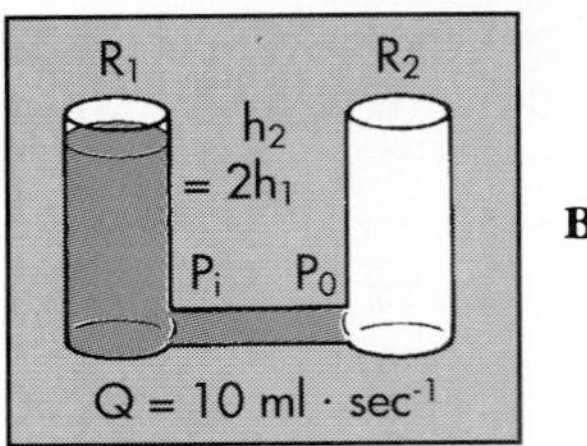

B, When the fluid level in R_1 is increased twofold, the flow increases proportionately.

C

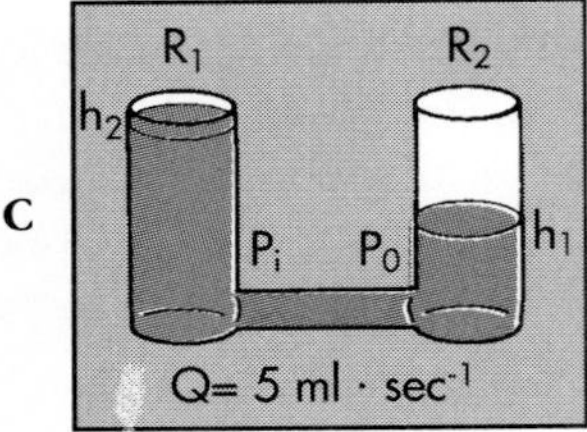

C, Flow from R_1 to R_2 is proportional to the difference between the pressures in R_1 and R_2.

D

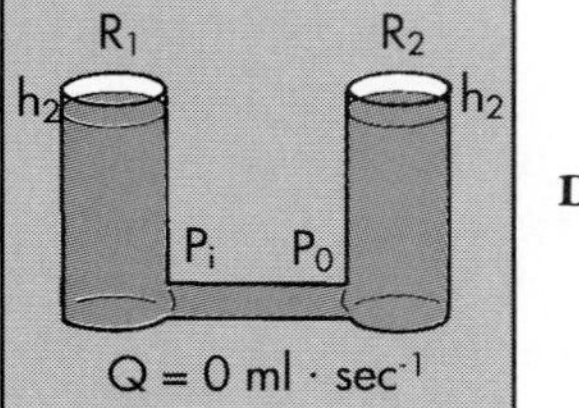

D, When pressure in R_2 rises to equal the pressure in R_1, flow ceases in the connecting tube.

Fig. 5-5 ■ The flow, V, of fluid through a tube connecting two reservoirs, R_1 and R_2, is proportional to the difference between the pressure, P_i, at the inflow end and the pressure, P_o, at the outflow end of the tube.

tained at h_2 (as in panel *C*), the flow will again become 5 ml/s. Thus flow is directly proportional to the difference between inflow and outflow pressures:

$$Q \propto P_i - P_o \qquad (5)$$

If the fluid level in R_2 attains the same height as in R_1, flow will cease (panel *D*).

For any given pressure difference between the two ends of a tube, the flow will depend on the dimensions of the tube. Consider the tube connected to the reservoir in Fig. 5-6, *A*. With length l_1 and radius r_1, the flow Q_1 is observed to be 10 ml/s.

The tube connected to the reservoir in panel *B* has the same radius, but is twice as long. Under these conditions the flow Q_2 is found to be 5 ml/s, or only half as great as Q_1. Conversely, for a tube half as long as l_1 the flow would be twice as great as Q_1. In other words, flow is inversely proportional to the length of the tube:

$$Q \propto 1/l \qquad (6)$$

The tube connected to the reservoir in Fig. 5-6, *C* is the same length as l_1, but the radius is twice as great. Under these conditions, the flow Q_3 is found to increase to a value of 160 ml/s, which is sixteen times greater than Q_1. The precise measurements of Poiseuille revealed that flow varies directly as the fourth power of the radius:

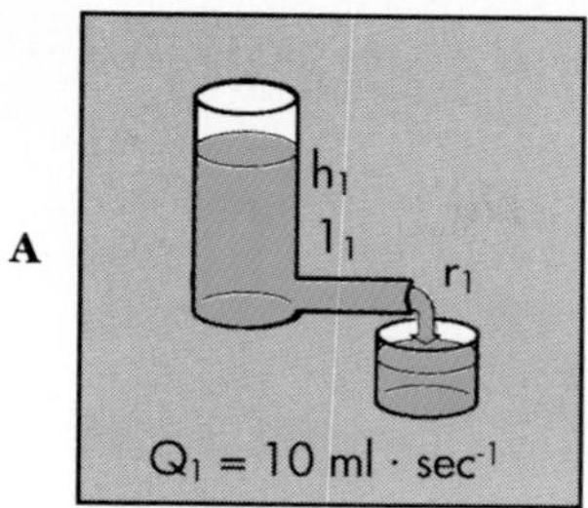

A, Reference condition: for a given pressure, length, radius, and viscosity, let the flow (V_1) equal 10 ml·s^{-1}.

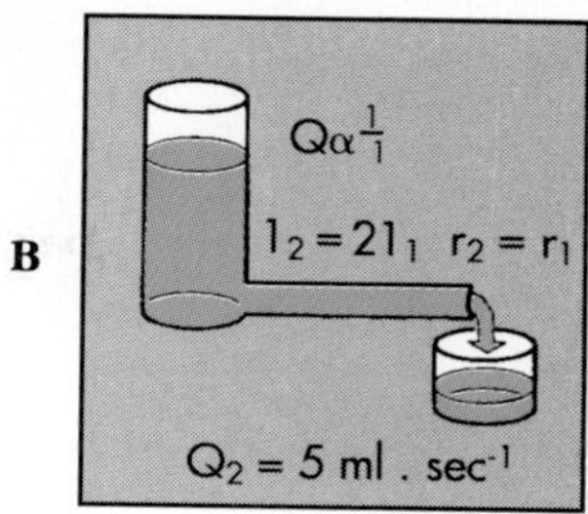

B, If tube length doubles, flow decreases by 50%.

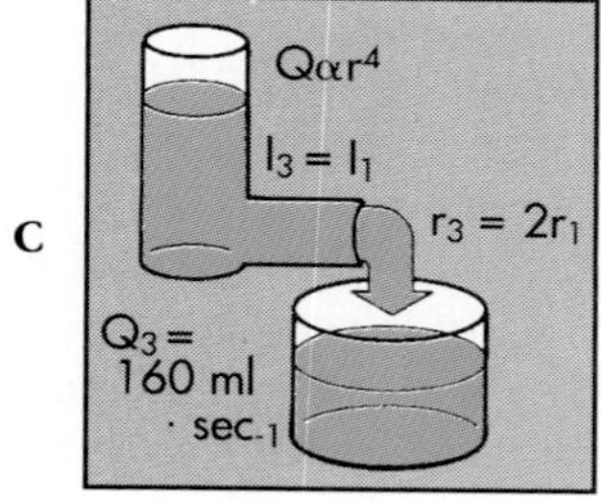

C, If tube radius doubles, flow increases 16-fold.

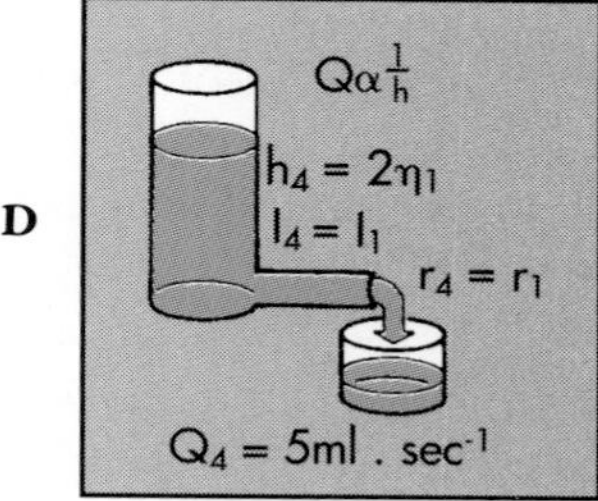

D, If viscosity doubles, flow decreases by 50%.

Fig. 5-6 ■ The flow, *V*, of fluid through a tube is inversely proportional to the length, l, and the viscosity, η, and is directly proportional to the fourth power of the radius, *r*.

$$Q \propto r^4 \tag{7}$$

Thus, in the example above, because $r_3 = 2r_1$, Q_3 will be proportional to $(2r_1)^4$, or $16r_1^4$; therefore, Q_3 will equal $16Q_1$.

Finally, for a given pressure difference and for a cylindrical tube of given dimensions, the flow will vary as a function of the nature of the fluid itself. This flow-determining property of fluids is termed **viscosity**, η, which has been defined by Newton as the ratio of **shear stress** to the **shear rate** of the fluid.

These terms may be comprehended most clearly by considering the flow of a homogeneous fluid between parallel plates. In Fig. 5-7 let the bottom plate (the bottom of a large basin) be stationary, and let the upper plate move at a constant velocity along the upper surface of the fluid. The **shear stress**, τ, is defined as the ratio of F:A, where F is the force applied to the upper plate in the direction of its motion along the upper surface of the fluid and A is the area of the upper plate in contact with the fluid. The shear rate is du/dy, where u is the velocity of a minute fluid element in the direction parallel to the motion of the upper plate and y is the distance of that fluid element above the bottom, stationary plate.

For a movable plate traveling with constant

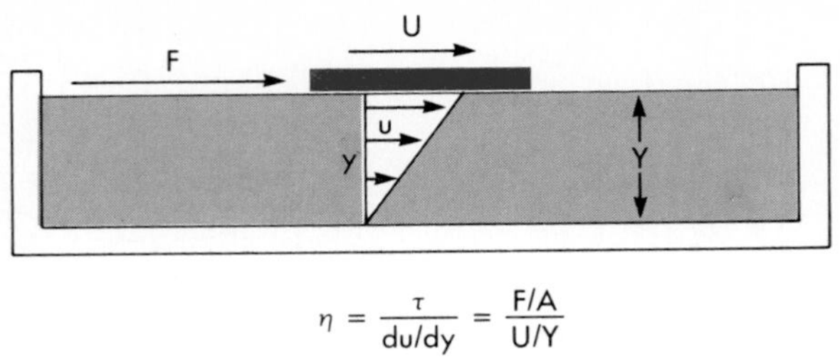

$$\eta = \frac{\tau}{du/dy} = \frac{F/A}{U/Y}$$

Fig. 5-7 ■ For a newtonian fluid, the viscosity, η, is defined as the ratio of shear stress, τ, to shear rate, *du/dy*. For a plate of contact area, *A*, moving across the surface of a liquid, τ equals the ratio of the force, *F*, applied in the direction of motion to the contact area, *A*, and *du/dy* equals the ratio of the velocity of the plate, *U*, to the depth of the liquid, *Y*.

velocity across the surface of a homogeneous fluid, the velocity profile of the fluid will be linear. The fluid layer in contact with the upper plate will adhere to it and therefore will move at the same velocity, U, as the plate. Each minute element of fluid between the plates will move at a velocity, u, proportional to its distance, y, from the lower plate. Therefore, the shear rate will be U/Y, where Y is the total distance between the two plates. Since viscosity, η, is defined as the ratio of shear stress, τ, to the shear rate du/dy, in the example illustrated in Fig. 5-7,

$$\eta = (F/A)/(U/Y) \qquad (8)$$

Thus the dimensions of viscosity are dynes/cm^2 divided by (cm/s)/cm, or dyne-s-cm^{-2}. In honor of Poiseuille, 1 dyne-s-cm^{-2} has been termed a **poise**. The viscosity of water at 20° C is approximately 0.01 **poise**, or 1 centipoise. In the case of certain nonhomogeneous fluids, notably suspensions such as blood, the ratio of the shear stress to the shear rate is not constant; such fluids are said to be **nonnewtonian**.

With regard to the flow of newtonian fluids through cylindrical tubes, the flow will vary inversely as the viscosity. Thus in the example of flow from the reservoir in Fig. 5-6, *D,* if the viscosity of the fluid in the reservoir were doubled, then the flow would be halved (5 ml/s instead of 10 ml/s).

In summary, for the steady, laminar flow of a newtonian fluid through a cylindrical tube, the flow, Q, varies directly as the pressure difference, $P_i - P_o$, and the fourth power of the radius, r, of the tube, and it varies inversely as the length, l, of the tube and the viscosity, η, of the fluid. The full statement of **Poiseuille's law** is

$$Q = \frac{\pi(P_i - P_o)r^4}{8\eta l} \qquad (9)$$

where π/8 is the constant of proportionality.

■ RESISTANCE TO FLOW

In electrical theory the resistance, R, is defined as the ratio of voltage drop, E, to current flow, I. Similarly, in fluid mechanics the hydraulic resistance, R, may be defined as the ratio of pressure drop, $P_i - P_o$, to flow, Q; P_i and P_o are the pressures at the inflow and outflow ends, respectively, of the hydraulic system. For the steady, laminar flow of a newtonian fluid through a cylindrical tube, the physical components of hydraulic resistance may be appreciated by rearranging Poiseuille's law to give the **hydraulic resistance equation**

$$R = \frac{P_i - P_o}{Q} = \frac{8\eta l}{\pi r^4} \qquad (10)$$

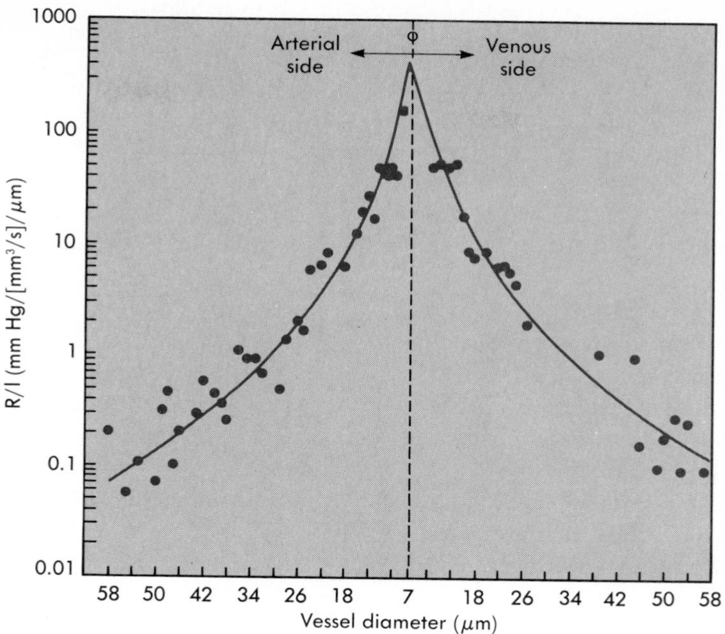

Fig. 5-8 ■ The resistance per unit length (R/l) for individual small blood vessels in the cat mesentery. The capillaries, diameter 7 μm, are denoted by the vertical dashed line. Resistances of the arterioles are plotted to the left and resistances of the venules are plotted to the right of the vertical dashed line. The solid circles represent the actual data. The two curves through the data represent the following regression equations for the arteriole and venule data, respectively: (a) arterioles, $R/l = 1.02 \times 10^6 D^{-4.04}$, and (b) venules, $R/l = 1.07 \times 10^6 D^{-3.94}$. Note that for both types of vessels, the resistance per unit length is inversely proportional to the fourth power (within 1%) of the vessel diameter (D). (Redrawn from Lipowsky, H.H., Kovalcheck, S., and Zweifach, B.W.: Circ. Res. 43:738, 1978. By permission of the American Heart Association, Inc.)

Thus, when Poiseuille's law applies, the resistance to flow depends only on the dimensions of the tube and on the characteristics of the fluid.

The principal determinant of the resistance to blood flow through any individual vessel within the circulatory system is its caliber. The resistance to flow through small blood vessels in cat mesentery has been measured, and the resistance per unit length of vessel (R/l) is plotted against the vessel diameter in Fig. 5-8. The resistance is highest in the capillaries (diameter 7 μm), and it diminishes as the vessels increase in diameter on the arterial and venous sides of the capillaries. The values of R/l were found to be virtually proportional to the fourth power of the diameter for the larger vessels on both sides of the capillaries.

Changes in vascular resistance induced by natural stimuli occur by changes in radius. The principal changes are achieved by alterations in the contraction of the circular smooth muscle cells in the vessel wall. However, changes in internal pressure also alter the caliber of the blood vessels, and therefore alter the resistance to blood flow through those vessels. The blood vessels are elastic tubes. Hence, the greater the **transmural pressure** (i.e., the difference between the internal and external pressures), the greater will be the caliber of the vessel, and the less will be its hydraulic resistance.

From Fig. 1-2 it may be noted that the greatest upstream to downstream drop in internal pressure occurs in the arterioles. Because the total flow is the same through the various series components of the circulatory system, it follows that the greatest resistance to flow resides in the arterioles. For example, if R_a represents the resistance of the arterioles, and R_x represents the resistance of any other component of the vascular system in series with the arterioles, then by the definition of hydraulic resistance (equation 10),

$$R_a = (P_i - P_o)_a / Q_a \text{ for the arterioles, and}$$

$$R_x = (P_i - P_o)_x / Q_x \text{ for the other component.}$$

But because the two components are in series, $Q_a = Q_x$, as stated above. Therefore

$$R_a / R_x = (P_i - P_o)_a / (P_i - P_o)_x \tag{11}$$

That is, the ratio of the pressure drop across the length of the arterioles to the pressure drop across the length of any other series component of the vascular system is equal to the ratio of the hydraulic resistances of these two vascular components. The reason why the highest resistance does not reside in the capillaries (as might otherwise be suspected from Fig. 5-8) is related to the relative numbers of parallel capillaries and parallel arterioles, as explained below (p. 124). The arterioles are vested with a thick coat of circularly arranged smooth muscle fibers, by means of which the lumen radius may be varied. From the hydraulic resistance equation, wherein R varies inversely as r^4, it is clear that small changes in radius will alter resistance greatly.

In the cardiovascular system the various types of vessels listed along the horizontal axis in Fig. 1-2 lie in series with one another. Furthermore, the individual members of each category of vessels are ordinarily arranged in parallel with one another (see Fig. 1-3). For example, the capillaries throughout the body are in most instances parallel elements, with the notable exceptions of the renal vasculature (wherein the peritubular capillaries are in series with the glomerular capillaries) and the splanchnic vasculature (wherein the intestinal and hepatic capillaries are aligned in series). Formulas for the total hydraulic resistance of components arranged in series and in parallel have been derived in the same manner as those for similar combinations of electrical resistances.

Three hydraulic resistances, R_1, R_2, and R_3, are arranged in series in the schema depicted in Fig. 5-9. The pressure drop across the entire system—that is, the difference between inflow pressure, P_i, and outflow pressure, P_o—consists of the sum of the pressure drops across each of the individual resistances (equation *a*). Under steady-state conditions, the flow, Q, through any given cross section must equal the flow through any other cross section. By dividing each component in equation *a* by Q (equation *b*), it becomes evident from the definition of resistance that the total resistance, R_t, of the entire system equals the sum of the individual resistances, that is,

$$R_t = R_1 + R_2 + R_3 \tag{12}$$

For resistances in parallel, as illustrated in Fig. 5-10, the inflow and outflow pressures are the same for all tubes. Under steady-state conditions, the total flow, Q_t, through the system equals the sum of the flows through the individual parallel elements (equation *a*). Because the pressure gradient $(P_i - P_o)$ is identical for all parallel elements, each term in equation *a* may be divided by that pressure gradient to yield equation *b*. From the definition of resistance, equation *c* may be derived. This states that the reciprocal of the total resistance, R_t,

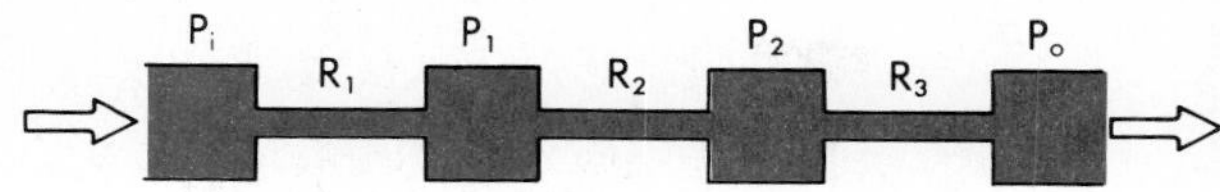

$$\text{(a)}\ P_i - P_o = (P_i - P_1) + (P_1 - P_2) + (P_2 - P_o)$$

$$\text{(b)}\ \frac{P_i - P_o}{Q} = \frac{(P_i - P_1)}{Q} + \frac{(P_1 - P_2)}{Q} + \frac{(P_2 - P_o)}{Q}$$

$$\text{(c)}\ R_t = R_1 + R_2 + R_3$$

Fig. 5-9 For resistances (R_1, R_2, and R_3) arranged in series, the total resistance R_t, equals the sum of the individual resistances.

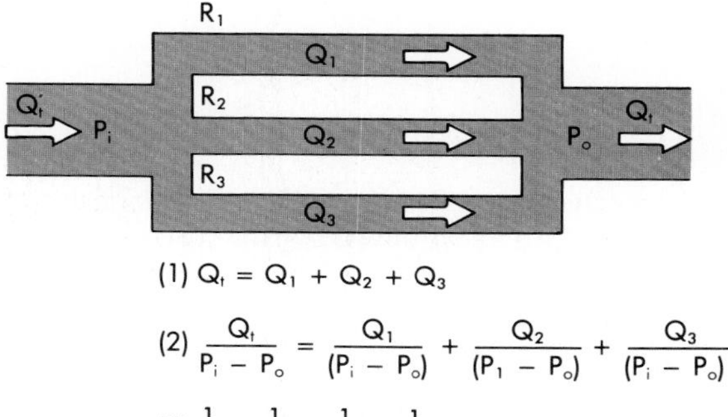

$$\text{(1)}\ Q_t = Q_1 + Q_2 + Q_3$$

$$\text{(2)}\ \frac{Q_t}{P_i - P_o} = \frac{Q_1}{(P_i - P_o)} + \frac{Q_2}{(P_1 - P_o)} + \frac{Q_3}{(P_i - P_o)}$$

$$\text{(3)}\ \frac{1}{R_t} = \frac{1}{R_1} + \frac{1}{R_2} + \frac{1}{R_3}$$

Fig. 5-10 ■ For resistances (R_1, R_2, and R_3) arranged in parallel, the reciprocal of the total resistance, R_t, equals the sum of the reciprocals of the individual resistances.

equals the sum of the reciprocals of the individual resistances, that is,

$$\frac{1}{R_t} = \frac{1}{R_1} + \frac{1}{R_2} + \frac{1}{R_3} \qquad (13)$$

Stated in another way, if we define hydraulic **conductance** as the reciprocal of resistance, it becomes evident that, for tubes in parallel, the total conductance is the sum of the individual conductances.

By considering a few simple illustrations, some of the fundamental properties of parallel hydraulic systems become apparent. For example, if the resistance of the three parallel elements in Fig. 5-10 were all equal, then

$$R_1 = R_2 = R_3$$

Therefore,

$$1/R_t = 3/R_1$$

and

$$R_t = R_1/3$$

Thus the total resistance is less than any of the individual resistances. After further consideration, it becomes evident that for any parallel arrangement, the total resistance must be less than that of *any* individual component. For example, consider a system in which a very high-resistance tube is added in parallel to a low-resistance tube. The total resistance must be less than that of the low-resistance component by itself, because the high-resistance component affords an additional pathway, or conductance, for fluid flow.

As a physiological illustration of these principles, consider the relationship between the **total peripheral resistance** (TPR) of the entire systemic vascular bed and the resistance of one of its components, such as the renal vasculature. In an individual with a cardiac output of 5000 ml/min and an arterial pressure of 100 mm Hg, the TPR will be 0.02 mm Hg/ml/min, or 0.02 PRU (peripheral resistance units). Blood flow through one kidney would be approximately 600 ml/min. Renal resistance would therefore be 100 mm Hg/600 ml/min, or 0.17 PRU, which is 8.5 times as great as the TPR.

From Fig. 1-2 it seems paradoxical that the resistance to flow through the arterioles (as manifested by the pressure drop between the arterial and capillary ends of these vessels) is considerably greater than that through certain other vascular components, despite the fact

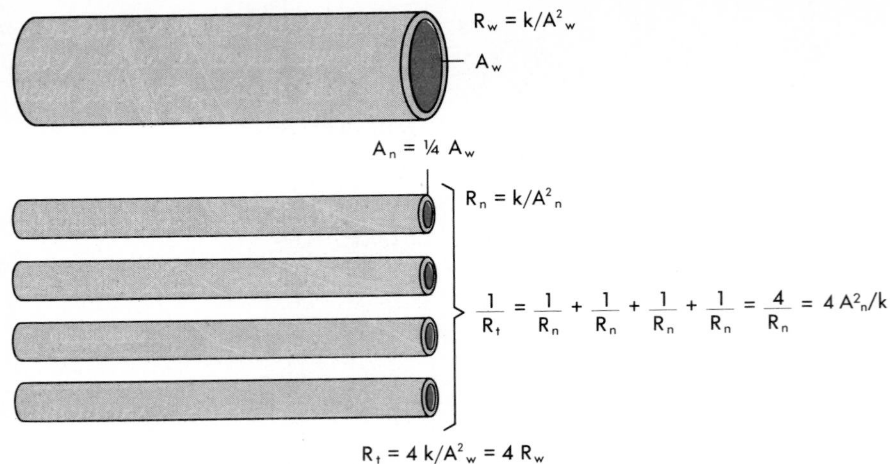

Fig. 5-11 ■ When four narrow tubes, each of area A_n, are connected in parallel, the total cross-sectional area equals the area A_w, of a wide tube of area such that $A_w = 4A_n$. Although the total areas are equal, the total resistance, R_t, to flow through the parallel narrow tubes is four times as great as the resistance, R_w, through the single wide tube.

that the total cross-sectional area of the arteri-oies exceeds that for these same vascular components. For example, the total cross-sectional area of the arterioles greatly exceeds that of the large arteries, yet the resistance to flow through the arterioles exceeds that through the large arteries.

Consideration of simple models of tubes in parallel will help resolve this apparent paradox. In Fig. 5-11 the resistance to flow through one wide tube of cross-sectional area A_w is compared with that through four narrower tubes in parallel, each of area A_n. The total cross-sectional area of the parallel system of four narrow tubes equals the area of the wide tube; that is,

$$A_w = 4A_n \quad (14)$$

Because resistance, R, is inversely proportional to the fourth power of the radius, r, and since

$$A = \pi r^2 \quad (15)$$

for cylindrical tubes, it follows that

$$R = k/A^2 \quad (16)$$

The proportionality constant, k, is related to tube length and fluid viscosity, both of which will be held constant in the example under consideration. From equation 16, the resistances of the wide tube, R_w, and a single narrow tube, R_n, are

$$R_w = k/A_w^2 \quad (17)$$

$$R_n = k/A_n^2 \quad (18)$$

From equation 13,

$$\frac{1}{R_t} = \frac{1}{R_n} + \frac{1}{R_n} + \frac{1}{R_n} + \frac{1}{R_n} = \frac{4}{R_n} \quad (19)$$

Substituting the value of R_n in equation 18,

$$1/R_t = 4A_n^2/k \quad (20)$$

Rearranging,

$$R_t = k/4A_n^2 \quad (21)$$

From equations 14 and 17,

$$R_t = 4k/A_w^2 = 4R_w \quad (22)$$

Hence the resistance of four such tubes in parallel is four times as great as that of a single tube of equal total cross-sectional area.

If a similar calculation is made for eight such tubes in parallel, with each tube having one fourth the cross-sectional area of the single wide tube, it will be found that the total resistance will equal $2R_w$. In this circumstance the resistance to flow through eight such narrow tubes in parallel will still be twice as great as that through the single tube, despite the fact that the total cross-sectional area for the eight narrow tubes is twice as great as for the single wide tube. This is analogous to the relationship that exists between resistance and area in the circulatory system when comparing the arterioles with the large arteries. Despite the fact that the total cross-sectional area of all the arterioles greatly exceeds that of all the large arteries, the resistance to flow through the arterioles is considerably greater than that through the large arteries.

If the example is carried still further, it will be found that sixteen such narrow tubes in parallel, now with four times the total cross-sectional area of the single wide tube, will exert a resistance to flow just equal to the resistance through the wide tube. Any number of these narrow tubes in excess of sixteen, then, will have a lower resistance than that of the single wide tube. This is analogous to the situation for the arterioles and capillaries. The resistance to flow through a single capillary is much greater than that through a single arteriole (see Fig. 5-8). Yet the number of capillaries so greatly exceeds the number of arterioles, as reflected by the relative difference in total cross-sectional areas, that the pressure drop across the arterioles is considerably greater than the pressure drop across the capillaries (see Fig. 1-2).

■ LAMINAR AND TURBULENT FLOW

Under certain conditions, the flow of a fluid in a cylindrical tube will be **laminar** (sometimes called **streamlined**), as illustrated in Fig. 5-12. At the entrance of the tube all the fluid elements will have the same linear velocities, regardless of their radial positions. In progressing along the tube, however, the thin layer of fluid in contact with the wall of the tube adheres to the wall and hence is motionless. The layer of fluid just central to this external lamina must shear against this motionless layer and therefore moves slowly, but with a finite velocity. Similarly, the adjacent, more central layer travels still more rapidly. Close to the tube inlet the fluid layers near the axis of the tube still move with the same velocity, and do not shear against one another. However, at a distance from the tube inlet equal to several tube diameters, laminar flow becomes **fully developed**; that is, the velocity profiles do not change with longitudinal distance along the tube. In fully developed laminar flow the longitudinal velocity profile is that of a paraboloid (Fig. 5-13). The velocity of the fluid adjacent to the wall is zero, whereas the velocity at the center of the stream is maximum and equal to twice the mean velocity of flow across the entire cross section of the tube. In laminar flow, fluid elements remain in one lamina, or streamline, as the fluid progresses longitudinally along the tube.

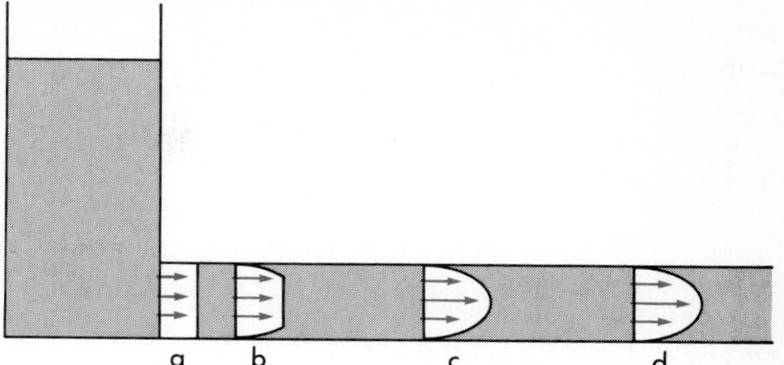

Fig. 5-12 ■ Laminar flow in a cylindrical tube. At the inlet, *a*, the velocities are equal at all radial distances from the center of the tube. Near the inlet, *b*, the velocity profile is flat near the center of the tube, but a velocity gradient is established near the wall. When flow becomes fully developed, *c* and *d*, the velocity profile is parabolic.

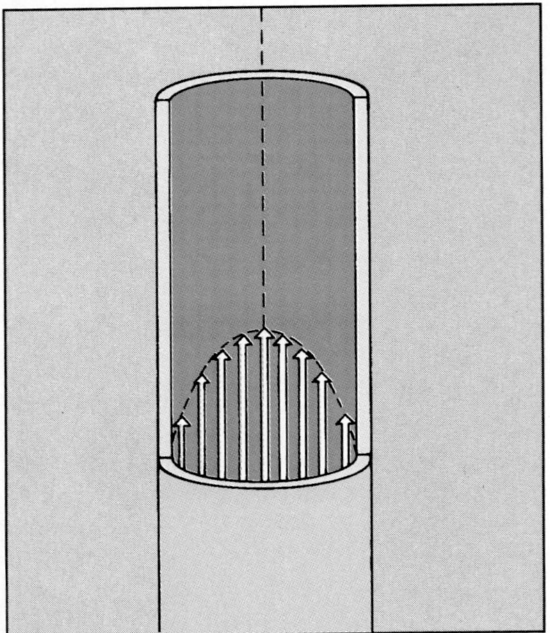

Fig. 5-13 ■ In laminar flow all elements of the fluid move in streamlines that are parallel to the axis of the tube; movement does not occur in a radial or circumferential direction. The layer of fluid in contact with the wall is motionless; the fluid that moves along the axis of the tube has the maximal velocity.

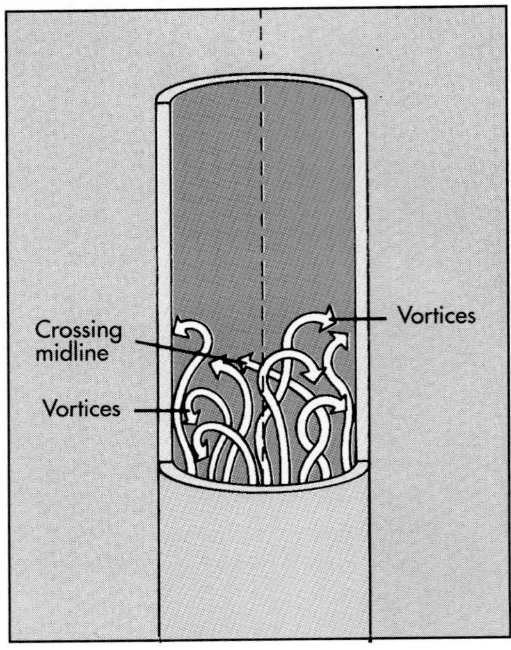

Fig. 5-14 ■ In turbulent flow the elements of the fluid move irregularly in axial, radial, and circumferential directions. Vortices frequently develop.

Irregular motions of the fluid elements may develop in the flow of fluid through a tube; this flow is called **turbulent.** Under such conditions fluid elements do not remain confined to definite laminae but rapid, radial mixing occurs (Fig. 5-14). A considerably greater pressure is required to force a given flow of fluid through the same tube when the flow is turbulent than when it is laminar. In turbulent flow the pressure drop is approximately proportional to the square of the flow rate, whereas in laminar flow, the pressure drop is proportional to the first power of the flow rate. Hence, to produce a given flow, a pump such as the heart must do considerably more work if turbulence develops.

Whether turbulent or laminar flow will exist in a tube under given conditions may be predicted on the basis of a dimensionless number called **Reynold's number**, N_R. This number represents the ratio of inertial to viscous forces. For a fluid flowing through a cylindrical tube,

$$N_R = \rho D \bar{v}/\eta \qquad (23)$$

where D is the tube diameter, $\bar{v}$ is the mean velocity, ρ is the density, and η is the viscosity. For $N_R < 2000$, the flow will usually be laminar; for $N_R > 3000$, the flow will be turbulent. Various possible conditions may develop in the transition range of N_R between 2000 and 3000. Because flow tends to be laminar at low N_R and turbulent at high N_R, the definition of N_R indicates that large diameters, high velocities, and low viscosities predispose to turbulence. In addition to these factors, abrupt variations in tube dimensions or irregularities in the tube walls may produce turbulence.

Turbulence is usually accompanied by audible vibrations. When turbulent flow exists within the cardiovascular system, it is usually detected as a **murmur**. The factors listed above that predispose to turbulence may account for murmurs heard clinically. In severe anemia **functional cardiac murmurs** (murmurs not caused by structural abnormalities) are frequently detectable. The physical basis for such murmurs resides in (1) the reduced viscosity of blood in anemia, and (2) the high flow velocities associated with the high cardiac output that usually prevails in anemic patients.

Blood clots, or **thrombi,** are much more likely to develop in turbulent than in laminar flow. One of the problems with the use of artificial valves in the surgical treatment of valvular heart disease is that thrombi may occur in association with the prosthetic valve. The thrombi may be dislodged and occlude a crucial blood vessel. It is thus important to design such valves to avert turbulence.

■ SHEAR STRESS ON THE VESSEL WALL

In Fig. 5-7, an external force was applied to a plate floating on the surface of a liquid in a large basin. This force, exerted parallel to the surface, caused a shearing stress on the liquid below, thereby producing a differential motion of each layer of liquid relative to the adjacent layers. At the bottom of the basin, the flowing liquid exerted a shearing stress on the surface of the basin in contact with the liquid. By rearranging the equation for viscosity stated in Fig. 5-7, it is apparent that the shear stress, τ, equals η (du/dy); that is, the shear stress equals the product of the viscosity and the shear rate. Hence, the greater the rate of flow, the greater the shear stress that the liquid exerts on the walls of the container in which it flows.

For precisely the same reasons, the rapidly flowing blood in a large artery tends to pull the endothelial lining of the artery along with it. This force (**viscous drag**) is proportional to the shear rate (du/dy) of the layers of blood near the wall. For a flow regimen that obeys Poiseuille's law,

$$\tau = 4\eta Q/\pi r^3 \tag{24}$$

The greater the rate of blood flow (Q) in the artery, the greater will be du/dy near the arterial wall, and the greater will be the viscous drag (τ).

In certain types of arterial disease, particularly in patients with hypertension, the subendothelial layers tend to degenerate locally, and small regions of the endothelium may lose their normal support. The viscous drag on the arterial wall may cause a tear between a normally supported and an unsupported region of the endothelial lining. Blood m y then flow from the vessel lumen, through the rift in the lining and dissect between the various layers of the artery. Such a lesion is called a **dissecting aneurysm**. It occurs most commonly in the proximal portions of the aorta and is extremely serious. One reason for its predilection for this site is the high velocity of blood flow, with the associated large values of du/dy at the endothelial wall. The shear stress at the vessel wall also influences many other vascular functions, such as the permeability of the vascular walls to large molecules, the biosynthetic activity of the endothelial cells, the integrity of the formed elements in the blood, and the coagulation of the blood.

■ RHEOLOGICAL PROPERTIES OF BLOOD

The viscosity of a newtonian fluid, such as water, may be determined by measuring the rate of flow of the fluid at a given pressure gradient through a cylindrical tube of known length and radius. As long as the fluid flow is laminar, the viscosity may be computed by substituting these values into Poiseuille's equation. The viscosity of a given newtonian fluid at a specified temperature will be constant over a wide range of tube dimensions and flows. However, for a nonnewtonian fluid, the viscosity calculated by substituting into Poiseuille's equation may vary considerably as a function of tube dimensions and flows. Therefore, in considering the rheological properties of a suspension such as blood, the term **viscosity** does not have a unique meaning. The terms **anomalous viscosity** and **apparent viscosity** are frequently applied to the value of viscosity obtained for blood under the particular conditions of measurement.

Rheologically, blood is a suspension of formed elements, principally erythrocytes, in a relatively homogeneous liquid, the blood plasma. For this reason the apparent viscosity of blood varies as a function of the **hematocrit ratio** (ratio of volume of red blood cells to volume of whole blood). In Fig. 5-15 the upper curve represents the ratio of the apparent viscosity of whole blood to that of plasma over a range of hematocrit ratios from 0% to 80%, measured in a tube 1 mm in diameter. The viscosity of plasma is 1.2 to 1.3 times that of water. Fig. 5-15 (upper curve) shows that blood, with a normal hematocrit ratio of 45%, has an apparent viscosity 2.4 times that of plasma. In severe anemia, blood viscosity is low. With increasing hematocrit ratios the slope of the curve increases progressively; it is especially steep at the upper range of erythrocyte concentrations. A rise in hematocrit ratio from 45% to 70%, which occurs in **polycythemia**, increases the apparent viscosity more than twofold, with a proportionate effect on the resistance to blood flow. The effect of such a change in hematocrit ratio on peripheral resistance may be appreciated when it is recognized that even in the most severe cases of essential hypertension, the total peripheral resistance rarely increases by more than a factor of two. In hypertension, the increase in peripheral resistance is achieved by arteriolar vasoconstriction.

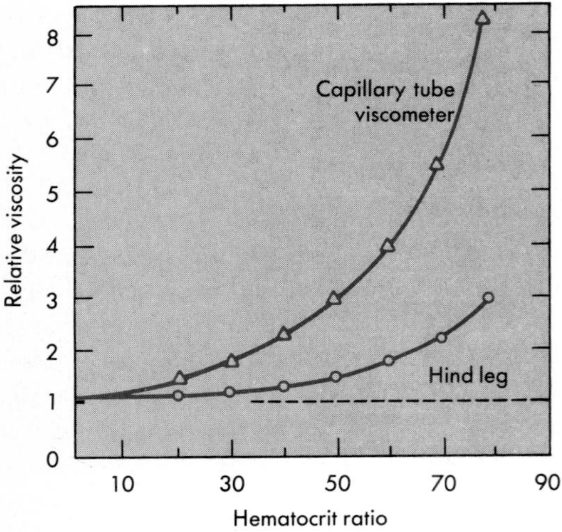

Fig. 5-15 ■ Viscosity of whole blood, relative to that of plasma, increases at a progressively greater rate as the hematocrit ratio increases. For any given hematocrit ratio the apparent viscosity of blood is less when measured in a biological viscometer (such as the hind leg of a dog) than in a conventional capillary tube viscometer. (Redrawn from Levy, M.N., and Share, L.: Circ. Res. 1:247, 1953.)

For any given hematocrit ratio the apparent viscosity of blood depends on the dimensions of the tube employed in estimating the viscosity. Fig. 5-16 demonstrates that the apparent viscosity of blood diminishes progressively as tube diameter decreases below a value of about 0.3 mm. The diameters of the highest resistance blood vessels, the arterioles, are considerably less than this critical value. This phenomenon therefore reduces the resistance to flow in the blood vessels that possess the greatest resistance.

The apparent viscosity of blood, when measured in living tissues, is considerably less than when measured in a conventional capillary tube viscometer with a diameter greater than 0.3 mm. In the lower curve of Fig. 5-15, the apparent relative viscosity of blood was assessed by using the hind leg of an anesthetized dog as a biological viscometer. Over the entire range of hematocrit ratios, the apparent viscosity was less as measured in the living tissue than in the capillary tube viscometer (upper curve), and the disparity was greater the higher the hematocrit ratio.

The influence of tube diameter on apparent viscosity is ascribable in part to the change in actual composition of the blood as it flows through small tubes. The composition changes because the red blood cells tend to accumulate in the faster axial stream, whereas the blood component that flows in the slower marginal layers is mainly plasma. To illustrate this phenomenon, a reservoir such as R_1 in Fig. 5-5, *C* has been filled with blood possessing a given hematocrit ratio. The blood in R_1 was constantly agitated to prevent settling and was permitted to flow through a narrow capillary

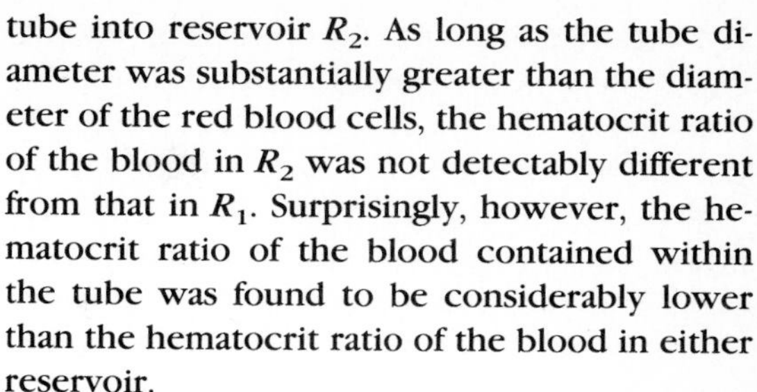

tube into reservoir R_2. As long as the tube diameter was substantially greater than the diameter of the red blood cells, the hematocrit ratio of the blood in R_2 was not detectably different from that in R_1. Surprisingly, however, the hematocrit ratio of the blood contained within the tube was found to be considerably lower than the hematocrit ratio of the blood in either reservoir.

In Fig. 5-17, the relative hematocrit is the ratio of the hematocrit in the tube to that in the reservoir at either end of the tube. For tubes of 500 μm diameter or greater, the relative hematocrit ratio was close to 1. However, as the tube diameter was diminished below 500 μm, the relative hematocrit ratio progressively diminished; for a tube diameter of 30 μm, the relative hematocrit ratio was only 0.6.

That this situation results from a disparity in the relative velocities of the red cells and plasma can be appreciated on the basis of the following analogy. Consider the flow of automobile traffic across a bridge that is 3 miles long. Let the cars move in one lane at a speed

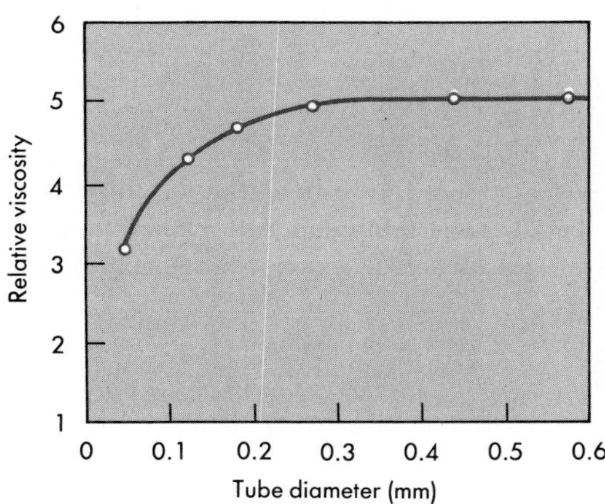

Fig. 5-16 ■ Viscosity of blood, relative to that of water, increases as a function of tube diameter up to a diameter of about 0.3 mm. (Redrawn from Fåhraeus, R., and Lindqvist, T.: Am. J. Physiol. 96:562, 1931.)

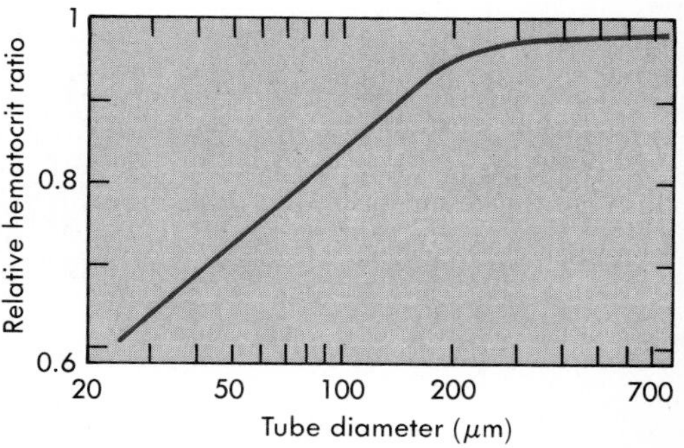

Fig. 5-17 ■ The "relative hematocrit ratio" of blood flowing from a feed reservoir through capillary tubes of various calibers, as a function of the tube diameter. The relative hematocrit is the ratio of the hematocrit of the blood in the tubes to that of the blood in the feed reservoir. (Redrawn from Barbee, J.H., and Cokelet, G.R.: Microvasc. Res. 3:6, 1971.)

of 60 miles per hour and the trucks in another lane at 20 miles per hour, as illustrated in Fig. 5-18. If one car and one truck start out across the bridge each minute, then except for the initial few minutes of traffic flow across the bridge one car and one truck will arrive at the other end each minute. Yet if one counts the actual number of cars and trucks on the bridge at any moment, there will be three times more of the slower moving trucks than of the more rapidly traveling cars.

Because the axial portions of the bloodstream contain a greater proportion of red cells and they move with a greater velocity, the red cells tend to traverse the tube in less time than does the plasma. Therefore, the red cells correspond to the rapidly moving cars in the analogy, and the plasma corresponds to

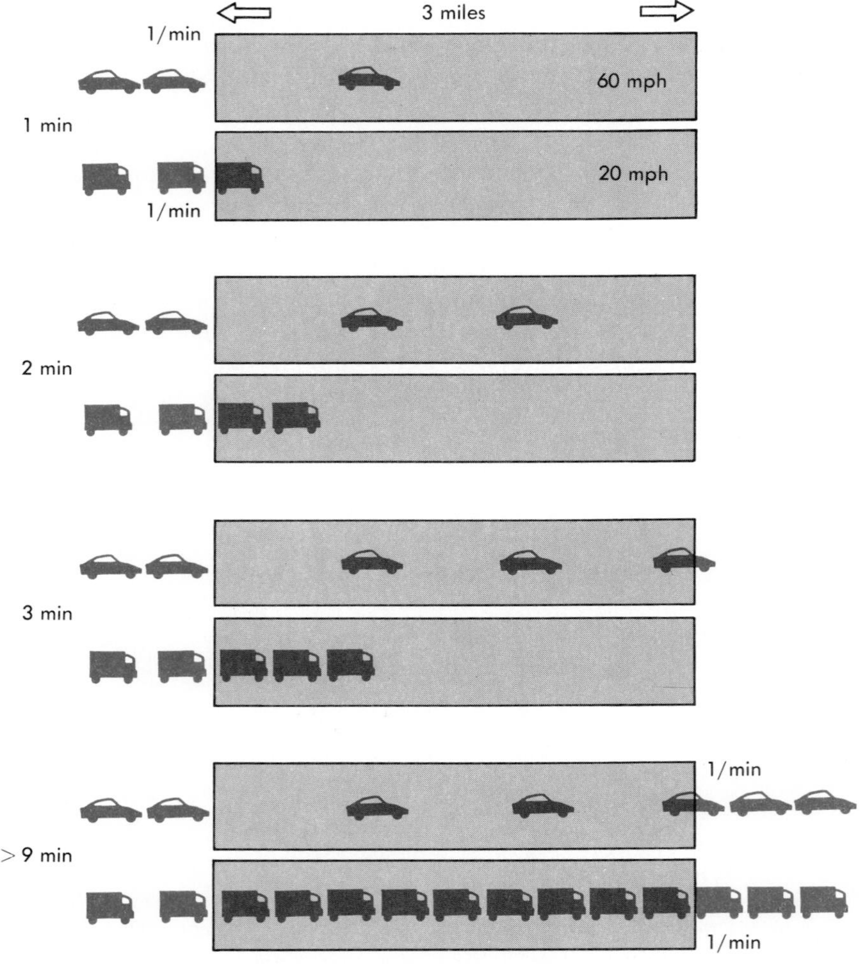

Fig. 5-18 ■ When the car velocity is three times as great as the truck velocity, the ratio of the number of cars to trucks on a bridge will be 1:3, even though one of each type of vehicle enters and leaves the bridge each minute.

the slowly moving trucks. Measurement of transit times through various organs have shown that red cells do travel faster than the plasma. Furthermore, the hematocrit ratios of the blood contained in various tissues are lower than those in blood samples withdrawn from large arteries or veins in the same animal (Fig. 5-19).

The physical forces responsible for the drift of the erythrocytes toward the axial stream and away from the vessel walls are not fully understood. One factor is the great flexibility of the red blood cells. At low flow (or shear) rates, comparable to those in the microcirculation, rigid particles do not migrate toward the axis of a tube, whereas flexible particles do migrate. The concentration of flexible particles near the tube axis is enhanced by increasing the shear rate.

The apparent viscosity of blood diminishes as the shear rate is increased (Fig. 5-20), a phenomenon called **shear thinning**. The greater tendency of the erythrocytes to accumulate in the axial laminae at higher flow rates is partly responsible for this nonnewtonian behavior. However, a more important factor is that at very slow rates of shear, the suspended cells tend to form aggregates, which would increase viscosity. As the flow is increased, this aggregation would decrease and so also would the apparent viscosity (see Fig. 5-20).

The tendency for the erythrocytes to aggregate at low flows depends on the concentration in the plasma of the larger protein molecules, especially fibrinogen. For this reason, the changes in blood viscosity with shear rate are much more pronounced when the concentration of fibrinogen is high. Also, at low flow

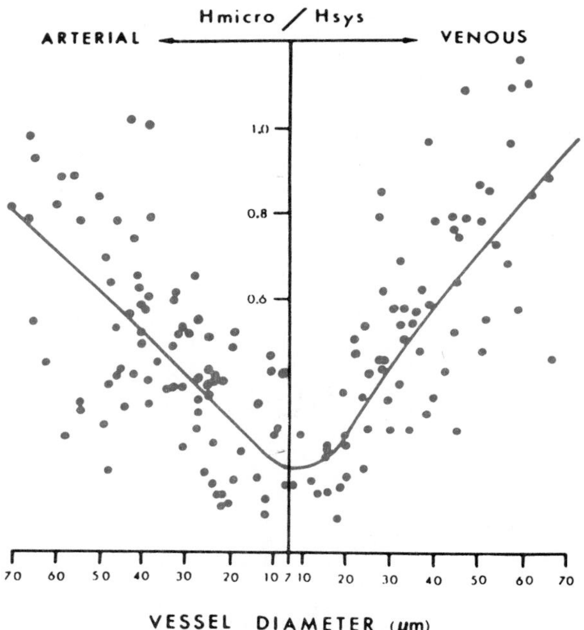

Fig. 5-19 ■ The hematocrit ratio (H_{micro}) of the blood in various sized arterial and venous microvessels in the cat mesentery, relative to the hematocrit ratio (H_{sys}) in the large systemic vessels. The hematocrit ratio is least in the capillaries and tiny venules. (Modified from Lipowsky, H.H. et al.: Microvasc. Res. 19:297, 1980.)

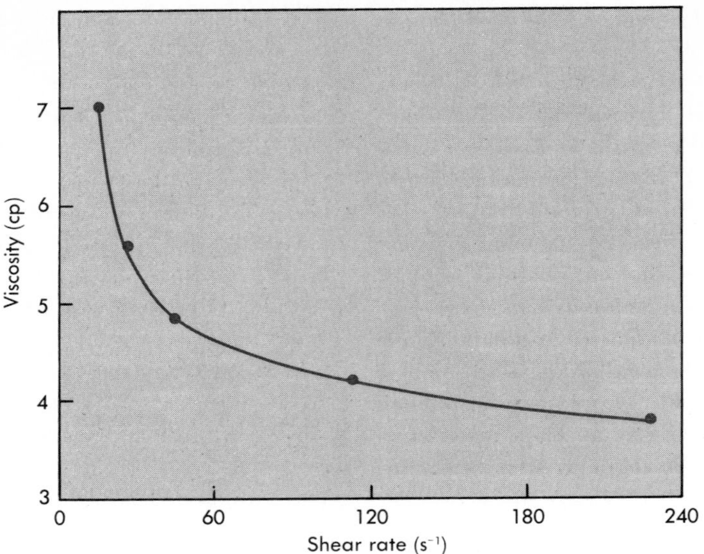

Fig. 5-20 ▪ Decrease in the viscosity of blood (centipoise) at increasing rates of shear. The shear rate refers to the velocity of one layer of fluid relative to that of the adjacent layers and is directionally related to the rate of flow. (Redrawn from Amin, T.M., and Sirs, J.A.: Q. J. Exp. Physiol. 70:37, 1985.)

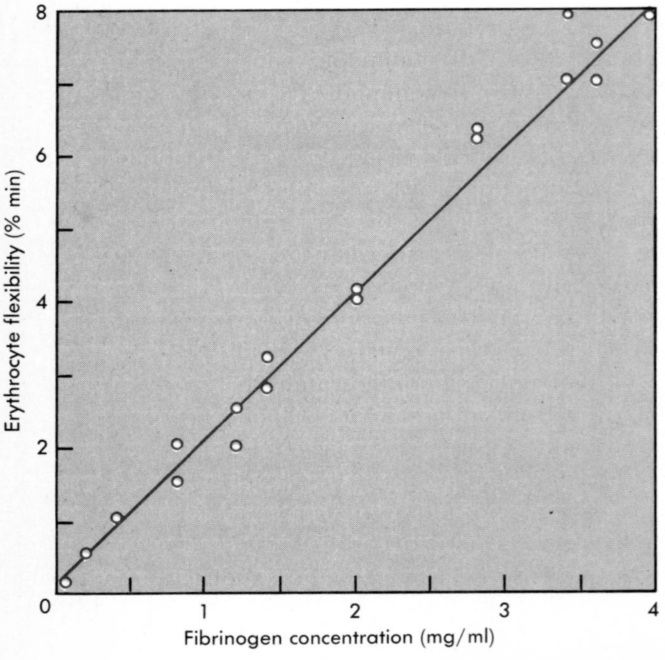

Fig. 5-21 ▪ The effect of the plasma fibrinogen concentration on the flexibility of human erythrocytes. (Redrawn from Amin, T.M., and Sirs, J.A.: Q. J. Exp. Physiol. 70:37, 1985.)

rates, the leukocytes tend to adhere to the endothelial cells of the microvessels, thereby increasing the apparent viscosity.

The deformability of the erythrocytes is also a factor in shear thinning, especially at high hematocrit ratios. The mean diameter of human red blood cells is about 8 μm, yet they are able to pass through openings with a diameter of only 3 μm. As blood that is densely packed with erythrocytes is caused to flow at progressively greater rates, the erythrocytes become more and more deformed, which diminishes the apparent viscosity of the blood. The flexibility of human erythrocytes is enhanced as the concentration of fibrinogen in the plasma increases (Fig. 5-21). If the red blood cells become hardened, as they are in certain spherocytic anemias, shear thinning may become much less prominent.

■ SUMMARY

1. The vascular system is composed of two major subdivisions in series with one another: the systemic circulation and the pulmonary circulation.
2. Each subdivision comprises a number of types of vessels (e.g., arteries, arterioles, capillaries) that are aligned in series with one another. In general, the vessels of a given type are arranged in parallel with each other.
3. The mean velocity (v) of blood flow in a given type of vessel is directly proportional to the total blood flow (Q_t) being pumped by the heart, and it is inversely proportional to the cross-sectional area (A) of all the parallel vessels of that type; i.e., $v = Q_t/A$.
4. The laterally directed pressure in the bloodstream decreases as the flow velocity increases; the decrement in lateral pressure is proportional to the square of the velocity. The changes are insignificant, however, except when flow is very large.
5. When blood flow is relatively steady and laminar in vessels larger than arterioles, the flow (Q) is proportional to the pressure drop down the vessel ($P_i - P_o$) and to the fourth power of the radius (r), and it is inversely proportional to the length (l) of the vessel and to the viscosity (η) of the fluid; i.e., $Q = \pi(P_i - P_o)r^4/8\eta l$ (Poiseuille's law).
6. For resistances aligned in series, the total resistance equals the sum of the individual resistances.
7. For resistances aligned in parallel, the reciprocal of the total resistance equals the sum of the reciprocals of the individual resistances.
8. Flow tends to become turbulent when flow velocity is high, when fluid viscosity is low, when tube diameter is large, or when the wall of the vessel is very irregular.
9. Blood flow is nonnewtonian in very small vessels; i.e., Poiseuille's law is not applicable. The apparent viscosity of the blood diminishes as shear rate (flow) increases and as the tube dimensions decrease.

■ BIBLIOGRAPHY

Journal articles

Amin, T.M., and Sirs, J.A.: The blood rheology of man and various animal species, Q. J. Exp. Physiol. 70:37, 1985.

Carroll, R.J., and Falsetti, H.L.: Retrograde coronary artery flow in aortic valve disease, Circulation 54:494, 1976.

Chien, S.: Role of blood cells in microcirculatory regulation, Microvasc. Res. 29:129, 1985.

Cokelet, G.R., and Goldsmith, H.L.: Decreased hydrodynamic resistance in the two-phase flow of blood through small vertical tubes at low flow rates, Circ. Research 68:1, 1991.

Goldsmith, H.L.: The microrheology of human blood, Microvasc. Res. 31:121, 1986.

Klanchar, M., Tarbell, J.M., and Wang, D.-M.: In vitro study of the influence of radial wall motion on wall shear stress in an elastic tube model of the aorta, Circ. Res. 66:1624, 1990.

Lipowsky, H.H., Usami, S., and Chien, S.: In vivo measurements of "apparent viscosity" and microvessel hematocrit in the mesentery of the cat, Microvasc. Res. 19:297, 1980.

McKay, C.B., and Meiselman, H.J.: Osmolality-mediated Fahraeus and Fahraeus-Lindqvist effects for human RBC suspensions, Am. J. Physiol. 254:H238, 1988.

Sarelius, I.H., and Duling, B.R.: Direct measurement of microvessel hematocrit, red cell flux, velocity, and transit time, Am. J. Physiol. 243:H1018, 1982.

Secomb, T.W.: Flow-dependent rheological properties of blood in capillaries, Microvasc. Res. 34:46, 1987.

Sutera, S.P., Tilton, R.G., Larson, K.B., Kilo, C.J., and Williamson, J.R.: Vascular flow resistance in rabbit hearts: "apparent viscosity" of RBC suspensions, Microvasc. Res. 36:305, 1988.

Tangelder, G.J., Slaaf, D.W., Arts, T., and Reneman, R.S.: Wall shear rate in arterioles in vivo: least estimates from platelet velocity profiles, Am. J. Physiol. 254:H1059, 1988.

Thompson, T.N., La Celle, P.L., and Cokelet, G.R.: Perturbation of red blood cell flow in small tubes by white blood cells, Pflugers Arch. 413:372, 1989.

Winter, D.C., and Nerem, R.M.: Turbulence in pulsatile flows, Ann. Biomed. Eng. 12:357, 1984.

Zamir, M.: The role of shear forces in arterial branching, J. Gen. Physiol. 67:213, 1976.

Books and monographs

Chien, S., Usami, S., and Skalak, R.: Blood flow in small tubes. In Renkin, E.M., and Michel, C.C., editors: Handbook of physiology; Section 2: The cardiovascular system—Microcirculation, vol. IV, Bethesda, Md., 1984, American Physiological Society.

Cokelet, G.R., Meiselman, H.J., and Brooks, D.E., editors: Erythrocyte mechanics and blood flow, New York, 1980, Alan R. Liss, Inc.

Fung, Y.C.: Biodynamics: circulation, New York, 1984, Springer-Verlag New York, Inc.

Lowe, G.D.O.: Clinical blood rheology, vol. I, Boca Raton, 1988, C.R.C. Press, Inc.

Milnor, W.R.: Hemodynamics, Baltimore, 1982, Williams & Wilkins.

Taylor, D.E.M., and Stevens, A.L., editors: Blood flow: theory and practice, New York, 1983, Academic Press, Inc.

6 The Arterial System

■ HYDRAULIC FILTER

The principal function of the systemic and pulmonary arterial systems is to distribute blood to the capillary beds throughout the body. The arterioles, the terminal components of this system, regulate the distribution of flow to the various capillary beds. Between the heart and the arterioles, the aorta and pulmonary artery and their major branches constitute a system of conduits of considerable volume and distensibility. An arterial system composed of elastic conduits and high-resistance terminals constitutes a **hydraulic filter** analogous to the resistance-capacitance filters of electrical circuits.

Hydraulic filtering converts the intermittent output of the heart to a steady flow through the capillaries. This important function of the large elastic arteries has been likened to the **Windkessels** of antique fire engines. The Windkessel contained a large volume of trapped air. The compressibility of the trapped air converted the intermittent inflow of water to a steady outflow at the nozzle of the fire hose.

The analogous function of the large elastic arteries is illustrated in Fig. 6-1. The heart is an intermittent pump. The entire stroke volume is discharged into the arterial system during systole, which usually occupies approximately one third of the duration of the cardiac cycle. In fact, as described on p. 72, most of the stroke volume is pumped during the rapid ejection phase, which constitutes about half of the systole. Part of the energy of cardiac contraction is dissipated as forward capillary flow during systole; the remainder is stored as potential energy, in that much of the stroke volume is retained by the distensible arteries (Fig. 6-1, *A, B*). During diastole the elastic recoil of the arterial walls converts this potential energy into capillary blood flow. If the arterial walls were rigid, then capillary flow would cease during diastole (Fig. 6-1, *C, D*).

Hydraulic filtering minimizes the work load of the heart. More work is required to pump a given flow intermittently than steadily; the more effective the filtering, the less the excess work. A simple example will illustrate this point.

Consider first the steady flow of a fluid at a rate of 100 ml/s through a hydraulic system with a resistance of 1 mm Hg/ml/s. This combination of flow and resistance would result in a constant pressure of 100 mm Hg, as shown in Fig. 6-2, *A*. Neglecting any inertial effect, hydraulic work, W, may be defined as

$$W = \int_{t_1}^{t_2} P\,dV \tag{1}$$

Compliant arteries

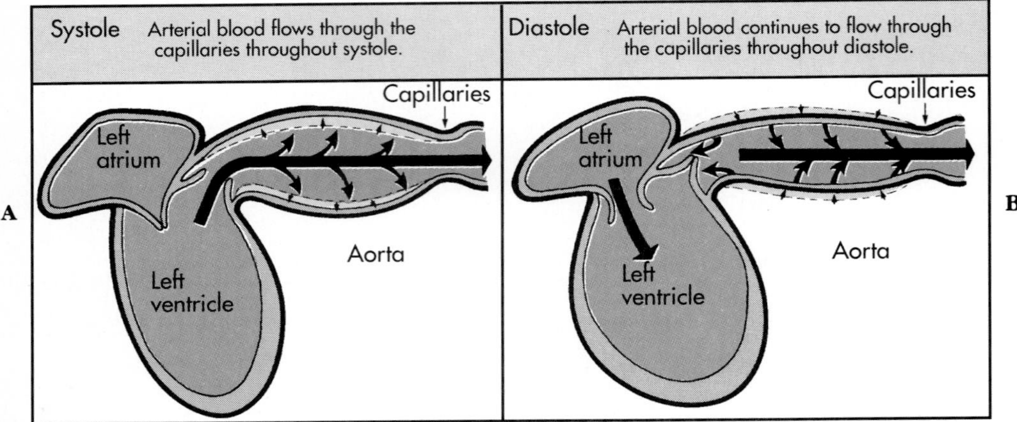

A, When the arteries are normally compliant, a substantial fraction of the stroke volume is stored in the arteries during ventricular systole. The arterial walls are stretched.

B, During ventricular diastole the previously stretched arteries recoil. The volume of blood that is displaced by the recoil furnishes continuous capillary flow throughout diastole.

Rigid arteries

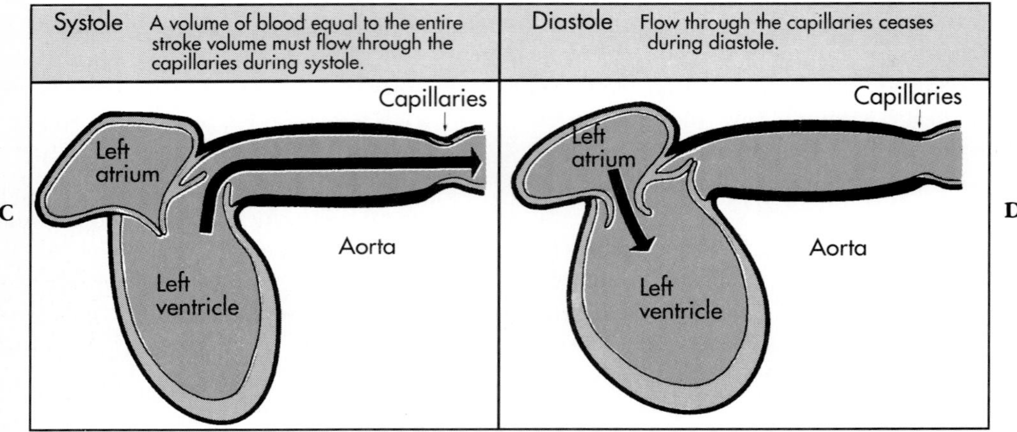

C, When the arteries are rigid, virtually none of the stroke volume can be stored in the arteries.

D, Rigid arteries cannot recoil appreciably during diastole.

Fig. 6-1 ■ When the arteries are normally compliant, blood flows through the capillaries throughout the cardiac cycle. When the arteries are rigid, blood flows through the capillaries during systole, but flow ceases during diastole.

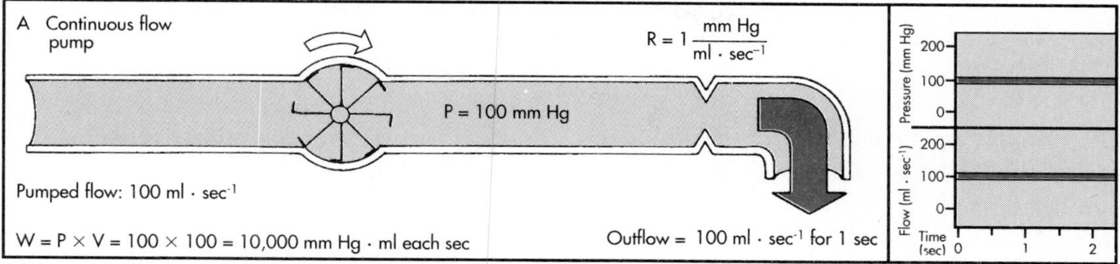

A, The flow is steady, and pressure will remain constant regardless of the distensibility of the conduit.

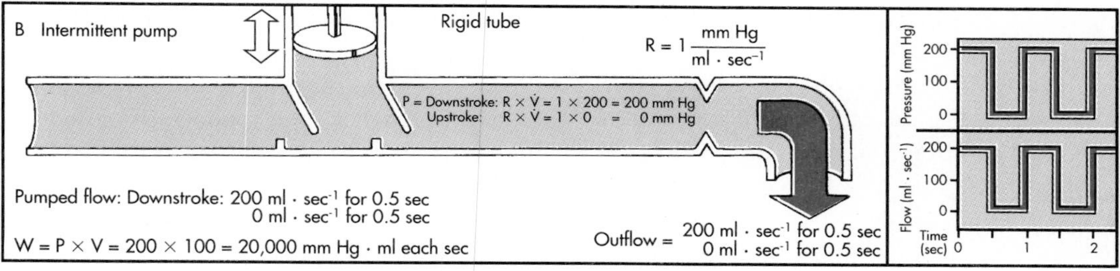

B, The flow produced by the pump is intermittent; it is steady for half the cycle and ceases for the remainder of the cycle. The conduit is rigid, and therefore the flow produced by the pump during its downstroke must exit through the resistance during the same 0.5 second that elapses during the downstroke. The pump must do twice as much work as the pump in **A.**

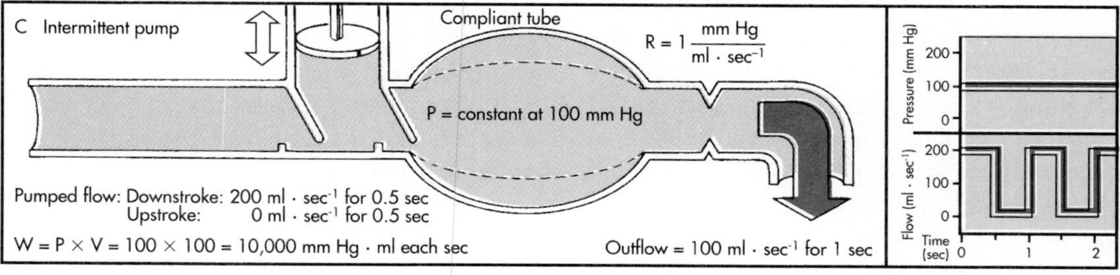

C, The pump operates as in **B,** but the conduit is infinitely distensible. This results in perfect filtering of the pressure; that is, the pressure is steady, and the flow through the resistance is also steady. The work equals that in **A.**

Fig. 6-2 ■ The relationships between pressure and flow for three hydraulic systems. In each the overall flow is 100 ml · sec^{-1} and the resistance is 1 mm Hg · ml^{-1} · sec.

that is, each small increment of volume, dV, pumped is multiplied by the pressure, P, existing at the time, and the products are integrated over the time interval of interest, $t_2 - t_1$, to give the total work, W. For steady flow,

$$W = PV \quad (2)$$

In the example in Fig. 6-2, *A,* the work done in pumping the fluid for 1 s would be 10,000 mm Hg-ml (or 1.33×10^7 dyne-cm).

Next, consider an intermittent pump that puts out the same volume per second, but pumps the entire volume at a steady rate over 0.5 s and then pumps nothing during the next 0.5 s. Hence, it pumps at the rate of 200 ml/s for 0.5, as shown in Fig. 6-2, *B* and *C.* In *B* the conduit is rigid and the fluid is incompressible, but the system has the same resistance as in *A.* During the pumping phase of the cycle (systole) the flow of 200 ml/s through a resistance of 1 mm Hg/ml/s would produce a pressure of 200 mm Hg. During the filling phase of the pump (diastole) the pressure would be 0 mm Hg in this rigid system. The work done during systole would be 20,000 mm Hg-ml, which is twice that required in the example shown in Fig. 6-2, *A.*

If the system were very distensible, hydraulic filtering would be very effective, and the pressure would remain virtually constant throughout the entire cycle (Fig. 6-2, *C*). Of the 100 ml of fluid pumped during the 0.5 s of systole, only 50 ml would be emitted through the high-resistance outflow end of the system during systole. The remaining 50 ml would be stored by the distensible conduit during systole and would flow out during diastole. Hence the pressure would be virtually constant at 100 mm Hg throughout the cycle. The fluid pumped during systole would be ejected at only half the pressure that prevailed in Fig. 6-2, *B,* and, therefore, the work would be only half as great. With nearly perfect filtering, as in Fig. 6-2, *C,* the work would be identical to that for steady flow (Fig. 6-2, *A*).

Naturally, the filtering accomplished by the systemic and pulmonic arterial systems is intermediate between the examples in Fig. 6-2, *B* and *C.* Ordinarily, the additional work imposed by intermittency of pumping, in excess of that for steady flow, is about 35% for the right ventricle and about 10% for the left ventricle. These fractions change, however, with variations in heart rate, peripheral resistance, and arterial distensibility.

■ ARTERIAL ELASTICITY

The elastic properties of the arterial wall may be appreciated by considering first the **static pressure—volume relationship** for the aorta. To obtain the curves shown in Fig. 6-3, aortas were obtained at autopsy from individuals in different age groups. All branches of the aorta were ligated and successive volumes of liquid were injected into this closed elastic system just as successive increments of water might be introduced into a balloon. After each increment of volume, the internal pressure was measured. In Fig. 6-3 the curve relating pressure to volume for the youngest age group (curve *a*) is sigmoidal. Although the curve is nearly linear over most of its extent, the slope decreases at the upper and lower ends. At any point, the slope (dV/dP) represents the aortic **compliance.** Thus in young individuals the aortic compliance is least at very high and low pressures and greatest over the usual range of pressure variations. This sequence of compliance changes resembles the familiar compliance changes encountered in inflating a balloon. The greatest difficulty in introducing air into the balloon is experienced at the beginning of inflation and again at near-maximum volume, just before rupture of the balloon. At intermediate volumes, the balloon is relatively easy to inflate.

It is also apparent from Fig. 6-3 that the curves become displaced downward and the slopes diminish as a function of advancing age. Thus, for any pressure above about 80 mm Hg, the compliance decreases with age, a manifestation of increased rigidity caused by progressive changes in the collagen and elastin contents of the arterial walls.

The above effects of the subject's age on the elastic characteristics of the arterial system were derived from aortas removed at autopsy (Fig. 6-3). Such age related changes have been confirmed in living subjects by ultrasound imaging techniques. These studies have disclosed that the increase in the diameter of the aorta produced by each cardiac contraction is much less in elderly persons than in young persons (Fig. 6-4). The effects of aging on the **elastic modulus** of the aorta in healthy subjects are

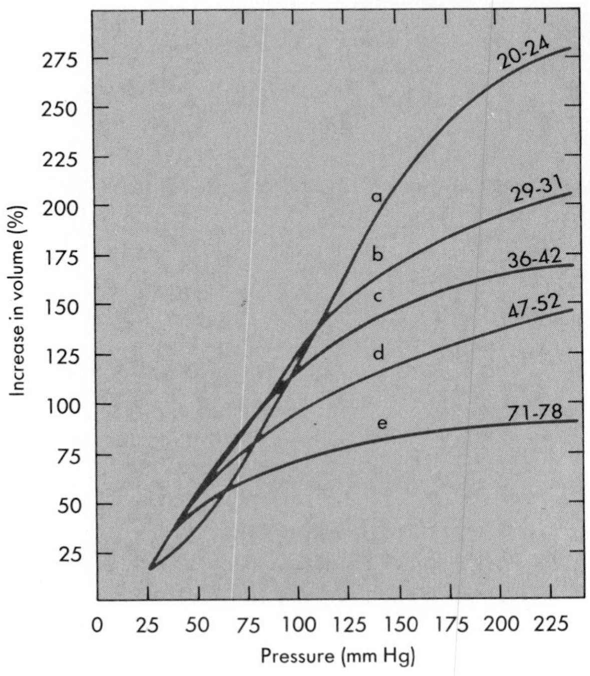

Fig. 6-3 ■ Pressure-volume relationships for aortas obtained at autopsy from humans in different age groups (denoted by the numbers at the right end of each of the curves). (Redrawn from Hallock, P., and Benson, I.C.: J. Clin. Invest. 16:595, 1937.)

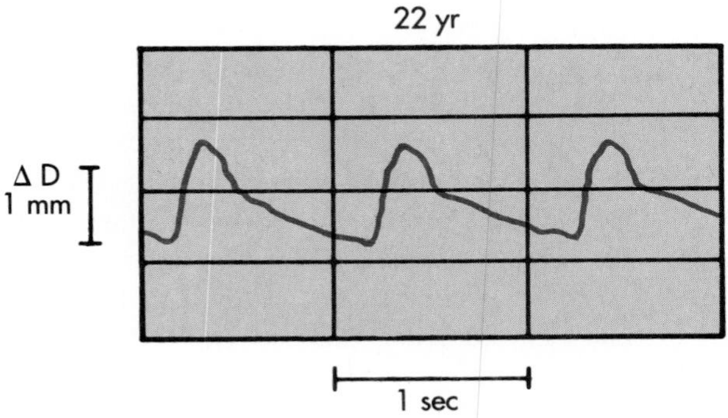

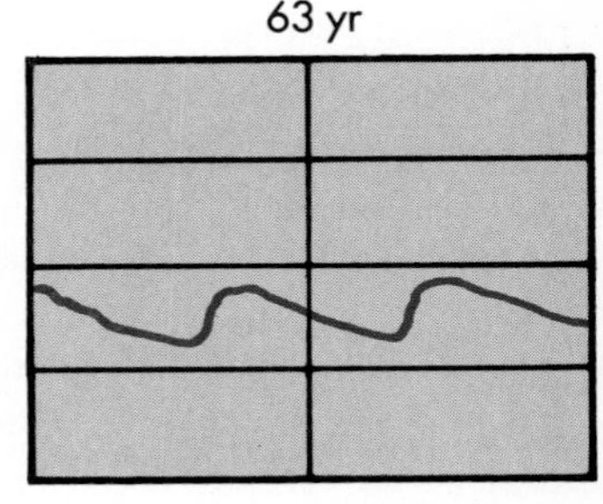

Fig. 6-4 ■ The pulsatile changes in diameter, measured ultrasonically, in a 22-year-old and in a 63-year-old man. (Modified from Imura, T., et al.: Cardiovasc. Res. 20:208, 1986.)

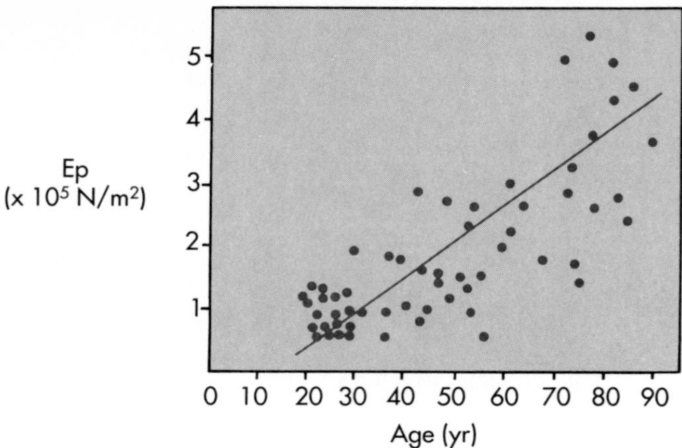

Fig. 6-5 ■ The effects of age on the elastic modulus (Ep) of the abdominal aorta in a group of 61 human subjects. (Modified from Imura, T., et al: Cardiovasc. Res. 20:208, 1986.)

shown in Figure 6-5. The elastic modulus, E_p, is defined as

$$E_p = \Delta P/(\Delta D/D) \quad (3)$$

where ΔP is the aortic pulse pressure (Fig. 6-6), D is the mean aortic diameter during the cardiac cycle, and ΔD is the maximum change in aortic diameter during the cardiac cycle.

The fractional change in diameter ($\Delta D/D$) of the aorta during the cardiac cycle reflects its change in volume as the left ventricle ejects its stroke volume into the aorta each systole. Thus, E_p is **inversely** related to compliance, which is the ratio of ΔV to ΔP. Consequently, the **increase** in elastic modulus with aging (see Fig. 6-5) and the **decrease** in compliance with aging (see Fig. 6-3) both reflect the stiffening of the arterial walls as individuals age.

The heart is unable to eject its stroke volume into a rigid arterial system as rapidly as into a more compliant system. As compliance diminishes, peak arterial pressure occurs progressively later in systole. Hence, the rapid ejection phase of systole is significantly prolonged as aortic compliance decreases.

■ DETERMINANTS OF THE ARTERIAL BLOOD PRESSURE

The determinants of the pressure within the arterial system cannot be evaluated precisely. Yet the arterial blood pressure is routinely measured in patients, and it provides a useful clue to their cardiovascular status. We will therefore take a simplified approach to explain the principal determinants of the arterial blood pressure. To accomplish this, the determinants of the **mean arterial pressure** (defined in the next section) will first be analyzed. The **systolic** and **diastolic arterial pressures** will then be considered as the upper and lower limits of periodic oscillations about this mean pressure. Finally, the changes in arterial pressure as the pulse wave progresses from the origin of the aorta toward the capillaries will be discussed.

The determinants of the arterial blood pressure will be arbitrarily subdivided into "physical" and "physiological" factors (Fig. 6-7). The arterial system will be assumed to be a static, elastic system, and the only two "physical" factors considered will be the **blood volume**

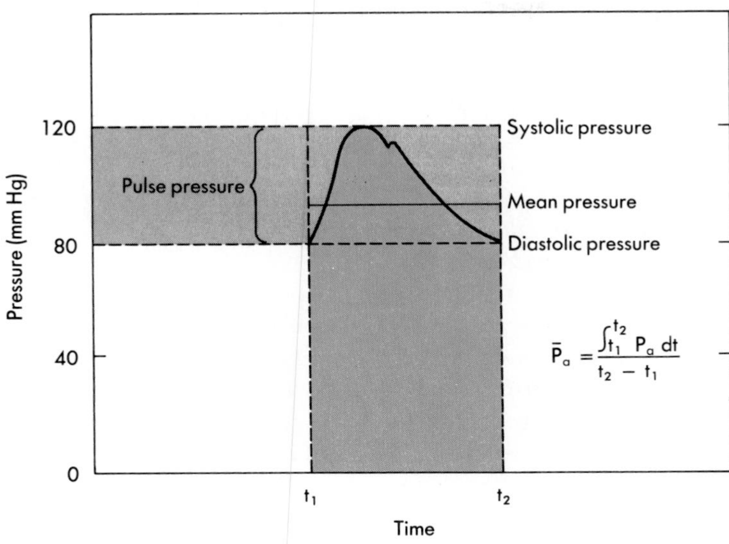

Fig. 6-6 ■ Arterial systolic, diastolic, pulse, and mean pressures. The mean arterial pressure $(\bar{P}_a)$ represents the area under the arterial pressure curve *(shaded area)* divided by the cardiac cycle duration $(t_2 - t_1)$.

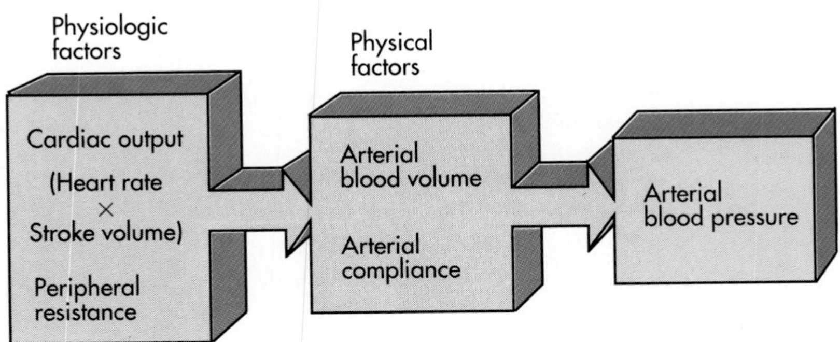

Fig. 6-7 ■ The arterial blood pressure is determined directly by two major physical factors, the arterial blood volume and the arterial compliance. These physical factors are affected in turn by certain physiologic factors, primarily the heart rate, stroke volume, cardiac output (heart rate × stroke volume), and peripheral resistance.

within the arterial system and the **elastic characteristics** (compliance) of the system. Certain "physiological" factors will be considered, namely, **cardiac output,** which equals **heart rate × stroke volume**) and **peripheral resistance.** Such physiological factors will be shown to operate through one or both of the physical factors, however.

Mean Arterial Pressure

The **mean arterial pressure** is the pressure in the arteries, averaged over time. It may be obtained from an arterial pressure tracing by measuring the area under the curve and dividing this area by the time interval involved, as shown in Fig. 6-6. The mean arterial pressure, P_a, usually can be approximated satisfactorily from the measured values of the systolic (P_s) and diastolic (P_d) pressures by means of the following formula:

$$\bar{P}_a \cong P_d + \frac{1}{3}(P_s - P_d) \tag{4}$$

The mean pressure will be considered to depend only on the mean blood volume in the arterial system and on the arterial compliance (see Fig. 6-7). The arterial volume, V_a, in turn, depends on the rate of inflow, Q_h, from the heart into the arteries **(cardiac output)** and the rate of outflow, Q_r, from the arteries through the resistance vessels **(peripheral runoff);** expressed mathematically,

$$dV_a/dt = Q_h - Q_r \tag{5}$$

If arterial inflow exceeds outflow, then arterial volume increases, the arterial walls are stretched more, and pressure rises. The converse happens when arterial outflow exceeds inflow. When inflow equals outflow, arterial pressure remains constant.

Cardiac Output. The change in pressure in response to an alteration of cardiac output can be better appreciated by considering some simple examples. Under control conditions, let cardiac output be 5 L/min and mean arterial pressure ($\bar{P}_a$) be 100 mm Hg (Fig. 6-8, *A*). From the definition of total peripheral resistance

$$R = (\bar{P}_a - \bar{P}_{ra})/Q_r \tag{6}$$

If $\bar{P}_{ra}$ (mean right atrial pressure) is negligible compared with $\bar{P}_a$,

$$R \cong \bar{P}_a/Q_r \tag{7}$$

Therefore, in the example, R is 100/5, or 20 mm Hg/L/min.

Now let cardiac output, Q_h, suddenly increase to 10 L/min (Fig. 6-8, *B*). Instantaneously, $\bar{P}_a$ will be unchanged. Because the outflow, Q_r, from the arteries depends on $\bar{P}_a$ and R, Q_r also will remain unchanged at first. Therefore, Q_h, now 10 L/min, will exceed Q_r, still only 5 L/min. This will increase the mean arterial blood volume ($\bar{V}_a$). From equation 5, when $Q_h > Q_r$, then $d\bar{V}_a/dt > 0$; that is, volume is increasing.

Because $\bar{P}_a$ depends on the mean arterial blood volume, V_a, and the arterial compliance, C_a, an increase in $\bar{V}_a$, will raise the $\bar{P}_a$. By definition

$$C_a = d\bar{V}_a/d\bar{P}_a \tag{8}$$

Therefore,

$$d\bar{V}_a = C_a d\bar{P}_a \tag{9}$$

and

$$\frac{d\bar{V}_a}{dt} = C_a\frac{d\bar{P}_a}{dt} \tag{10}$$

From equation 2,

$$\frac{d\bar{P}_a}{dt} = \frac{Q_h - Q_r}{C_a} \tag{11}$$

Hence P_a will rise when $Q_h > Q_r$, will fall when $Q_h < Q_r$ and will remain constant when $Q_h = Q_r$.

In this example, in which Q_h is suddenly increased to 10 L/min, $\bar{P}_a$ will continue to rise as long as Q_h exceeds Q_r. It is evident from equation 7 that Q_r will not attain a value of 10 L/min until $\bar{P}_a$ reaches a level of 200 mm Hg, as

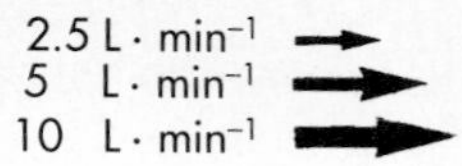

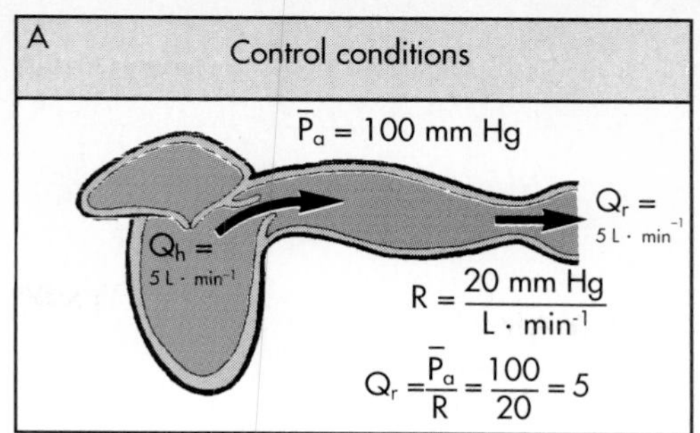

A, Under control conditions $\dot{Q}_h = 5\ L \cdot min^{-1}$, $\overline{P}_a = 100$ mm Hg, and R = 20 mm Hg · L^{-1} min. $\dot{Q}_r$ must equal $\dot{Q}_h$, and therefore the mean blood volume $(\overline{V}_a)$ in the arteries will remain constant from heartbeat to heartbeat.

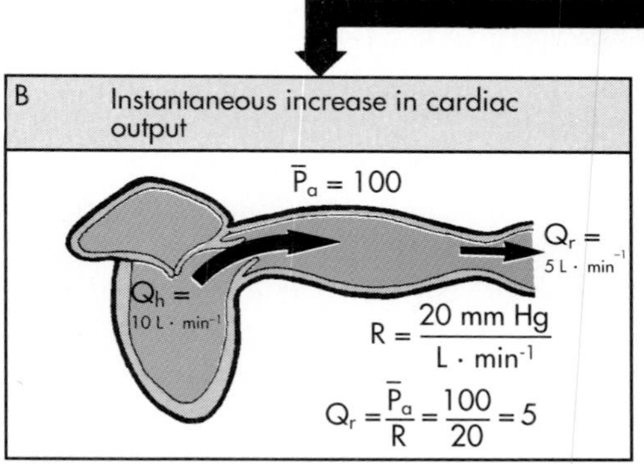

B, If Q_h suddenly increases to 10 L · min^{-1}, Q_h will initially exceed Q_r, and therefore $\overline{P}_a$ will begin to rise rapidly.

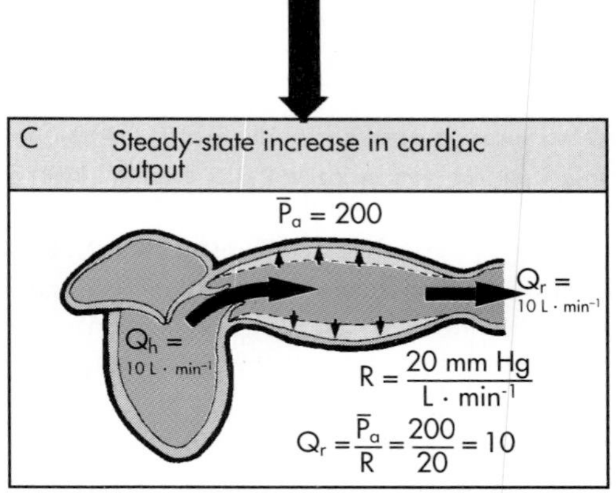

C, The disparity between Q_h and Q_r progressively increases arterial blood volume. The volume continues to increase until $\overline{P}_a$ reaches a level of 200 mm Hg.

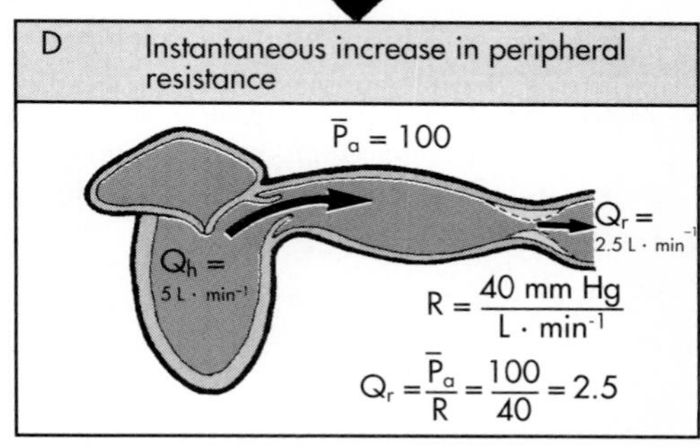

D, If R abruptly increases to 40 mm Hg · L^{-1} · min, Q_r suddenly decreases and therefore Q_h exceeds Q_r. Thus $\overline{P}_a$ will rise progressively.

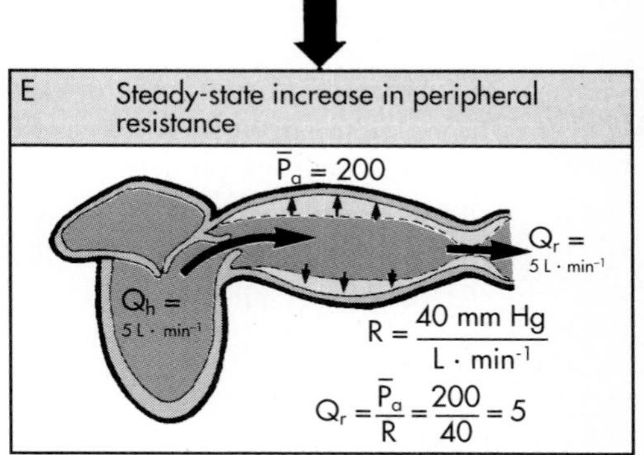

E, The excess of Q_h over Q_r accumulates blood in the arteries. Blood continues to accumulate until $\overline{P}_a$ rises to a level of 200 mm Hg.

Fig. 6-8 ■ The relationship of mean arterial blood pressure $(\overline{P}_a)$ to cardiac output $(\dot{Q}_h)$, peripheral runoff (Q_r), and peripheral resistance *(R)* under control conditions **(A)**, in response to an increase in cardiac output **(B and C)**, and in response to an increase in peripheral resistance **(D** and **E)**.

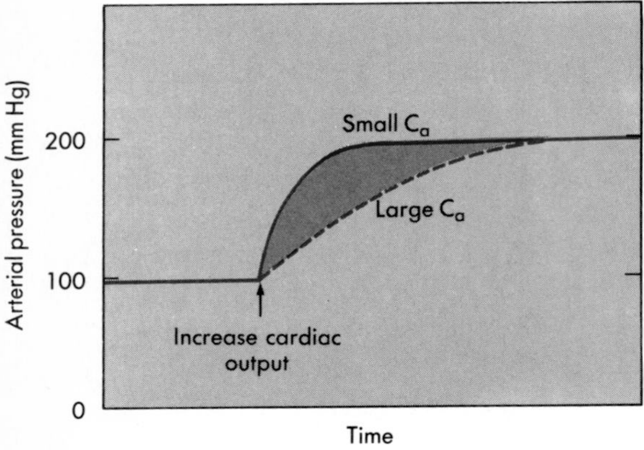

Fig. 6-9 ■ When cardiac output is suddenly increased, the arterial compliance *(C_a)* determines the **rate** at which the mean arterial pressure will attain its new, elevated value, but will not determine the **magnitude** of the new pressure.

long as R remains constant at 20 mm Hg/L/min. Hence, as $\overline{P}_a$ approaches 200, Q_r will almost equal Q_h and $\overline{P}_a$ will rise very slowly. When Q_h is first raised, however, Q_h is greatly in excess of Q_r, and therefore $\overline{P}_a$ will rise sharply. The pressure-time tracing in Fig. 6-9 indicates that, regardless of the value of C_a, the slope gradually diminishes as pressure rises, to approach a final value asymptotically.

Furthermore, the **height** to which $\overline{P}_a$ will rise is independent of the elastic characteristics of the arterial walls. $\overline{P}_a$ must rise to a level such that $Q_r = Q_h$. It is apparent from equation 6 that Q_r depends only on pressure gradient and resistance to flow. Hence C_a determines only the **rate** at which the new equilibrium value of $\overline{P}_a$ will be approached, as illustrated in Fig. 6-9. When C_a is small (rigid vessels), a relatively slight increment in $\overline{V}_a$ (caused by a transient excess of Q_h over Q_r) increases $\overline{P}_a$ greatly. Hence $\overline{P}_a$ attains its new equilibrium level quickly. Conversely, when C_a is large, then considerable volumes can be accommodated with relatively small pressure changes. Therefore the new equilibrium value of $\overline{P}_a$ is reached at a slower rate.

Peripheral Resistance. Similar reasoning may now be applied to explain the changes in $\overline{P}_a$ that accompany alterations in peripheral resistance. Let the control conditions be identical with those of the preceding example, that is, $Q_h = 5$, $\overline{P}_a = 100$, and $R = 20$ (see Fig. 6-8, *A*). Then let R suddenly be increased to 40 (Fig. 6-8, *D*). Instantaneously, $\overline{P}_a$ will be unchanged. With $\overline{P}_a = 100$ and $R = 40$, $Q_r = \overline{P}_a/R = 2.5$ L/min. If Q_h remains constant at 5 L/min, $Q_h \geq Q_r$, and $\overline{V}_a$ will increase; hence $\overline{P}_a$ will rise. $\overline{P}_a$ will continue to rise until it reaches 200 mm Hg (see Fig. 6-8, *E*). At this level, $Q_r = 200/40 = 5$ L/min, which equals Q_h. $\overline{P}_a$ will then remain at this new elevated equilibrium level as long as Q_h and R do not change again.

It is clear, therefore that *the level of the mean arterial pressure depends on cardiac output and peripheral resistance.* It is immaterial whether any change in cardiac output is accomplished by an alteration of heart rate, of stroke volume, or of both. Any change in heart rate that is balanced by a concomitant, oppositely directed change in stroke volume will not alter Q_h. Hence $\overline{P}_a$ will not be affected.

Pulse Pressure

If we assume that the arterial pressure, P_a, at any moment depends on the two physical factors (see Fig. 6-7) arterial blood volume, V_a, and arterial capacitance, C_a, it can be shown that the arterial **pulse pressure** (difference between systolic and diastolic pressures) is principally a function of **stroke volume** and **arterial compliance.**

Stroke Volume. The effect of a change in stroke volume on pulse pressure may be analyzed under conditions in which C_a remains virtually constant over a substantial range of pressures. C_a is constant over any linear region of the pressure-volume curve (Fig. 6-10). Volume is plotted along the vertical axis, and pressure is plotted along the horizontal axis; the slope, dV/dP, equals the compliance, C_a.

In an individual with such a linear $P_a:V_a$ curve, the arterial pressure would oscillate about some mean value ($\overline{P}_A$ in Fig. 6-10) that depends entirely on cardiac output and peripheral resistance, as explained previously. This mean pressure corresponds to some mean arterial blood volume, $\overline{V}_A$. The coordinates $\overline{P}_A$, $\overline{V}_A$ define point $\overline{A}$ on the graph. During diastole, peripheral runoff from the arterial system occurs in the absence of ventricular ejection of blood, and P_a and V_a diminish to minimum values, P_1 and V_1, just before the next ventricular ejection. P_1 is then, by definition, the *diastolic pressure.*

During the rapid ejection phase of systole, the volume of blood introduced into the arterial system exceeds the volume that exits through the arterioles. Arterial pressure and volume therefore rise from point A_1 toward point A_2 in Fig. 6-10. The maximum arterial volume, V_2, is reached at the end of the rapid ejection phase (Fig. 3-13), and this volume corresponds to a peak pressure, P_2, which is the *systolic pressure.*

The *pulse pressure* is the difference between systolic and diastolic pressures ($P_2 - P_1$ in Fig. 6-10), and it corresponds to some **arterial volume increment,** $V_2 - V_1$. *This increment equals the volume of blood discharged by the left ventricle during the rapid ejection phase minus the volume that has run off to the periphery during this same phase of the cardiac cycle.* When a normal heart beats at a normal frequency, the volume increment during the rapid ejection phase is a large fraction of the stroke volume (about 80%). It is this increment that will raise arterial volume rapidly from V_1 to V_2 and hence will cause the arterial pressure to rise from the diastolic to the systolic level (P_1 to P_2 in Fig. 6-10). During the remainder of the cardiac cycle, peripheral runoff will greatly exceed cardiac ejection. During diastole, of course, cardiac ejection equals zero. The resultant arterial blood volume decrement will cause volumes and pressures to fall from point A_2 back to point A_1.

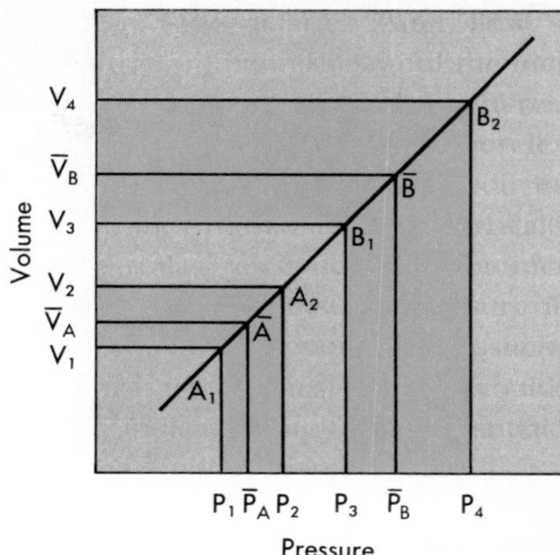

Fig. 6-10 ■ Effect of a change in stroke volume on pulse pressure in a system in which arterial compliance constant over the range of pressures and volumes involved. A larger volume increment ($V_4 - V_3$ as compared to $V_2 - V_1$) results in a greater mean pressure ($\overline{P}_B$ as compared to $\overline{P}_A$) and a greater pulse pressure ($P_4 - P_3$ as compared to $P_2 - P_1$).

If stroke volume is now doubled, while heart rate and peripheral resistance remain constant, the mean arterial pressure will be doubled, to $\overline{B}$ in Fig. 6-10. Thus the arterial pressure will now oscillate each heartbeat about this new value of the mean arterial pressure. A normal, vigorous heart will eject this greater stroke volume during a fraction of the cardiac cycle approximately equal to the fraction that prevailed at the lower stroke volume. Therefore, the arterial volume increment, $V_4 - V_3$, will be a large fraction of the new stroke volume, and hence it will be approximately twice as great as the previous volume increment ($V_2 - V_1$). With a linear P_a:V_a curve, the greater volume increment will be reflected by a **pulse pressure** ($P_4 - P_3$) that will be approximately **twice as great** as the original pulse pressure ($P_2 - P_1$). With a rise in both mean and pulse pressures, inspection of Fig. 6-10 reveals that the rise in systolic pressure (from P_2 to P_4) exceeds the rise in diastolic pressure (from P_1 to P_3). Thus, an increase in stroke volume raises systolic pressure more than it raises diastolic pressure.

Arterial Compliance. To assess how arterial compliance affects pulse pressure, the relative effects of a given volume increment ($V_2 - V_1$ in Fig. 6-11) in a young person (curve *A*) and in an elderly person (curve *B*) will be compared. Let cardiac output and total peripheral resistance be the same in both people; therefore, $\overline{P}_a$ will be the same. It is apparent from Fig. 6-11 that the same volume increment ($V_2 - V_1$) will cause a greater pulse pressure ($P_4 - P_1$) in the less distensible arteries of the elderly individual than in the more compliant arteries of the young one ($P_3 - P_2$). For the reasons enunciated on p. 138, this will impose a greater work load on the left ventricle of the elderly person than on that of the young person, even if the stroke volumes, total peripheral resistances (TPR), and mean arterial pressures are equivalent.

Fig. 6-12 displays the effects of changes in arterial compliance and in peripheral resistance, R_p, on the arterial pressure in an isolated cat heart preparation. As the compliance was reduced from 43 to 14 to 3.6 units, the pulse pressure increased significantly. In this preparation, the stroke volume decreased as the compliance was diminished. This accounts for the failure of the mean arterial pressure to remain constant at the different levels of arterial compliance. The effects of changes in peripheral resistance in this same preparation are described in the next section.

Total Peripheral Resistance and Arterial Diastolic Pressure. It is often stated that increased TPR affects mainly the level of

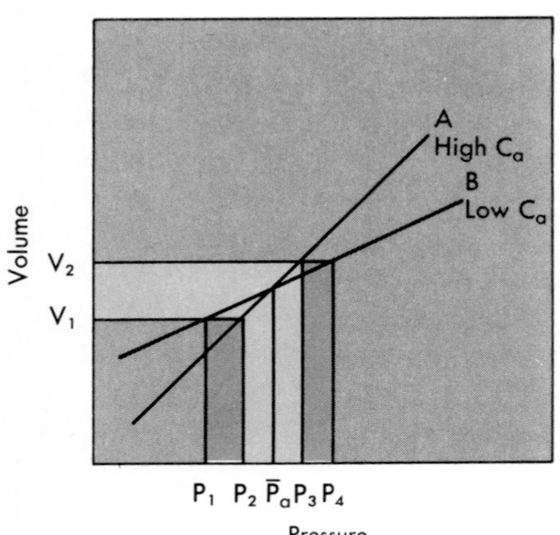

Fig. 6-11 ■ For a given volume increment *($V_2 - V_1$)* a reduced arterial compliance (curve *B* as compared to curve *A*) results in an increased pulse pressure *($P_4 - P_1$* as compared to *$P_3 - P_2$)*.

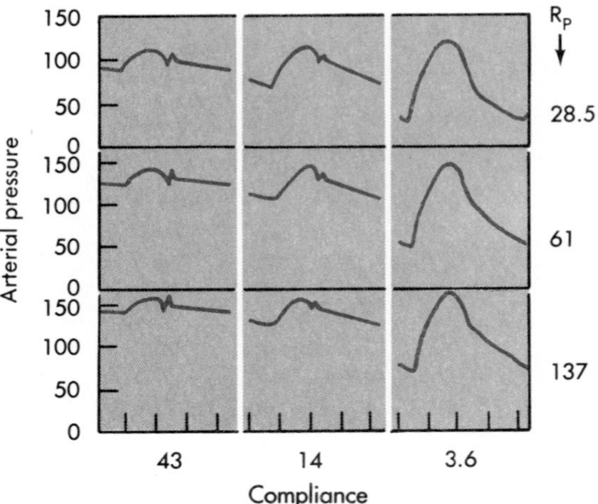

Fig. 6-12 ■ The changes in aortic pressure induced by changes in arterial compliance and peripheral resistance *(R_p)* in an isolated cat heart preparation. (Modified from Elizinga, G., and Westerhof, N.: Circ. Res. 32:178, 1973. By permission of the American Heart Association, Inc.)

the diastolic arterial pressure. The validity of such an assertion deserves close scrutiny. First, let TPR be increased in an individual with a linear P_a:V_a curve, as depicted in Fig. 6-13, *A*. If heart rate and stroke volume remain constant, then an increase in TPR will increase $\overline{P}_a$ proportionately (from P_2 to P_5). If the volume increments ($V_2 - V_1$ and $V_4 - V_3$) are equal at both levels of TPR, then the pulse pressures ($P_3 - P_1$ and $P_6 - P_4$) will also be equal. Hence systolic (P_6) and diastolic (P_4) pressures will have been elevated by exactly the same amounts from their respective control levels (P_3 and P_1).

Chronic *hypertension*, a condition characterized by a persistent elevation of TPR, occurs more commonly in older persons than in younger persons. The P_a:V_a curve for a hypertensive patient would therefore resemble that shown in Fig. 6-13, *B*, which is like the curves in Fig. 6-3 for older individuals.

The curve in Fig. 6-13, *B*, reveals that C_a is less at higher than at lower pressures. As before, if cardiac output remains contant, an increase in TPR would increase $\overline{P}_a$ proportionately (from P_2 to P_5). For equivalent increases in TPR, the elevation of pressure from P_2 to P_5 will be the same in panel A as in panel B, for reasons discussed on p. 144. If the volume increment ($V_4 - V_3$ in Fig. 6-13, *B*) at elevated TPR were equal to the control increment ($V_2 - V_1$), the pulse pressure ($P_6 - P_4$) in the hypertensive range would greatly exceed that ($P_3 - P_1$) at normal pressure levels. In other words, a given volume increment will produce a greater pressure increment (i.e., pulse pressure) when the arteries are more rigid than when they are more compliant. Hence the rise in systolic pressure ($P_6 - P_3$) will exceed the increase in diastolic pressure ($P_4 - P_1$). *Thus, an increase in peripheral resistance will raise systolic pressure more than it will raise diastolic pressure.*

These hypothetical changes in arterial pressure closely resemble those actually seen in patients with hypertension. Diastolic pressure is indeed elevated in such individuals, but ordinarily not more than 10 to 40 mm Hg above the average normal level of 80 mm Hg, whereas it is not uncommon for systolic pres-

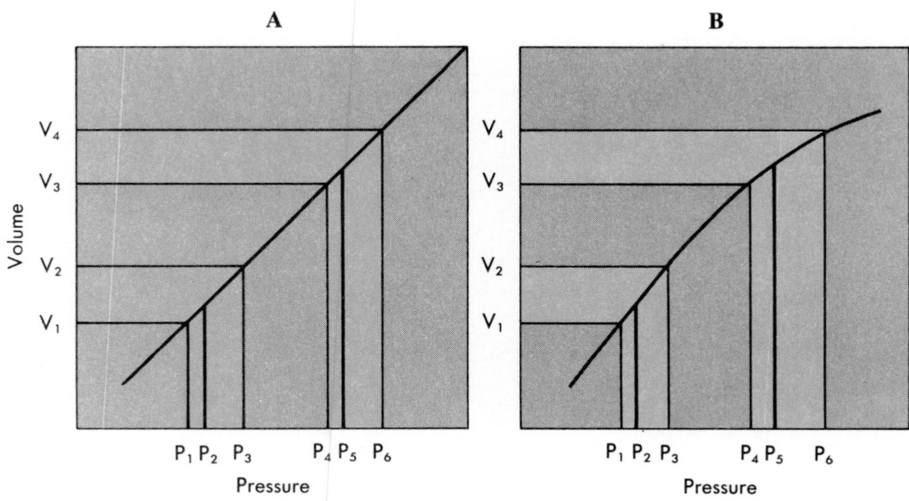

Fig. 6-13 ■ Effect of a change in TPR (volume increment remaining constant) on pulse pressure when the pressure-volume curve for the arterial system is rectilinear, **A**, or curvilinear, **B**.

sures to be elevated by 50 to 150 mm Hg above the average normal level of 120 mm Hg. The combination of an increased resistance and diminished arterial compliance would be represented in Fig. 6-12 by a shift in direction from the top left panel to the bottom right panel; that is, both the mean pressure and the pulse pressure would be increased significantly. These results also coincide with the changes predicted by Fig. 6-13, *B.*

■ PERIPHERAL ARTERIAL PRESSURE CURVES

The radial stretch of the ascending aorta brought about by left ventricular ejection initiates a pressure wave that is propagated down the aorta and its branches. The pressure wave travels much faster than does the blood itself. It is this pressure wave that one perceives by palpating a peripheral artery.

The velocity of the pressure wave varies inversely with the vascular compliance. Accurate measurement of the transmission velocity has provided valuable information about the elastic characteristics of the arterial tree. In general, transmission velocity increases with age, confirming the observation that the arteries become less compliant with advancing age (Figs. 6-3 and 6-5). Also, velocity increases progressively as the pulse wave travels from the ascending aorta toward the periphery. This indicates that vascular compliance is less in the more distal than in the more proximal portions of the arterial system, a fact that has been confirmed by direct measurement.

The arterial pressure contour becomes distorted as the wave is transmitted down the arterial system; the changes in configuration of the pulse with distance are shown in Fig. 6-14. Aside from the increasing delay in the onset of the initial pressure rise, three major changes occur in the arterial pulse contour as the pressure wave travels distally. First, the high-frequency components of the pulse, such as the incisura (that is, the notch that appears at the end of ventricular ejection), are damped out and soon disappear. Second, the systolic portions of the pressure wave become narrowed and elevated. In the curves shown in Fig. 6-14, the systolic pressure at the level of the knee was 39 mm Hg greater than that recorded in the aortic arch. Third, a hump may appear on the diastolic portion of the pressure wave. These changes in contour are pronounced in young individuals, but they diminish with age. In elderly patients the pulse wave may be

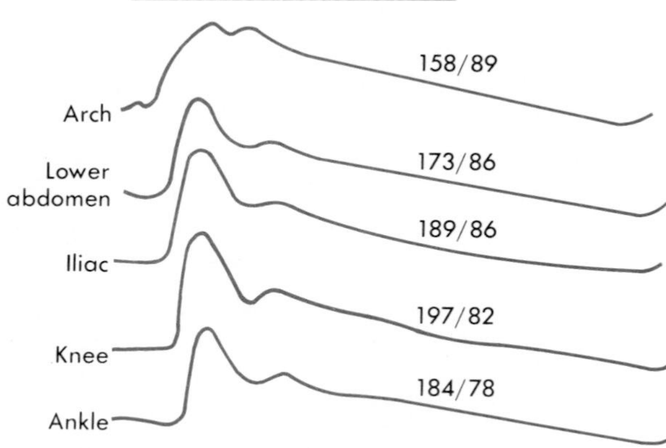

Fig. 6-14 ■ Arterial pressure curves recorded from various sites in an anesthetized dog. (From Remington, J.W., and O'Brien, L.J.: Am. J. Physiol. 218:437, 1970.)

transmitted virtually unchanged from the ascending aorta to the periphery.

The damping of the high-frequency components of the arterial pulse is largely caused by the viscoelastic properties of the arterial walls. The precise mechanism for the peaking of the pressure wave is controversial. Probably several factors contribute, including (1) reflection, (2) tapering, (3) resonance, and (4) changes in transmission velocity with pressure level. Relative to the first of these mechanisms, whenever significant changes in configuration or in dimensions occur (such as at points of branching), pressure waves are reflected backward. Hence pressure at any time and location is determined by the algebraic summation of an antegrade incident wave and retrograde reflected waves. The second factor, tapering, alters the pulse contour because the lumen progressively narrows beyond each successive branch. A pressure wave becomes amplified as it progresses down a tapered tube. With respect to resonance, the arterial tree resonates at certain frequencies, and other frequencies are effectively damped. Finally, as stated previously, transmission velocity varies inversely with arterial compliance. Furthermore, compliance varies inversely with pressure level (see Fig. 6-3). Hence the points on the pressure curve at the higher pressures tend to travel faster than those at lower pressures. Thus the peak of the arterial pressure curve tends to catch up with the beginning of the same curve. This contributes to the peaking and narrowing of the curve in more distal vessels.

■ BLOOD PRESSURE MEASUREMENT IN HUMANS

In hospital intensive care units, needles or catheters may be introduced into peripheral arteries of patients, and arterial blood pressure can then be measured **directly** by means of strain gauges. Ordinarily, however, the blood pressure is estimated **indirectly** by means of a **sphygmomanometer.** This instrument consists of an inextensible cuff containing an inflatable bag. The cuff is wrapped around the extremity (usually the arm, occasionally the thigh) so that the inflatable bag lies between the cuff and the skin, directly over the artery to be compressed. The artery is occluded by inflating the bag, by means of a rubber squeeze bulb, to a pressure in excess of arterial systolic pressure. The pressure in the bag is measured by means of a mercury or an aneroid manometer. Pressure is released from the bag at a rate of 2 or 3 mm Hg per heartbeat by means of a needle valve in the inflating bulb (Fig. 6-15).

When blood pressure readings are taken from the arm, the systolic pressure may be estimated by palpating the radial artery at the wrist **(palpatory method).** When pressure in the bag exceeds the systolic level, no pulse will be perceived. As the pressure falls just below the systolic level (Fig. 6-15, *A*), a spurt of blood will pass through the brachial artery under the cuff during the peak of systole and a slight pulse will be felt at the wrist.

The **auscultatory method** is a more sensitive and therefore a more precise method for measuring systolic pressure, and it also permits the estimation of the diastolic pressure level. The practitioner listens with a stethoscope applied to the skin of the antecubital space over the brachial artery. While the pressure in the bag exceeds the systolic pressure, the brachial artery is occluded and no sounds are heard (Fig. 6-15, *B*). When the inflation pressure falls just below the systolic level (120 mm Hg in Fig. 6-15, *A*), a small spurt of blood escapes through the cuff and slight tapping sounds (called **Korotkoff sounds**) are heard with each heartbeat. The pressure at which the first sound is detected represents the **systolic pressure.** It usually corresponds closely with the directly measured systolic pressure.

As inflation pressure continues to fall, more blood escapes under the cuff per beat and the

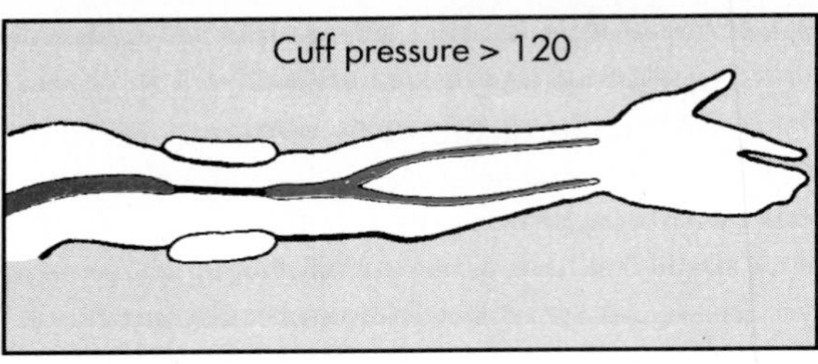

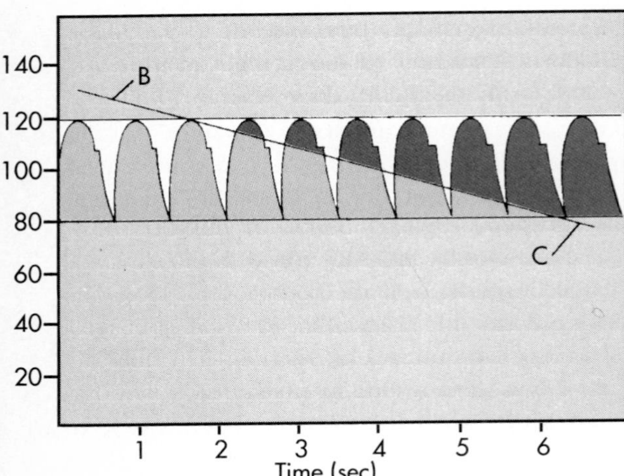

A, Consider that the arterial blood pressure is being measured in a patient whose blood pressure is 120/80 mm Hg. The pressure (represented by the *oblique line*) in a cuff around the patient's arm is allowed to fall from greater than 120 mm Hg (point *B*) to below 80 mm Hg (point *C*) in about 6 seconds.

B, When the cuff pressure exceeds the systolic arterial pressure (120 mm Hg), no blood progresses through the arterial segment under the cuff, and no sounds can be detected by a stethoscope bell placed on the arm distal to the cuff.

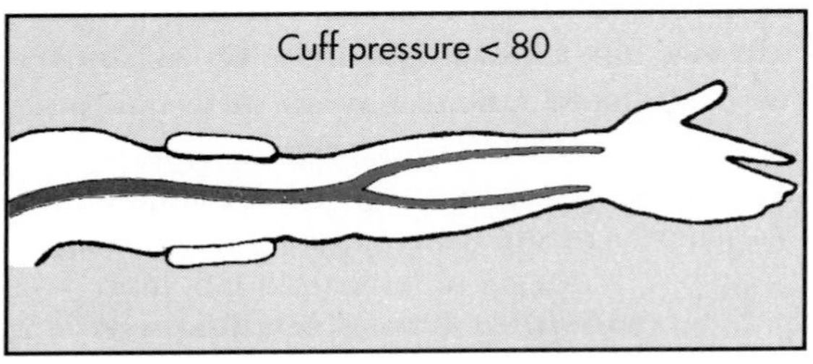

C, When the cuff pressure falls below the diastolic arterial pressure, arterial flow past the region of the cuff is continuous, and no sounds are audible. When the cuff pressure is between 120 and 80 mm Hg, spurts of blood traverse the artery segment under the cuff with each heartbeat, and the Korotkoff sounds are heard through the stethoscope.

Fig. 6-15 ■ Measurement of arterial blood pressure with a sphygmomanometer.

sounds become louder thuds. As the inflation pressure approaches the diastolic level, the Korotkoff sounds become muffled. As they fall just below the diastolic level (80 mm Hg in Fig. 6-15, *A*), the sounds disappear; this indicates the **diastolic pressure.** The origin of the Korotkoff sounds is related to the spurt of blood passing under the cuff and meeting a static column of blood; the impact and turbulence generate audible vibrations. Once the inflation pressure is less than the diastolic pressure, flow is continuous in the brachial artery and sounds are no longer heard (Fig. 6-15, *C*).

■ SUMMARY

1. The arteries serve not only to conduct blood from the heart to the capillaries, but also to store some of the ejected blood during each cardiac systole so that flow can

continue through the capillaries during cardiac diastole.

2. The aging process diminishes the compliance of the arteries.
3. The less compliant the arteries, the more work the heart must do to pump a given cardiac output.
4. The mean arterial pressure varies directly with the cardiac output and total peripheral resistance.
5. The arterial pulse pressure varies directly with the stroke volume but inversely with the arterial compliance.
6. The contour of the systemic arterial pressure wave is distorted as it travels from the ascending aorta to the periphery. The high frequency components of the wave are damped, the systolic components are narrowed and elevated, and a hump may appear in the diastolic component of the wave.
7. When blood pressure is measured by a sphygmomanometer in humans, (a) the systolic pressure is manifested by the occurrence of a tapping sound that originates in the artery distal to the cuff as the cuff pressure falls below the peak arterial pressure, which permits spurts of blood to pass through the compressed artery, and (b) the diastolic pressure is manifested by the disappearance of the sound as the cuff pressure falls below the minimum arterial pressure, which permits flow through the artery to become continuous.

■ BIBLIOGRAPHY

Journal articles

Alexander, J., Jr., Burkhoff, D., Schipke, J., and Sagawa, K.: Influence of mean pressure on aortic impedance and reflections in the systemic arterial system, Am. J. Physiol. 257:H969, 1989.

Blank, S.G., West, J.E., Müller, F.B., Cody, R.J., Harshfield, G.A., Pecker, M.S., Laragh, J.H., and Pickering, T.G.: Wideband external pulse recording during cuff deflation: a new technique for evaluation of the arterial pressure pulse and measurement of blood pressure, Circ. 77:1297, 1988.

Burattini, R., Gnudi, G., Westerhof, N., and Fioretti, S.: Total systemic arterial compliance and aortic characteristic impedance in the dog as a function of pressure: a model based study, Computers Biomed. Res. 20:154, 1987.

Burkhoff, D., Alexander, J., Jr., and Schipke, J.: Assessment of Windkessel as a model of aortic input impedance, Am. J. Physiol. 255:H742, 1988.

Campbell, K.B., Lee, L.C., Frasch, H.F., and Noordergraaf, A.: Pulse reflection sites and effective length of the arterial system, Am. J. Physiol. 256:H1684, 1989.

Finkelstein, S.M., and Collins, V.R.: Vascular hemodynamic impedance measurement, Prog. Cardiovasc. Dis. 24:401, 1982.

Imura, T., Yamamoto, K., Kanamori, K., Mikami, T., and Yasvda, H.: Non-invasive ultrasonic measurement of the elastic properties of the human abdominal aorta, Cardiovasc. Res. 20:208, 1986.

Isnard, R.N., Pannier, B.M., Laurent, S., London, G.M., Diebold, B., and Safar, M.E.: Pulsatile diameter and elastic modulus of the aortic arch in essential hypertension: a noninvasive study, J. Am. Coll. Cardiol. 13:399, 1989.

Kenner, T.: Arterial blood pressure and its measurement, Basic Res. Cardiol. 83:107, 1988.

Laskey, W.K., Parker, H.G., Ferrari, V.A., Kussmaul, W.G., and Noordergraaf, A.: Estimation of total systemic arterial compliance in humans, J. Appl. Physiol. 69:112, 1990.

McIlroy, M.B., and Targett, R.C.: Model of the systemic arterial bed showing ventricular-systemic arterial coupling, Am. J. Physiol. 254:H609, 1988.

O'Rourke, M.F.: Vascular impedance in studies of arterial and cardiac function, Physiol. Rev. 62:570, 1982.

Piene, H.: Pulmonary arterial impedance and right ventricular function, Physiol. Rev. 66:606, 1986.

Zuckerman, B.D., Weisman, H.F., and Yin, F.C.P.: Arterial hemodynamics in a rabbit model of atherosclerosis, Am. J. Physiol. 257:H891, 1989.

Books and monographs

Bauer, R.D., and Busse, R., editors: Arterial system: dynamics, control theory and regulation, Heidelberg, 1978, Springer-Verlag.

Dobrin, P.B.: Vascular mechanics. In Handbook of physiology; Section 2: The cardiovascular system—peripheral circulation and organ blood flow, vol. III, Bethesda, Md., 1983, American Physiological Society.

Fung, Y.C.: Biodynamics: circulation, Heidelberg, 1984, Springer-Verlag.

Milnor, W.R.: Hemodynamics, Baltimore, 1982, Williams & Wilkins.

Taylor, D.E.M., and Stevens, A.L., editors: Blood flow: theory and practice, New York, 1983, Academic Press, Inc.

7 The Microcirculation and Lymphatics

The entire circulatory system is geared to supply the body tissues with blood in amounts commensurate with their requirements for oxygen and nutrients. The capillaries, consisting of a single layer of endothelial cells, permit rapid exchange of water and solutes with interstitial fluid. The muscular arterioles, which are the major **resistance vessels,** regulate regional blood flow to the capillary beds, and the venules and veins serve primarily as collecting channels and storage, or **capacitance, vessels.**

The arterioles, which range in diameter from about 5 to 100 μm, have a thick smooth muscle layer, a thin adventitial layer, and an endothelial lining (Fig. 1-1). The arterioles give rise directly to the capillaries (5 to 10 μm diameter) or in some tissues to **metarterioles** (10 to 20 μm diameter), which then give rise to capillaries (see Fig. 7-1). The metarterioles can serve either as thoroughfare channels to the venules, bypassing the capillary bed, or as conduits to supply the capillary bed. There are often cross connections between arterioles and between venules, as well as in the capillary network. Arterioles that give rise directly to capillaries regulate flow through their cognate capillaries by constriction or dilation. The capillaries form an interconnecting network of tubes of different lengths with an average length of 0.5 to 1 mm.

Capillary distribution varies from tissue to tissue. In metabolically active tissues, such as cardiac and skeletal muscle and glandular structures, capillaries are numerous, whereas in less active tissues, such as subcutaneous tissue or cartilage, **capillary density** is low. Also, all capillaries are not of the same diameter, and because some capillaries have diameters less than that of the erythrocytes, it is necessary for the cells to become temporarily deformed in their passage through these capillaries. Fortunately, the normal red cells are quite flexible and readily change their shape to conform with that of the small capillaries.

Blood flow in the capillaries is not uniform and depends chiefly on the contractile state of the arterioles. The average velocity of blood flow in the capillaries is approximately 1 mm/s; however, it can vary from zero to several millimeters per second in the same vessel within a brief period. These changes in capillary blood flow may be of random type or may show rhythmical oscillatory behavior of different frequencies that are caused by contraction and relaxation **(vasomotion)** of the precapillary vessels. This vasomotion is to some extent an intrinsic contractile behavior of the vascular smooth muscle and is independent of external input. Furthermore, changes in **transmural pressure** (intravascular minus extravascular pressure) influence the contractile state of the precapillary vessels. An increase in transmural pressure, whether produced by an increase in venous pressure or by dilation of arterioles, results in contraction of the terminal arterioles at the points of origin of the capillaries, whereas a decrease in transmural pressure elicits precapillary vessel relaxation (see myogenic response, p. 176). In addition, humoral and possibly neural factors also affect vasomotion. For example, when the precapillary vessels contract in response to increased transmural pressure, the contractile response can be overridden and vasomotion abolished. This effect is accomplished by metabolic (humoral) factors (p. 178) when the oxygen supply becomes too low for the requirements of the parenchymal tissue, as occurs in muscle during exercise.

Although reduction of transmural pressure will induce relaxation of the terminal arterioles, blood flow through the capillaries obviously cannot increase if the reduction in intravascular pressure is caused by severe constriction of the parent arterioles, metarterioles, or small arteries. Large arterioles and metarterioles also exhibit vasomotion, but in the con-

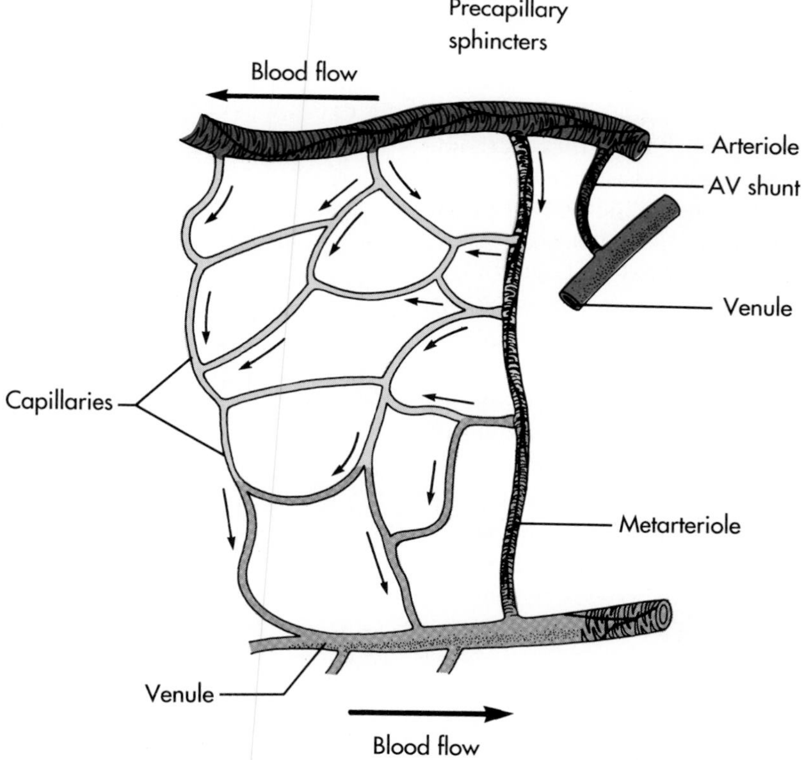

Fig. 7-1 ■ Composite schematic drawing of the microcirculation. The circular structures on the arteriole and venule represent smooth muscle fibers, and the branching solid lines represent sympathetic nerve fibers. The arrows indicate the direction of blood flow.

traction phase they usually do not completely occlude the lumen of the vessel and arrest blood flow as may occur with contraction of the terminal arterioles. Thus *flow rate may be altered by contraction and relaxation of small arteries, arterioles, and metarterioles.*

Because blood flow through the capillaries provides for exchange of gases and solutes between blood and tissue, it has been termed **nutritional flow,** whereas blood flow that bypasses the capillaries in traveling from the arterial to the venous side of the circulation has been termed **nonnutritional,** or **shunt flow** (see Fig. 7-1). In some areas of the body (e.g., fingertips) true arteriovenous shunts exist (p. 232). However, in many tissues, such as muscle, evidence of anatomical shunts is lacking. Nevertheless, nonnutritional flow can occur and has been termed a physiologic shunting. It is the result of a greater flow of blood through previously open capillaries with either no change or an increase in the number of closed capillaries. In tissues that have metarterioles, shunt flow may be continuous from arteriole to venule during low metabolic activity when many precapillary vessels are closed. When metabolic activity increases in such tissues and more precapillary vessels open, blood passing through the metarterioles is readily available for capillary perfusion.

The true capillaries are devoid of smooth muscle and are therefore incapable of active constriction. Nevertheless, the endothelial cells that form the capillary wall contain actin and myosin and can alter their shape in response to certain chemical stimuli. Evidence is lacking, however, that changes in endothelial cell shape regulate blood flow through the capillaries. Hence, changes in capillary diameter are passive and are caused by alterations in precapillary and postcapillary resistance.

The thin-walled capillaries can withstand high internal pressures without bursting because of their narrow lumen. This can be explained in terms of the **law of Laplace** and is illustrated in the following comparison of wall tension of a capillary with that of the aorta (Table 1). The Laplace equation is

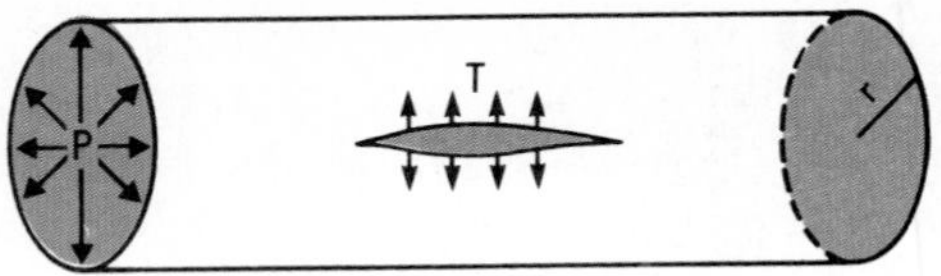

Fig. 7-2 ■ Diagram of a small blood vessel to illustrate the law of Laplace—T = Pr, where P = intraluminal pressure, r = radius of the vessel, and T = wall tension as the force per unit length tangential to the vessel wall, tending to pull apart a theoretical longitudinal slit in the vessel.

$$T = Pr$$

where

T = Tension in the vessel wall

P = Transmural pressure

r = Radius of the vessel

Wall tension is the force per unit length tangential to the vessel wall that opposes the distending force (Pr) that tends to pull apart a theoretical longitudinal slit in the vessel (Fig. 7-2). Transmural pressure is essentially equal to intraluminal pressure, because extravascular pressure is negligible. The Laplace equation applies to very thin wall vessels, such as capillaries. Wall thickness must be taken into consideration when the equation is applied to thick wall vessels, such as the aorta. This is done by dividing Pr (pressure × radius) by wall thickness (w). The equation now becomes

$$\sigma \text{ (wall stress)} = Pr/w$$

To convert pressure in mm Hg (height of Hg column) to dynes per square centimeter, P = hρg, where h = the height of Hg column in centimeters, ρ = the density of Hg in g/cm^3, g = gravitational acceleration in cm/s^2, σ = force per unit area, and w = wall thickness.

Thus at normal aortic and capillary pressures

Table 1 ■ Vessel wall tension in the aorta and a capillary

	Aorta	*Capillary*
Radius (r)	1.5 cm	5×10^{-4} cm
Height of Hg column (h)	10 cm Hg	2.5 cm Hg
ρ	13.6 g/cm^3	13.6 g/cm^3
g	980 cm/s^2	980 cm/s^2
$\bar{P}$	$10 \times 13.6 \times 980 = 1.33 \times 10^5$ dyne/cm^2	$2.5 \times 13.6 \times 980 = 3.33 \times 10^4$ dyne/cm^2
w	0.2 cm	1×10^{-4} cm
T = Pr	$(1.33 \times 10^5)(1.5) = 2 \times 10^5$ dyne/cm	$(3.33 \times 10^4)(5 \times 10^{-4}) = 16.7$ dyne/cm
$\sigma = \frac{Pr}{w}$	$\frac{2 \times 10^5}{0.2} = 1 \times 10^6$ dyne/cm^2	$\frac{16.7}{1 \times 10^{-4}} = 1.67 \times 10^5$ dyne/cm^2

the wall tension of the aorta is about 12,000 times greater than that of the capillary (see Table 1). In a person standing quietly, capillary pressure in the feet may reach 100 mm Hg. Under such conditions capillary wall tension increases to 66.5 dynes/cm, a value that is still only one three-thousandth that of the wall tension in the aorta at the same internal pressure. However, σ (stress), which takes wall thickness into consideration, is only about tenfold greater in the aorta than in the capillary.

In addition to providing an explanation for the ability of capillaries to withstand large internal pressures, the preceding calculations also point out that in dilated vessels, wall tension increases even when internal pressure remains constant and may, under certain circumstances (for example, aneurysm of the aorta), be an important factor in rupture of the vessel. The above equation also indicates that as the wall of the vessel becomes thicker, the wall stress decreases. In **hypertension** (high blood pressure) the arterial vessel walls thicken (hypertrophy of the vascular smooth muscle), thereby minimizing the arterial wall stress and hence the possibility of vessel rupture.

The diameter of the resistance vessels is determined by the balance between the contractile force of the vascular smooth muscle and the distending force produced by the intraluminal pressure. The greater the contractile activity of the vascular smooth muscle of an arteriole, the smaller its diameter, until a point is reached, in the case of small arterioles, when complete occlusion of the vessel occurs. This is caused by infolding of the endothelium and by trapping of the cells in the vessel. With progressive reduction in the intravascular pressure, vessel diameter decreases as does tension in the vessel wall (law of Laplace). When perfusion pressure is reduced, a point is reached where blood flow ceases even though there is still a positive pressure gradient. This phenomenon has been referred to as the **critical closing pressure,** and its mechanism is still controversial. This critical closing pressure is low when vasomotor activity is reduced by inhibition of sympathetic nerve activity to the vessel, and it is increased when vasomotor tone is enhanced by activation of the vascular sympathetic nerve fibers. It has been suggested that flow stops because of vessel collapse when vascular smooth muscle contractile stress exceeds the stress associated with vessel radius, wall thickness, and intraluminal pressure (law of Laplace).

■ VASOACTIVE ROLE OF ENDOTHELIUM

For many years it was thought that the endothelium was an inert single layer of cells that served solely as a passive filter to permit passage of water and small molecules across the blood vessel wall and to retain blood cells and large molecules (proteins) within the vascular compartment. Recently it has been demonstrated that the endothelium is a source of sub-

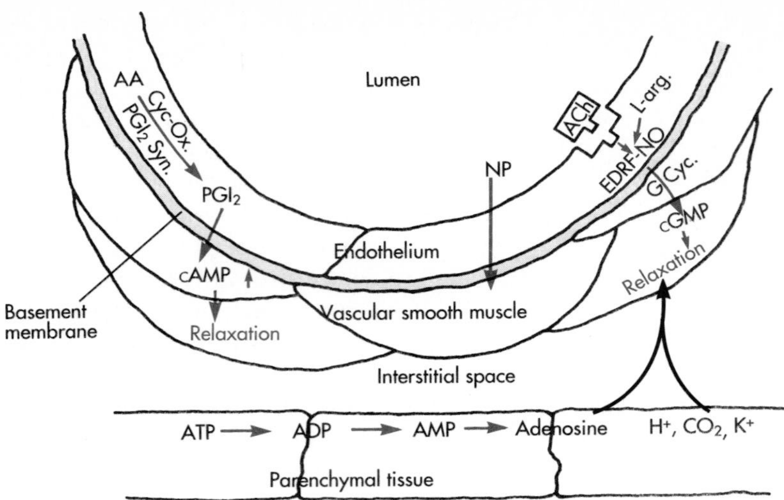

Fig. 7-3 ■ Endothelial and nonendothelial mediated vasodilation. Prostacyclin (PI_2) is formed from arachidonic acid (AA) by the action of cyclooxygenase (Cyc Ox) and prostacyclin synthetase (Pr Syn) in the endothelium and elicits relaxation of the adjacent vascular smooth muscle via increases in cyclic adenosine monophosphate (cAMP). Stimulation of the endothelial cells with acetylcholine (ACh) or other agents (see text) results in the formation and release of an endothelial-derived relaxing factor (EDRF), one of which is probably nitric oxide (NO). The EDRF stimulates guanylate cyclase (G Cyc) to increase cyclic guanosine monophosphate (cGMP) in the vascular smooth muscle to produce relaxation. The vasodilator agent nitroprusside (NP) acts directly on the vascular smooth muscle. Substances such as adenosine, hydrogen ions (H^+), CO_2 and potassium ions (K^+) can arise in the parenchymal tissue and elicit vasodilation by direct action on the vascular smooth muscle (see Chapter 8).

stances that elicit contraction or relaxation of the vascular smooth muscle.

As shown in Fig. 7-3, prostacyclin can relax vascular smooth muscle via an increase in the cyclic adenosine monophosphate (cAMP) concentration. **Prostacyclin** is formed in the endothelium from arachidonic acid and the process is catalyzed by prostacyclin synthetase. To what extent this occurs in vivo is not known, but the prostacyclin may be released by shear stress caused by the pulsatile blood flow. The primary function of prostacyclin is to inhibit platelet adherence to the endothelium and platelet aggregation, thereby to prevent intravascular clot formation.

Of far greater importance in endothelial-mediated vascular dilation is the formation and release of the **endothelial-derived relaxing factor (EDRF)** (see Fig. 7-3). Stimulation of the endothelial cells in vivo, in isolated arteries, or in culture by acetylcholine or several other agents (ATP, bradykinin, serotonin, substance P, histamine) causes the production and release of EDRF. In blood vessels from which the endothelium has been mechanically removed, these agents do not elicit vasodilation. The EDRF (probably synthesized from L-arginine) activates guanylate cyclase in the vascular smooth muscle to increase the cyclic guanosine monophosphate (cGMP) concentration, which produces relaxation, possibly by decreasing cytosolic free Ca^{++}. Strong evidence indicates that one form of EDRF is nitric oxide (NO), but at least one other form (a hyperpolarizing factor) has been demonstrated. EDRF release can be stimulated by the shear stress of blood flow on the endothelium, but the physiologic role of EDRF in the local regulation of blood flow remains to be elucidated. The drug nitroprusside also increases cGMP, which produces vasodilation but it acts directly on the vascular smooth muscle and is not endothelial-mediated (see Fig. 7-3). Vasodilator agents such as adenosine, hydrogen ions, CO_2, and potassium may be released from parenchymal tissue and act locally on the resistance vessels (see Fig. 7-3).

The endothelium can also synthesize an **endothelial-derived contracting factor (EDCF),** but little is known about its function. It is apparently not **endothelin,** a small vasoconstrictor peptide that has been isolated from endothelial cells.

■ PASSIVE ROLE OF ENDOTHELIUM

Transcapillary Exchange

Solvent and solute move across the capillary endothelial wall by three processes: diffusion, filtration, and by endothelial vesicles (pinocytosis).

The permeability of the capillary endothelial membrane is not the same in all body tissues. For example, the liver capillaries are quite permeable, and albumin escapes at a rate several-fold greater than from the less permeable muscle capillaries. Also, there is not uniform permeability along the whole capillary; the venous ends are more permeable than the arterial ends, and permeability is greatest in the venules. The greater permeability at the venous end of the capillaries and in the venules is due to the greater number of pores in these regions of the microvessels.

The sites where filtration occurs have been a controversial subject for a number of years. A little water flows through the capillary endothelial cell membranes but most of the water flows through apertures **(pores)** in the endothelial wall of the capillaries (Figs. 7-4 and 7-5). Calculations based on the transcapillary movement of solutes of small molecular size led to the prediction of pore diameters of about 4 nm. However, electron microscopy failed to reveal pores, and the clefts at the junctions of endothelial cells appeared to be fused at the tight junctions (see Figs. 7-4 and 7-5). However, studies on cardiac and skeletal muscle with horseradish peroxidase, a protein with a molecular weight of 40,000, have demonstrated that many of the clefts between adjacent endothelial cells are open. Electron microscopy revealed filling of the clefts with peroxidase from the lumen side of the capillaries with a gap at the narrowest point of about 4 nm, providing morphological support of the physiologic evidence for the existence of capillary pores. The clefts (pores) are sparse and represent only about 0.02% of the capillary surface area. In cerebral capillaries, where a blood-brain barrier to many small molecules exists, peroxidase studies do not reveal any pores. Transcapillary movement of solute (large and small molecules) may occur through channels formed by the fusion of vesicles (**vesicular channels**) across the endothelial cells (see Fig. 7-5). However, the existence of such channels has been seriously questioned. The basement membrane, a layer of fine fibrillar material around the capillaries, retards the passage of large molecules (greater than 10 nm radius).

In addition to clefts, some of the more porous capillaries (for example, in kidney, intestine) contain **fenestrations** (see Fig. 7-5) 20 to 100 nm wide, whereas others (such as in the liver) have a **discontinuous endothelium** (see Fig. 7-5). The fenestrations that appear to be sealed by a thin diaphragm are quite permeable to horseradish peroxidase and a number of other tracers. Hence larger mole-

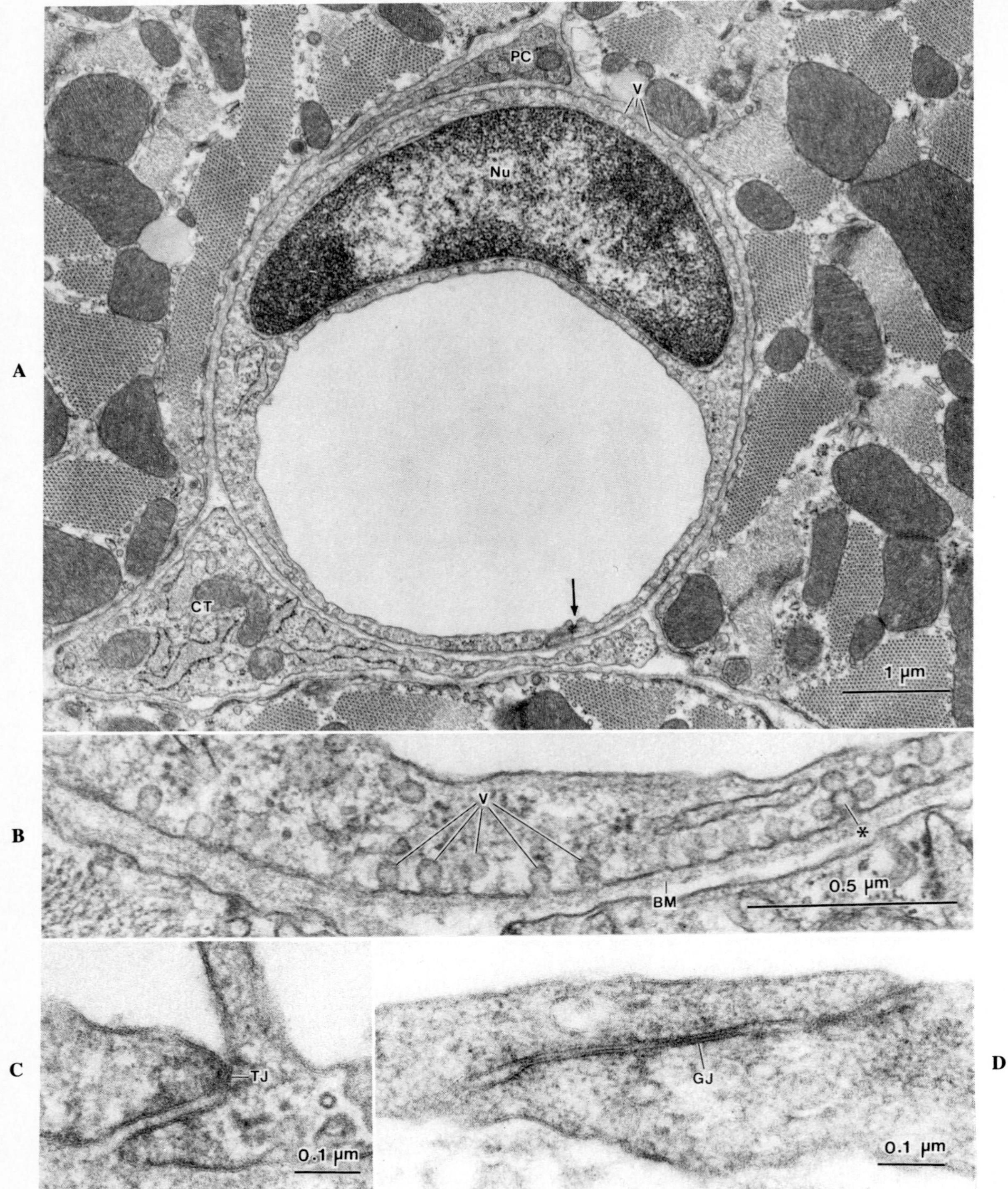

Fig. 7-4 ■ For legend see opposite page.

Fig. 7-4 ■ **A,** Cross-sectioned capillary in mouse ventricular wall. Luminal diameter is approximately 4 μm. In this thin section, the capillary wall is formed by a single endothelial cell (*Nu,* endothelial nucleus), which forms a junctional complex *(arrow)* with itself. The thin pericapillary space is occupied by a pericyte *(PC)* and a connective tissue *(CT)* cell ("fibroblast"). Note the numerous endothelial vesicles *(V).* **B,** Detail of endothelial cell in panel **A,** showing plasmalemmal vesicles *(V)* that are attached to the endothelial cell surface. These vesicles are especially prominent in vascular endothelium and are involved in transport of substances across the blood vessel wall. Note the complex alveolar vesicle (*). *BM,* Basement membrane. **C,** Junctional complex in a capillary of mouse heart. "Tight" junctions *(TJ)* typically form in these small blood vessels and appear to consist of fusions between apposed endothelial cell surface membranes. **D,** Interendothelial junction in a muscular artery of monkey papillary muscle. Although tight junctions similar to those of capillaries are found in these large blood vessels, extensive junctions that resemble gap junctions in the intercalated disks between myocardial cells often appear in arterial endothelium (example shown at *GJ*). (Micrographs courtesy Dr. Michael S. Forbes.)

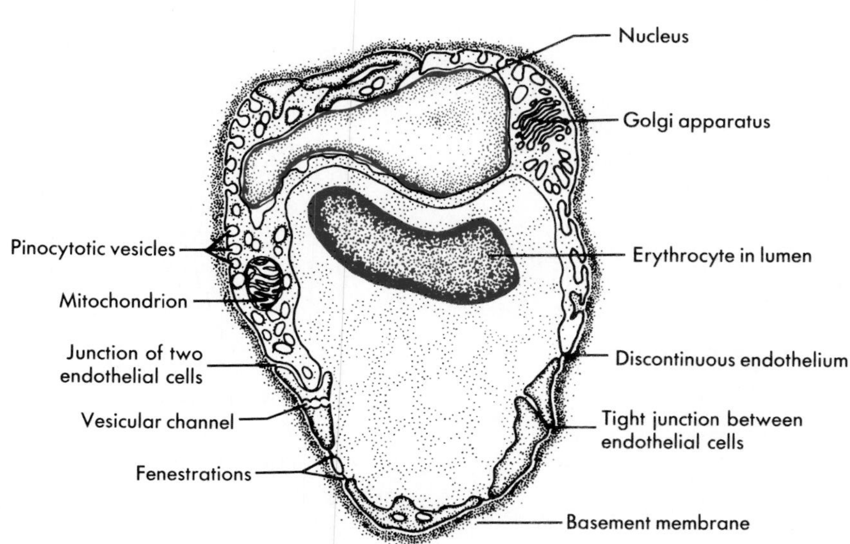

Fig. 7-5 ■ Diagrammatic sketch of an electron micrograph of a composite capillary in cross section.

cules can penetrate capillaries with fenestrations or gaps caused by discontinuous endothelium than can pass through the intercellular clefts of the endothelium.

Diffusion.

Under normal conditions only about 0.06 ml of water per minute moves back and forth across the capillary wall per 100 g of tissue as a result of filtration and absorption, whereas 300 ml of water per minute per 100 g of tissue do so by diffusion, a 5000-fold difference.

Relating filtration and diffusion to blood flow, we find that about 2% of the plasma passing through the capillaries is filtered. In contrast, the diffusion of water is 40 times greater than the rate that it is brought to the capillaries by blood flow. The transcapillary exchange of solutes is also primarily governed by diffusion. Thus *diffusion is the key factor in providing exchange of gases, substrates, and waste products between the capillaries and the tissue cells.*

The process of diffusion is described by Fick's law:

$$J = -DA\frac{dc}{dx}$$

where

J = Quantity of a substance moved per unit time (t)

D = Free diffusion coefficient for a particular molecule (the value is inversely related to the square root of the molecular weight)

A = Cross-sectional area of the diffusion pathway

$\frac{dc}{dx}$ = Concentration gradient of the solute

Fick's law is also expressed as:

$$J = -PS(C_o - C_i)$$

where

P = Capillary permeability of the substance

S = Capillary surface area

C_i = Concentration of the substance inside the capillary

C_o = Concentration of the substance outside the capillary

Hence, the PS product provides a convenient expression of available capillary surface, because permeability is rarely altered under physiological conditions.

In the capillaries, diffusion of lipid-insoluble molecules is not free but is restricted to the pores whose mean size can be calculated by measurement of the diffusion rate of an uncharged molecule whose free diffusion coefficient is known. Movement of solutes across the endothelium is quite complex and involves corrections for attractions between solute and solvent molecules, interactions between solute molecules, pore configuration, and charge on the molecules relative to charge on the endothelial cells. It is not simply a question of random thermal movements of molecules down a concentration gradient.

For small molecules, such as water, NaCl, urea, and glucose, the capillary pores offer little restriction to diffusion (low **reflection coefficient**), and diffusion is so rapid that the mean concentration gradient across the capillary endothelium is extremely small. With lipid-insoluble molecules of increasing size, diffusion through muscle capillaries becomes progressively more restricted, until diffusion becomes minimal with molecules of a molecular weight above about 60,000. With small molecules the only limitation to net movement across the capillary wall is the rate at which blood flow transports the molecules to the capillary **(flow limited).**

When transport across the capillary is flow limited, the concentration of a small molecular solute in the blood reaches equilibrium with its concentration in the interstitial fluid near the origin of the capillary from the cognate arteriole. If an inert small molecule tracer is infused intraarterially, its concentration falls to negligible levels near the arterial end of the capillary (Fig. 7-6, *A*). If the flow is large, the small molecule tracer will be detectable farther downstream in the capillary. A somewhat larger molecule moves farther along the capil-

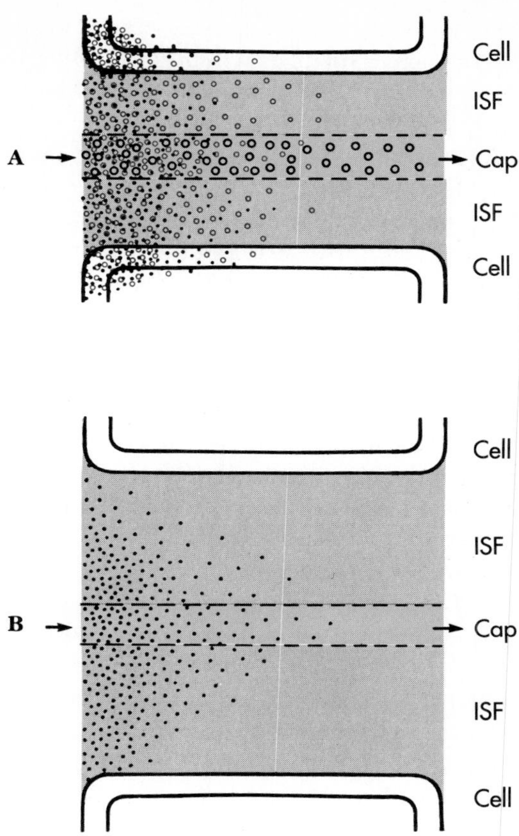

Fig. 7-6 ■ Flow and diffusion-limited transport from capillaries *(Cap)* to tissue. **A,** Flow-limited transport. The smallest water-soluble inert tracer particles *(black dots)* reach negligible concentrations after passing only a short distance down the capillary. Larger particles *(colored circles)* with similar properties travel farther along the capillary before reaching insignificant intracapillary concentrations. Both substances cross the interstitial fluid *(ISF)* and reach the parenchymal tissue (cell). Because of their size, more of the smaller particles are taken up by the tissue cells. The largest particles *(black circles)* cannot penetrate the capillary pores and hence do not escape from the capillary lumen except by pinocytotic vesicle transport. An increase in the volume of blood flow or an increase in capillary density will increase tissue supply for the diffusible solutes. Note that capillary permeability is greater at the venous end of the capillary (also in the venule, not shown) because of the larger number of pores in this region. **B,** Diffusion-limited transport. When the distance between the capillaries and the parenchymal tissue is large, as a result of edema or low capillary density, diffusion becomes a limiting factor in the transport of solutes from capillary to tissue even at high rates of capillary blood flow.

lary before reaching an insignificant concentration in the blood, and the number of still larger molecules that enter the arterial end of the capillary and cannot pass through the capillary pores is the same as the number leaving the venous end of the capillary (see Fig. 7-6, *A*).

With large molecules diffusion across the capillaries becomes the limiting factor **(diffusion limited).** In other words, capillary permeability to a large molecule solute limits its transport across the capillary wall (see Fig. 7-6, *A*). The diffusion of small lipid-insoluble molecules is so rapid that diffusion becomes limiting in blood-tissue exchange only when the distances between capillaries and parenchymal cells are large (for example, tissue edema or very low capillary density) (see Fig. 7-6, *B*). Furthermore, the rate of diffusion is uninfluenced by filtration in the direction opposite to the concentration gradient of the diffusible substance. In fact, filtration **or** absorption accelerates the movement of tracer ions from interstitial fluid to blood (**tissue clearance**). The reason for this enhanced tissue clearance is not known, but it may be the result of a stirring effect on the interstitial fluid or to changes in its structure (for example, gel to sol transformation or "canals" in a gel matrix).

Movement of lipid-soluble molecules across the capillary wall is not limited to capillary pores (only about 0.02% of the capillary surface), because such molecules can pass directly through the lipid membranes of the entire capillary endothelium. Consequently, *lipid-soluble molecules move with great rapidity between blood and tissue. The degree of lipid solubility (oil-to-water partition coefficient) provides a good index of the ease of transfer of lipid molecules through the capillary endothelium.*

Oxygen and carbon dioxide are both lipid soluble and readily pass through the endothelial cells. Calculations based on (1) the diffusion coefficient for O_2, (2) capillary density and diffusion distances, (3) blood flow, and (4) tissue O_2 consumption indicate that the O_2 supply of normal tissue at rest and during activity is not limited by diffusion or the number of open capillaries. Recent measurements of Po_2 and saturation of blood in the microvessels indicate that in many tissues O_2 saturation at the entrance of the capillaries has already decreased to a saturation of about 80% as a result of diffusion of O_2 from arterioles and small arteries. Such studies also have shown that CO_2 loading and the resultant intravascular shifts in the oxyhemoglobin dissociation curve occur in the precapillary vessels. These findings reflect not only the movement of gas to respiring tissue at the precapillary level, but also the direct flux of O_2 and CO_2 between adjacent arterioles, venules, and possibly arteries and veins **(countercurrent exchange).** This exchange of gas represents a diffusional shunt of gas around the capillaries, and, at low blood flow rates, it may limit the supply of O_2 to the tissue.

Capillary Filtration.

The direction and the magnitude of the movement of water across the capillary wall are determined by the algebraic sum of the hydrostatic and osmotic pressures that exist across the membrane. An increase in intracapillary hydrostatic pressure favors movement of fluid from the vessel to the interstitial space, whereas an increase in the concentration of osmotically active particles within the vessels favors movement of fluid into the vessels from the interstitial space.

Hydrostatic Forces. The hydrostatic pressure (blood pressure) within the capillaries is not constant and depends on the arterial pressure, the venous pressure, and the precapillary (arteriolar) and postcapillary (venules and small veins) resistances. An increase in arterial or venous pressure elevates capillary hydrostatic pressure, whereas a reduction in each has the opposite effect. An increase in arteriolar resistance or closure of arteries reduces capillary pressure, whereas greater venous resistance (venules and veins) increases capillary pressure.

Hydrostatic pressure is the principal force in capillary filtration. However, changes in the venous resistance affect capillary hydrostatic pressure more than do changes in arteriolar resistance. A given change in venous pressure produces a greater effect on capillary hydrostatic pressure than the same change in arterial pressure, and about 80% of an increase in venous pressure is transmitted back to the capillaries.

Despite the fact that capillary hydrostatic pressure (Pc) is variable from tissue to tissue (even within the same tissue), average values, obtained from many direct measurements in human skin, are about 32 mm Hg at the arterial end of the capillaries and 15 mm Hg at the venous end of the capillaries at the level of the heart (Fig. 7-7). When a person stands, the hydrostatic pressure is higher in the legs and lower in the head.

Tissue pressure, or more specifically interstitial fluid pressure (P_i) outside the capillaries, opposes capillary filtration, and it is $P_c - P_i$ that constitutes the driving force for filtration. The true value of P_i is still controversial. For years it was assumed to be close to zero in the normal (nonedematous) state. However, stud-

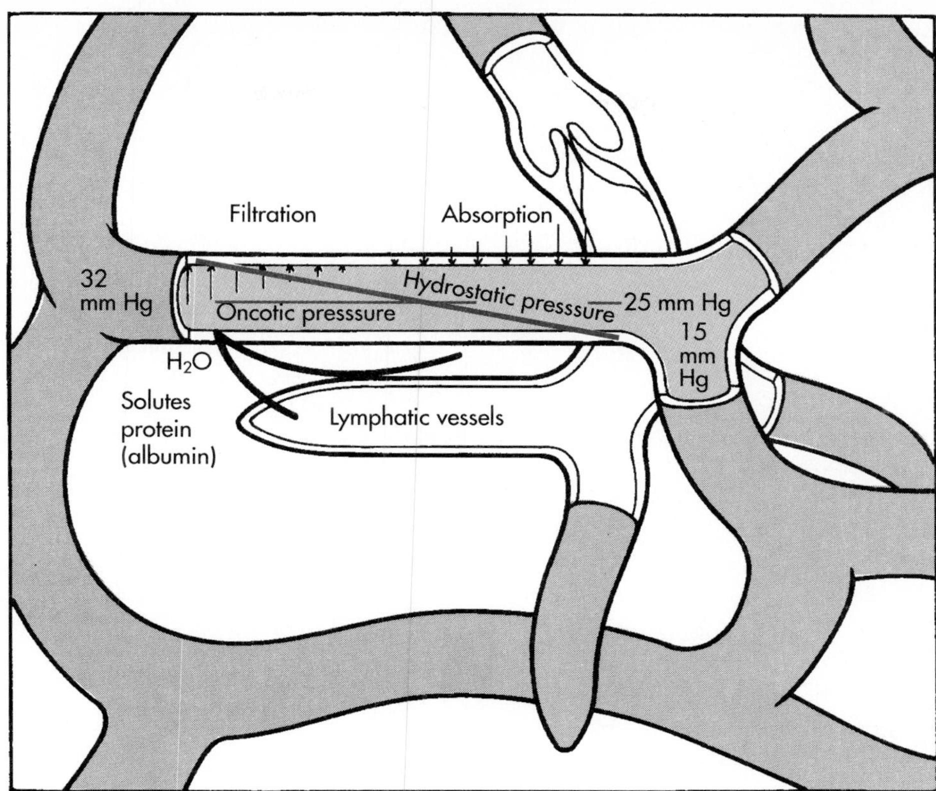

Fig. 7-7 ■ Schematic representation of the factors responsible for filtration and absorption across the capillary wall and the formation of lymph.

ies using perforated, plastic capsules implanted in the subcutaneous tissue, or wicks inserted through the skin, indicate a negative P_i of from -1 to -7 mm Hg. If the pressures recorded by these techniques are representative of interstitial fluid pressure in undisturbed tissue, then the hydrostatic driving force for capillary filtration is greater than the value of P_c.

Osmotic Forces. The key factor that restrains fluid loss from the capillaries is the osmotic pressure of the plasma proteins—usually termed the **colloid osmotic pressure** or **oncotic pressure** (π_p). The total osmotic pressure of plasma is about 6000 mm Hg, whereas the oncotic pressure is only about 25 mm Hg. However, this small oncotic pressure plays an important role in fluid exchange across the capillary wall, because the plasma proteins are essentially confined to the intravascular space, whereas the electrolytes that are responsible for the major fraction of plasma osmotic pressure are practically equal in concentration on both sides of the capillary endothelium. The relative permeability of solute to water influences the actual magnitude of the osmotic pressure. The **reflection coefficient** (σ) is the relative impediment to the passage of a substance through the capillary membrane. The reflection coefficient of water is zero and that of albumin (to which the endothelium is essentially impermeable) is 1. Filterable solutes have reflection coefficients between 0 and 1. Also, different tissues have different reflection coefficients for the same molecule, and therefore movement of a given solute across the endothelial wall varies with the tissue. The true oncotic pressure is defined by

$$\pi = \sigma RT\,(C_i - C_o)$$

where

σ = Reflection coefficient
R = Gas constant
T = Absolute temperature

C_i and C_o = Solute (essentially albumin) concentration inside and outside the capillary

Of the plasma proteins, albumin is preponderate in determining oncotic pressure. The average albumin molecule (molecular weight 69,000) is approximately half the size of the average globulin molecule (molecular weight 150,000) and is present in almost twice the concentration as the globulins (4.5 vs. 2.5 g/100 ml of plasma). Albumin also exerts a greater osmotic force than can be accounted for solely on the basis of the number of molecules dissolved in the plasma. Therefore it cannot be completely replaced by inert substances of appropriate molecular size such as dextran. This additional osmotic force becomes disproportionately greater at high concentrations of albumin (as in plasma) and is weak to absent in dilute solutions of albumin (as in interstitial fluid). One reason for this behavior of albumin is its negative charge at the normal blood pH and the attraction and retention of cations (principally Na^+) in the vascular compartment (the **Gibbs-Donnan effect**). Furthermore, albumin binds a small number of chloride ions, which increases its negative charge and, hence, its ability to retain more sodium ions inside the capillaries. The small increase in electrolyte concentration of the plasma over that of the interstitial fluid produced by the negatively charged albumin enhances its osmotic force to that of an ideal solution containing a solute of molecular weight of 37,000. If albumin did indeed have a molecular weight of 37,000, it would not be retained by the capillary endothelium because of its small size, and obviously could not function as a counterforce to capillary hydrostatic pressure. If, however, albumin did not have an enhanced osmotic force, it would require a concentration of about 12 g of albumin/100 ml of plasma to achieve a plasma oncotic pressure of 25 mm Hg. Such a high albumin concentration would greatly increase blood viscosity and the resistance to blood flow through the vascular system. The other factors that contribute to the nonlinearity of the relationship of albumin concentration to osmotic force are not known. About 65% of plasma oncotic pressure is attributable to albumin, about 15% to the globulins, and the remainder to other ill-defined components of the plasma.

Small amounts of albumin escape from the capillaries and enter the interstitial fluid, where they exert a very small osmotic force (0.1 to 5 mm Hg). This force, π_i, is small because of the low concentration of albumin in the interstitial fluid and because at low concentrations the osmotic force of albumin becomes simply a function of the number of albumin molecules per unit volume of interstitial fluid.

Balance of Hydrostatic and Osmotic Forces. The relationship between hydrostatic pressure and oncotic pressure and the role of these forces in regulating fluid passage across the capillary endothelium were expounded by Starling in 1896 and constitute the **Starling hypothesis.** It can be expressed by the equation:

$$\text{Fluid movement} = k[(P_c + \pi_i) - (P_i + \pi_p)]$$

where

P_c = Capillary hydrostatic pressure
P_i = Interstitial fluid hydrostatic pressure
π_p = Plasma protein oncotic pressure
π_i = Interstitial fluid oncotic pressure
k = Filtration constant for the capillary membrane

Filtration occurs when the algebraic sum is positive, and absorption occurs when it is negative.

Classically, it has been thought that filtration occurs at the arterial end of the capillary and absorption at its venous end because of the gradient of hydrostatic pressure along the capillary. This is true for the idealized capillary as depicted in Fig. 7-7, but direct observations have revealed that many capillaries show filtration for their entire length, whereas others show only absorption. In some vascular beds (for example, the renal glomerulus) hydrostatic pressure in the capillary is high enough to result in filtration along the entire length of the capillary. In other vascular beds, such as in the intestinal mucosa, the hydrostatic and oncotic forces are such that absorption occurs along the whole capillary. As discussed earlier in this chapter, capillary pressure is quite variable and depends on several factors, the principal one being the contractile state of the precapillary vessel. In the normal steady state, arterial pressure, venous pressure, postcapillary resistance, interstitial fluid hydrostatic and oncotic pressures, and plasma oncotic pressure are relatively constant, and change in precapillary resistance is the determining factor with respect to fluid movement across the wall for any given capillary. Because water moves so quickly across the capillary endothelium, the hydrostatic and osmotic forces are nearly in equilibrium along the entire capillary. Hence filtration and absorption in the normal state occur at very small degrees of imbalance of pressure across the capillary wall. Only a small percentage (2%) of the plasma flowing through the vascular system is filtered, and of this about 85% is absorbed in the capillaries and venules. The remainder returns to the vascular system as lymph fluid along with the albumin that escapes from the capillaries.

In the lungs the mean capillary hydrostatic pressure is only about 8 mm Hg. Because the plasma oncotic pressure is 25 mm Hg and the lung interstitial fluid pressure is approximately 15 mm Hg, the net force slightly favors reabsorption. Nevertheless, pulmonary lymph is formed and consists of fluid that is osmotically drawn out of the capillaries by the small amount of plasma protein that escapes through the capillary endothelium. Only in pathologic conditions, such as left ventricular failure or stenosis of the mitral valve, does pulmonary capillary hydrostatic pressure exceed plasma oncotic pressure. When this occurs, it may lead to pulmonary edema, a condition that can seriously interfere with gas exchange in the lungs.

Capillary Filtration Coefficient. The rate of movement of fluid across the capillary membrane (Q_f) depends not only on the algebraic sum of the hydrostatic and osmotic forces across the endothelium (ΔP), but also on the area of the capillary wall available for filtration (A_m), the distance across the capillary wall (Δx), the viscosity of the filtrate (η), and the filtration constant of the membrane (k). These factors may be expressed by the equation:

$$Q_f = \frac{kA_m\Delta P}{\eta\Delta x}$$

The dimensions are units of flow per unit of pressure gradient across the capillary wall per unit of capillary surface area. This expression, which describes the flow of fluid through a membrane (pores), is essentially Poiseuille's law for flow through tubes (p. 120).

Because the thickness of the capillary wall and the viscosity of the filtrate are relatively constant, they can be included in the filtration constant, k, and if the area of the capillary membrane is not known, the rate of filtration can be expressed per unit weight of tissue. Hence the equation can be simplified to

$$Q_f = k_t \Delta P$$

where k_t is the capillary filtration coefficient for a given tissue, and the units for Q_f are milliliters per minute per 100 g of tissue per millimeter of mercury pressure.

The rate of filtration and absorption are determined by the rate of change in tissue weight or volume at different mean capillary hydrostatic pressures that are altered by adjustment of arterial and venous pressures. At the isogravimetric or isovolumic point (constant weight or contant volume, respectively, as continuously measured with an appropriate scale or volume recorder), the hydrostatic and osmotic forces are balanced across the capillary wall and there is neither net filtration nor absorption. An abrupt increase in arterial pressure will increase capillary hydrostatic pressure and fluid will move from the capillaries to the interstitial fluid compartment. Because the pressure increment, the weight increase of the tissue per unit time, and the total weight of the tissue are known, the capillary filtration coefficient (or k_t) in milliliters per minute per 100 g of tissue per millimeter of mercury can be calculated. With the isogravimetric and isovolumic techniques, it is assumed that 80% of the increments in venous pressure are transmitted back to the capillaries, that precapillary and postcapillary resistances are constant when venous pressure is changed, and that the weight or volume change that occurs immediately after raising venous pressure is the result of vascular distension and not filtration. These assumptions may not always be correct; nevertheless, the filtration coefficient constitutes a useful index of capillary permeability and surface area.

In any given tissue the filtration coefficient per unit area of capillary surface, and hence capillary permeability, is not changed by different physiologic conditions, such as arteriolar dilation and capillary distension, or by such adverse conditions as hypoxia, hypercapnia, or reduced pH. With capillary injury (toxins, severe burns) capillary permeability increases, as indicated by the filtration coefficient, and significant amounts of fluid and protein leak out of the capillaries into the interstitial space.

Because capillary permeability is constant under normal conditions, the filtration coefficient can be used to determine the relative number of open capillaries (total capillary surface area available for filtration in tissue). For example, increased metabolic activity of contracting skeletal muscle induces relaxation of precapillary resistance vessels with opening of more capillaries **(capillary recruitment,** resulting in an increased filtering surface area).

Some protein is apparently required to maintain the integrity of the endothelial membrane. If the plasma proteins are replaced by nonprotein colloids so as to give the same oncotic pressure, the filtration coefficient is doubled and edema occurs. However, if as little as 0.2% albumin is added, normal permeability is restored. One reasonable explanation is that the albumin binds to certain sites on the endothelial membrane and alters pore dimensions.

Disturbances in Hydrostatic-Osmotic Balance. Changes in arterial pressure per se may have little effect on filtration, because the change in pressure may be countered by adjustments of the precapillary resistance vessels (autoregulation, p. 175), so that hydrostatic pressure in the open capillaries remains the same. However, with severe reduction in arterial pressure, as may occur in hemorrhage, there may be arteriolar constriction mediated by the sympathetic nervous system and a fall in venous pressure resulting from the blood loss. These changes will lead to a decrease in the capillary hydrostatic pressure. Furthermore, the low blood pressure in hemorrhage causes a decrease in blood flow (and hence O_2 supply) to the tissue with the result that vasodilator metabolites accumulate and induce relaxation of arterioles. Precapillary vessel relaxation is also engendered by the reduced transmural pressure. As a consequence of these several factors, absorption predominates over filtration and occurs at a larger capillary surface area. This is one of the compensatory mechanisms employed by the body to restore blood volume (p. 274).

An increase in venous pressure alone, as occurs in the feet when one changes from the lying to the standing position, would elevate capillary pressure and enhance filtration. However, the increase in transmural pressure causes precapillary vessel closure (myogenic mechanism, p. 176) so that the capillary filtration coefficient actually decreases. This reduction in capillary surface available for filtration protects against the extravasation of large amounts of fluid into the interstitial space (edema). With prolonged standing, particularly when associated with some elevation of venous pressure in the legs (such as that caused by tight garters or pregnancy) or with sustained increases in venous pressure as seen in congestive heart failure, filtration is greatly enhanced and exceeds the capacity of the lymphatic system to remove the capillary filtrate from the interstitial space.

A large amount of fluid can move across the capillary wall in a relatively short time. In a normal individual the filtration coefficient (k_t) for the whole body is about 0.0061 ml/min/100 g of tissue/mm Hg. For a 70 kg man, elevation of venous pressure of 10 mm Hg for 10 minutes would increase filtration from capillaries by 342 ml. This would not lead to edema formation, because the fluid is returned to the vascular compartment by the lymphatic vessels. When edema does develop, it usually appears in the dependent parts of the body, where the hydrostatic pressure is greatest, but its location and magnitude are also determined by the type of tissue. Loose tissues, such as the subcutaneous tissue around the eyes or in the scrotum, are more prone to collect larger quantities of interstitial fluid than are firm tissues, such as muscle, or encapsulated structures, such as the kidney.

The concentration of the plasma proteins may also change in different pathologic states and, hence, alter the osmotic force and movement of fluid across the capillary membrane. The plasma protein concentration is increased in dehydration (for example, water deprivation, prolonged sweating, severe vomiting, and diarrhea), and water moves by osmotic forces from the tissues to the vascular compartment. In contrast, the plasma protein concentration is reduced in nephrosis (a renal disease in which there is loss of protein in the urine) and edema may occur. When capillary injury is extensive, as in burns, intravascular fluid and plasma protein leak into the interstitial space. The protein that escapes from the vessel lumen increases the oncotic pressure of the interstitial fluid. This greater osmotic force outside the capillaries leads to additional fluid loss and possibly to severe dehydration of the patient.

Pinocytosis.

Some transfer of substances across the capillary wall can occur in tiny pinocytotic vesicles **(pinocytosis).** These vesicles (see Figs. 7-4 and 7-5), formed by a pinching off of the surface membrane, can take up substances on one side of the capillary wall, move by thermal kinetic energy across the cell, and deposit their contents at the other side. The amount of material that can be transported in this way is very small relative to that moved by diffusion. However, pinocytosis may be responsible for the movement of large lipid-insoluble molecules (30 nm) between blood and interstitial fluid. The number of pinocytotic vesicles in endothelium varies with the tissue (muscle $>$ lung $>$ brain) and increases from the arterial to the venous end of the capillary.

■ LYMPHATICS

The terminal vessels of the lymphatic system consist of a widely distributed closed-end network of highly permeable lymph capillaries that are similar in appearance to blood capillaries. However, they are generally lacking in tight junctions between endothelial cells and possess fine filaments that anchor them to the surrounding connective tissue. With muscular contraction these fine strands may distort the lymphatic vessel to open spaces between the endothelial cells and permit the entrance of protein and large particles and cells present in the interstitial fluid. The lymph capillaries drain into larger vessels that finally enter the right and left subclavian veins at their junctions with the respective internal jugular veins. Only cartilage, bone, epithelium, and tissues of the central nervous system are devoid of lymphatic vessels. The plasma capillary filtrate is returned to the circulation by virtue of tissue pressure, facilitated by intermittent skeletal muscle activity, contractions of the lymphatic vessels, and an extensive system of one-way valves. In this respect they resemble the veins, although even the larger lymphatic vessels have thinner walls than the corresponding veins and contain only a small amount of elastic tissue and smooth muscle.

The volume of fluid transported through the lymphatics in 24 hours is about equal to an animal's total plasma volume and the protein returned by the lymphatics to the blood in a day is about one fourth to one half of the circulating plasma proteins. This is the only means whereby protein (albumin) that leaves the vascular compartment can be returned to the blood, because back diffusion into the capillaries cannot occur against the large albumin concentration gradient. Were the protein not removed by the lymph vessels, it would accumulate in the interstitial fluid and act as an oncotic force to draw fluid from the blood capillaries to produce edema. In addition to returning fluid and protein to the vascular bed, the lymphatic system filters the lymph at the lymph nodes and removes foreign particles, such as bacteria. The largest lymphatic vessel, the **thoracic duct,** in addition to draining the lower extremities, returns protein lost through the permeable liver capillaries and carries substances absorbed from the gastrointestinal tract, principally fat in the form of chylomicrons, to the circulating blood.

Lymph flow varies considerably, being almost nil from resting skeletal muscle and increasing during exercise in proportion to the degree of muscular activity. It is increased by any mechanism that enhances the rate of blood capillary filtration, for example, increased capillary pressure or permeability or decreased plasma oncotic pressure. When either the volume of interstitial fluid exceeds the drainage capacity of the lymphatics or the lymphatic vessels become blocked, as may occur in certain disease states, interstitial fluid accumulates, chiefly in the more compliant tissues (for example, subcutaneous tissue) and gives rise to clinical edema.

■ SUMMARY

1. Blood flow through the capillaries is chiefly regulated by contraction and relaxation of the arterioles (resistance vessels).
2. The capillaries, which consist of a single layer of endothelial cells, can withstand high transmural pressure by virtue of their small diameter. According to the law of Laplace T (wall tension) = P (transmural pressure) × r (radius of the capillary).
3. The endothelium is the soure of endothelial-derived relaxing factor (EDRF) and prostacyclin, which relax vascular smooth muscles.

4. Movement of water and small solutes between the vascular and interstitial fluid compartments occur through capillary pores *mainly by diffusion* but also by filtration and absorption.
5. Because the rate of diffusion is about 40× greater than the blood flow in the tissue, exchange of small lipid insoluble molecules is **flow limited.** The larger the molecules the slower the diffusion until with large molecules the lipid insoluble molecules become **diffusion limited.** Molecules larger than about 60,000 kd are essentially confined to the vascular compartment.
6. Lipid-soluble substances such as CO_2 and O_2 pass directly through the lipid membranes of the capillary, and the ease of transfer is directly proportional to the degree of lipid solubility of the substance.
7. Capillary filtration and absorption are described by the Starling equation: Fluid movement $= k[(P_c + \pi_i) - (P_i + \pi_p)]$ where P_c = capillary hydrostatic pressure; P_i = interstitial fluid hydrostatic pressure; π_i = interstitial fluid oncotic pressure; π_p = plasma protein oncotic pressure. Filtration occurs when the algebraic sum is positive, and absorption occurs when it is negative.
8. Large molecules can move across the capillary wall in vesicles formed from the lipid membrane of the capillaries by a process called **pinocytosis.**
9. Fluid and protein that have escaped from the blood capillaries enter the lymphatic capillaries and are transported via the lymphatic system back to the blood vascular compartment.

■ BIBLIOGRAPHY

Journal articles

Bundgaard, M.: Transport pathways in capillaries—in search of pores, Ann. Rev. Physiol. 42:325, 1980.

Duling, B.R., and Klitzman, B.: Local control of microvascular function: role in tissue oxygen supply, Ann. Rev. Physiol. 42:373, 1980.

Feng, Q., and Hedner, T.: Endothelium-derived relaxing factor (EDRF) and nitric oxide II. Physiology, pharmacology and pathophysiological implications, Clin. Physiol. 10:503, 1990.

Furchgott, R.F., and Vanhoutte, P.M.: Endothelium-derived relaxing and contracting factors, FASEB J. 3:2007, 1989.

Gore, R.W., and McDonagh, P.F.: Fluid exchange across single capillaries, Ann. Rev. Physiol. 42:337, 1980.

Krogh, A.: The number and distribution of capillaries in muscles with calculation of the oxygen pressure head necessary for supplying the tissue, J. Physiol. 52:409, 1919.

Lewis, D.H., editor: Symposium on lymph circulation, Acta Physiol. Scand. Suppl. 463:9, 1979.

Rosell, S.: Neuronal control of microvessels, Ann. Rev. Physiol. 42:359, 1980.

Starling, E.H.: On the absorption of fluids from the connective tissue spaces, J. Physiol. 19:312, 1896.

Books and monographs

Bert, J.L., and Pearce, R.H.: The interstitium and microvascular exchange. In Handbook of physiology; Section 2: The cardiovascular system—microcirculation, vol. IV, Bethesda, Md., 1984, American Physiological Society.

Crone, C., and Levitt, D.G.: Capillary permeability to small solutes. In Handbook of physiology; Section 2: The cardiovascular system—microcirculation, vol. IV, Bethesda, Md., 1984, American Physiological Society.

Hudlicka, O.: Development of microcirculation: capillary growth and adaptation. In Handbook of physiology; Section 2: The cardiovascular system—microcirculation, vol. IV, Bethesda, Md., 1984, American Physiological Society.

Krogh, A.: The anatomy and physiology of capillaries, New York, 1959, Hafner Co.

Luscher, T.F., and Vanhoutte, P.M.: The endothelium: modulator of cardiovascular function, Boca Raton, Fla., 1990, CRC Press.

Michel, C.C.: Fluid movements through capillary walls. In Handbook of physiology, Section 2: The cardiovascular system—microcirculation, vol. IV, Bethesda, Md., 1984, American Physiological Society.

Mortillaro, N.A.: Physiology and pharmacology of the microcirculation, vol. 1, New York, 1983, Academic Press, Inc.

Renkin, E.M.: Control microcirculation and blood-tissue exchange. In Handbook of physiology; Section 2: The cardiovascular system—microcirculation, vol. IV, Bethesda, Md., 1984, American Physiological Society.

Shepro, D., and D'Amore, P.A.: Physiology and biochemistry of the vascular wall endothelium. In Handbook of physiology; Section 2: The cardiovascular system—microcirculation, vol. IV, Bethesda, Md., 1984, American Physiological Society.

Simionescu, M., and Simionescu, N.: Ultrastructure of the microvascular wall: functional correlations. In Handbook of physiology; Section 2: The cardiovascular system—microcirculation, vol. IV, Bethesda, Md., 1984, American Physiological Society.

Taylor, A.E., and Granger, D.N.: Exchange of macromolecules across the microcirculation. In Handbook of physiology; Section 2: The cardiovascular system—microcirculation, vol. IV, Bethesda, Md., 1984, American Physiological Society.

Wiedeman, M.P.: Architecture. In Handbook of physiology; Section 2: The cardiovascular system—microcirculation, vol. IV, Bethesda, Md., 1984, American Physiological Society.

Yoffey, J.M., and Courtice, F.C.: Lymphatics, lymph and the lymphomyeloid complex, London, 1970, Academic Press.

Zweifach, B.W., and Lipowsky, H.H.: Pressure-flow relations in blood and lymph microcirculation. In Handbook of physiology; Section 2: The cardiovascular system—microcirculation, vol. IV, Bethesda, Md., 1984, American Physiological Society.

8 The Peripheral Circulation and Its Control

The peripheral circulation is essentially under dual control, centrally through the nervous system and locally in the tissues by the environmental conditions in the immediate vicinity of the blood vessels. The relative importance of these two control mechanisms is not the same in all tissues. In some areas of the body, such as the skin and the splanchnic regions, neural regulation of blood flow predominates, whereas in others, such as the heart and brain, this mechanism plays a minor role.

The vessels chiefly involved in regulating the rate of blood flow throughout the body are called the **resistance vessels** (arterioles). These vessels offer the greatest resistance to the flow of blood pumped to the tissues by the heart and thereby are important in the maintenance of arterial blood pressure. Smooth muscle fibers constitute a large percentage of the composition of the walls of the resistance vessels (see Fig. 1-1). Therefore, the vessel lumen can be varied from one that is completely obliterated by strong contraction of the smooth muscle, with infolding of the endothelial lining, to one that is maximally dilated as a result of full relaxation of the vascular smooth muscle. Some resistance vessels are closed at any given moment in time and partial contraction **(tone)** of the vascular smooth muscle exists in the arterioles. Were all the resistance vessels in the body to dilate simultaneously, blood pressure would fall precipitously to very low levels.

■ VASCULAR SMOOTH MUSCLE

Vascular smooth muscle is the tissue responsible for the control of total peripheral resistance, arterial and venous tone, and the distribution of blood flow throughout the body. The smooth muscle cells are small, mononucleate, and spindle shaped. They are generally arranged in helical or circular layers around the larger blood vessels and in a single circular layer around arterioles (Fig. 8-1, *A* and *B*).). Also, parts of endothelial cells project into the vascular smooth muscle layer **(myoendothelial junctions)** at various points along the arterioles (Fig. 8-1, *C*). These projections suggest a functional interaction between endothelium and adjacent vascular smooth muscle. In general, the close association between action potentials and contraction observed in skeletal

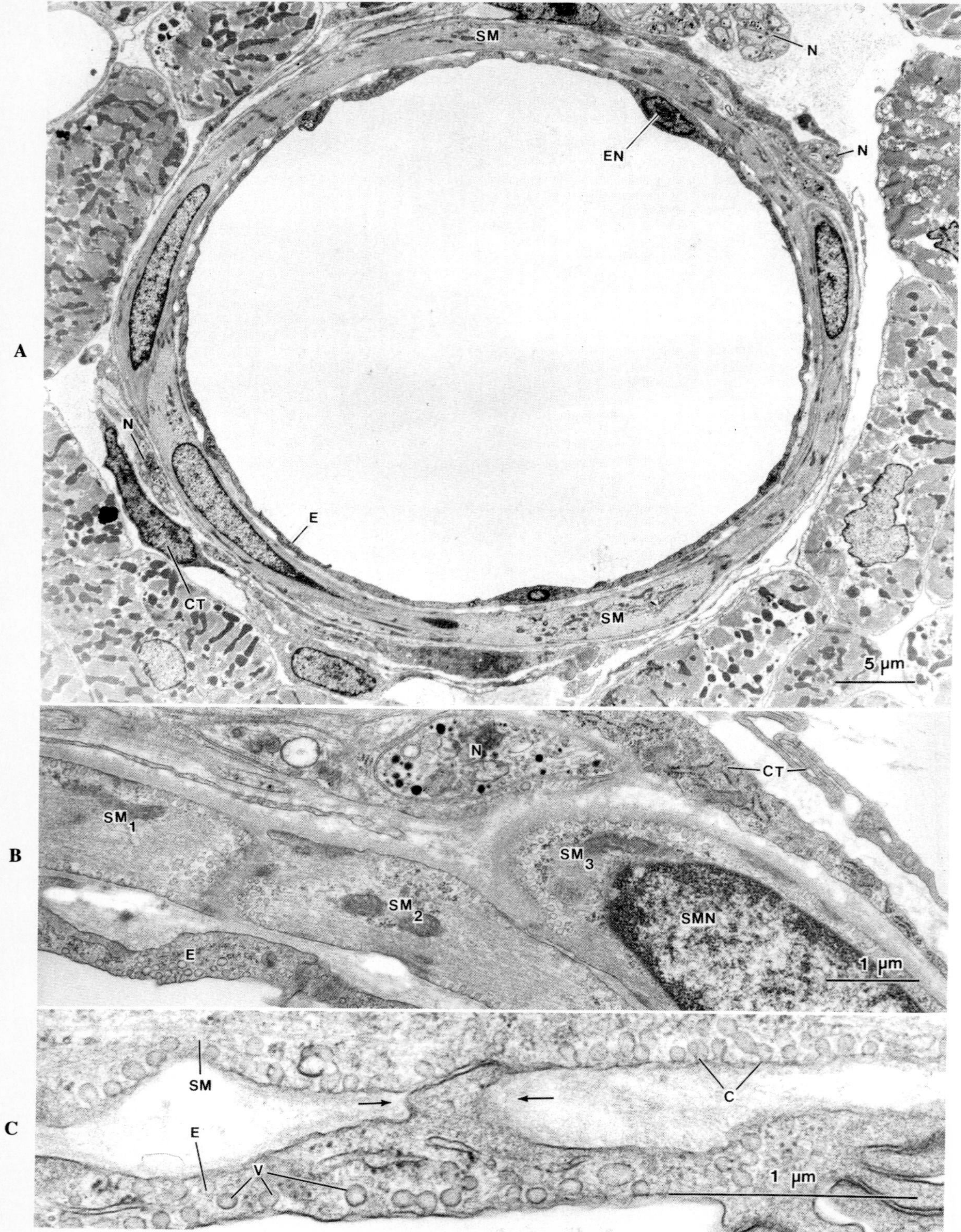

Fig. 8-1 ■ For legend see opposite page.

Fig. 8-1 ■ **A,** Low-magnification electron micrograph of an arteriole in cross section (inner diameter of approximately 40 μm) in cat ventricle. The wall of the blood vessel is composed largely of vascular smooth muscle cells *(SM)* whose long axes are directed approximately circularly around the vessel. A single layer of endothelial cells *(E)* forms the innermost portion of the blood vessel. Connective tissue elements *(CT)* such as fibroblasts and collagen make up the adventitial layer at the periphery of the vessel; nerve bundles also appear in this layer *(N). EN,* Endothelial cell nucleus. **B,** Detail of the wall of the blood vessel in panel **A.** This field contains a single endothelial layer *(E),* the medial smooth muscle layer (three smooth muscle cell profiles: SM_1, SM_2, SM_3), and the adventitial layer (containing nerves *[N]* and connective tissue *[CT]*). *SMN,* Smooth muscle nucleus. **C,** Another region of the arteriole, showing the area in which the endothelial *(E)* and smooth muscle *(SM)* layers are apposed. A projection of an endothelial cell (between arrows) is closely applied to the surface of the overlying smooth muscle, forming a "myoendothelial junction." Plasmalemmal vesicles are prominent in both the endothelium *(V)* and the smooth muscle cell (where such vesicles are known as "caveolae," *C*).

and cardiac muscle cells cannot be demonstrated in vascular smooth muscle, and vascular smooth muscle lacks transverse tubules.

Graded changes in membrane potential are often associated with increases or decreases in force. Contractile activity is generally elicited by neural or humoral stimuli. The behavior of smooth muscle in different vessels varies. For example, some vessels, particularly in the portal or mesenteric circulation, contain longitudinally oriented smooth muscle that is spontaneously active and that shows action potentials which are correlated with the contractions and the electrical coupling between cells.

The vascular smooth muscle cells contain large numbers of thin, actin filaments and comparatively small numbers of thick, myosin filaments. These filaments are aligned in the long axis of the cell but do not form visible sarcomeres with striations. Nevertheless, the sliding filament mechanism is believed to operate in this tissue, and phosphorylation of crossbridges regulates their rate of cycling. Compared to skeletal muscle, the smooth muscle contracts very slowly, develops high forces, maintains force for long periods of time with low ATP utilization, and operates over a considerable range of lengths under physiological conditions. Cell to cell conduction is via gap junctions as occurs in cardiac muscle. (see p. 55).

The interaction between myosin and actin, leading to contraction, is controlled by the myoplasmic Ca^{++} concentration as in other muscles, but the molecular mechanism whereby Ca^{++} regulates contraction differs. For example, smooth muscle lacks troponin and fast sodium channels. The increased myoplasmic Ca^{++} that elicits contraction can come through voltage gated calcium channels **(electromechanical coupling)** and through receptor-operated calcium channels **(pharmacomechanical coupling)** in the sarcolemma, and by release from the sarcoplasmic reticulum (Fig. 8-2). The cells relax when intracellular free Ca^{++} is pumped back into the sarcoplasmic reticulum and is extruded from the cell by the calcium pump in the cell membrane and by the Na-Ca exchanger.

The response to humoral stimuli, which is termed pharmacomechanical coupling, occurs without evidence of electrical excitation and is the predominant mechanism for eliciting contraction of vascular smooth muscle. In the category of pharmacological stimuli are such substances as catecholamines, histamine, acetyl-

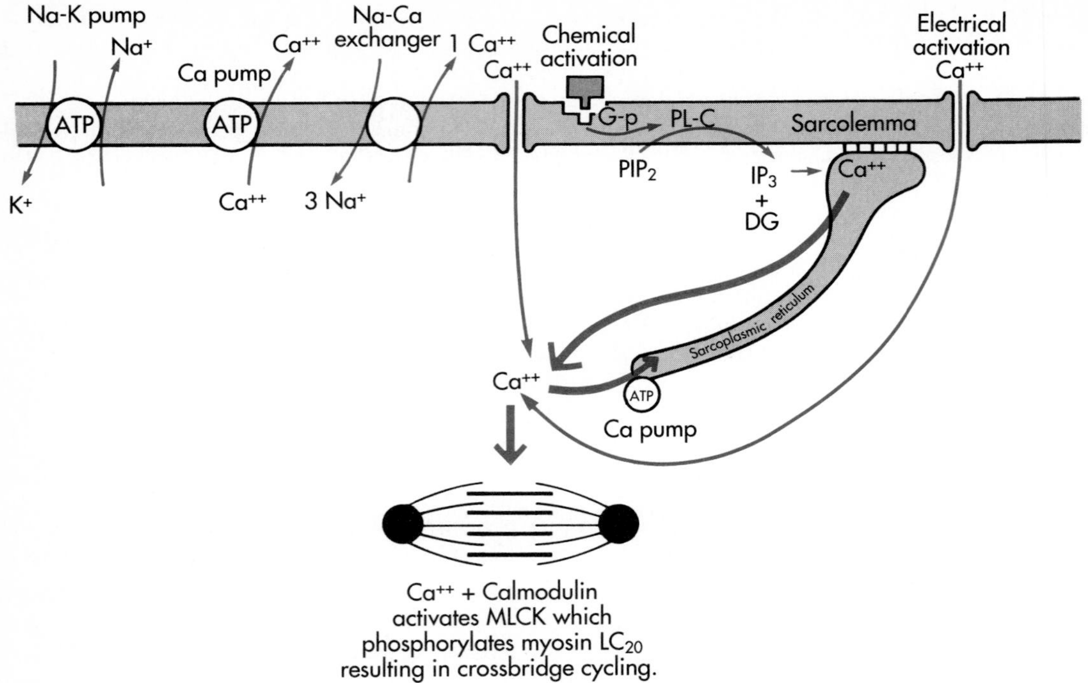

Fig. 8-2 ■ Excitation-contraction coupling in vascular smooth muscle. Calcium can enter the cell via electrically activated channels (electromechanical coupling) or via receptor-operated channels (chemical activation, termed pharmacomechanical coupling) in the sarcolemma. Calcium is also released from the sarcoplasmic reticulum in response to IP_3 stimulation and is taken back into the sarcoplasmic reticulum by a calcium pump. Calcium is extruded from the cell by a calcium pump and by the Na-Ca exchanger. G-p, guanine nucleotide binding protein; Pl-C, phospholipase C; PiP_2, phosphatidyl inositol bisphosphate; IP_3, inositol trisphosphate; D.G., diacylglycerol; MLCK, myosin light chain kinase.

choline, serotonin, angiotensin, adenosine, and prostaglandins.

As illustrated in Fig. 8-2 an agonist activates receptors in the vascular smooth muscle membrane. These receptors in turn activate phospholipase C in a reaction coupled to guanine nucleotide binding proteins (G proteins). The phospholipase C hydrolyzes phosphatidyl inositol bisphosphate in the membrane to yield diacylglycerol and inositol trisphosphate; the latter causes the release of Ca^{++} from the sarcoplasmic reticulum. The Ca^{++} binds to calmodulin, which in turn binds to myosin light chain kinase. This activated Ca^{++}-calmodulin-myosin kinase complex phosphorylates the light chains (20,000 dalton) of myosin. The phosphorylated myosin ATPase is then activated by actin, and the resulting crossbridge cycling initiates contraction.

Finally, the sensitivity of the contractile regulatory apparatus to Ca^{++} is increased by agonists. The mechanism for this enhanced sensitivity is still unclear but appears to involve G proteins. Relaxation occurs when the myosin light chain kinase is inactivated by dephosphorylation and the cytosolic Ca^{++} is lowered by

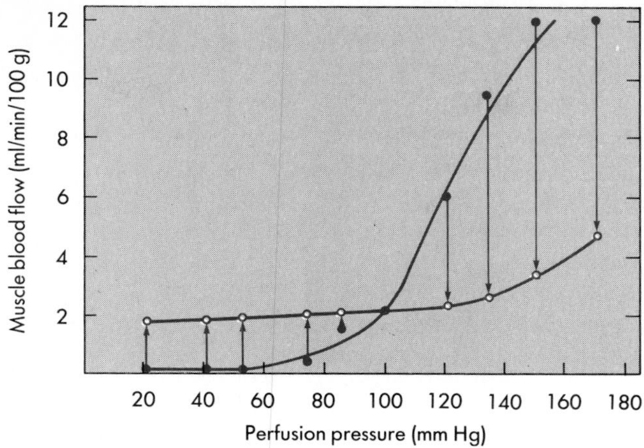

Fig. 8-3 ■ Pressure-flow relationship in the skeletal muscle vascular bed of the dog. The closed circles represent the flows obtained immediately after abrupt changes in perfusion pressure from the control level (point where lines cross). The open circles represent the steady-state flows obtained at the new perfusion pressure. (Redrawn from Jones, R.D., and Berne, R.M.: Circ. Res. 14:126, 1964.)

sarcoplasmic reticulum uptake and by Ca^{++} extrusion by the Ca pump and the Na-Ca exchanger. Local environmental changes alter the contractile state of vascular smooth muscle, and alterations such as increased temperature or increased carbon dioxide levels induce relaxation of this tissue.

Most of the arteries and veins of the body are supplied to different degrees solely by fibers of the sympathetic nervous system (see Fig. 8-1, *A* and *B*). These nerve fibers exert a tonic effect on the blood vessels, as evidenced by the fact that cutting or freezing the sympathetic nerves to a vascular bed (such as muscle) results in an increase in blood flow. Activation of the sympathetic nerves either directly or reflexly (p. 180 and 184) enhances vascular resistance. In contrast to the sympathetic nerves the parasympathetic nerves tend to decrease vascular resistance, but they innervate only a small fraction of the blood vessels in the body, mainly in certain viscera and pelvic organs.

■ INTRINSIC OR LOCAL CONTROL OF PERIPHERAL BLOOD FLOW

Autoregulation and Myogenic Regulation

In a number of different tissues the blood flow appears to be adjusted to the existing metabolic activity of the tissue. Furthermore, imposed changes in the perfusion pressure (arterial blood pressure) at constant levels of tissue metabolism, as measured by oxygen consumption, are met with vascular resistance changes that tend to maintain a constant blood flow. This mechanism is commonly referred to as **autoregulation** of blood flow and is illustrated graphically in Fig. 8-3. In the skeletal muscle preparation from which these data were gathered, the muscle was completely isolated from the rest of the animal and was in a resting state. From a control pressure of 100 mm Hg, the pressure was abruptly increased or decreased, and the blood flows observed immediately after changing the perfusion pressure are represented by the closed circles. Maintenance of the altered pressure at each new level was followed within 30 to 60 seconds by a return of flow to or toward the control levels; the open circles represent these steady-state flows. Over the pressure range of 20 to 120 mm Hg, the steady-state flow is relatively constant. Calculation of resistance across the vascular bed (pressure/flow) during steady-state conditions indicates that with elevation of perfusion pressure the resistance vessels constricted, whereas with reduction of perfusion pressure, they dilated.

The mechanism responsible for this constancy of blood flow in the presence of an altered perfusion pressure is not known, but it appears to be explained best by the **myogenic mechanism.**

According to the myogenic mechanism, the vascular smooth muscle contracts in response to stretch and relaxes with a reduction in tension. Therefore, the initial flow increment produced by an abrupt increase in perfusion pressure that passively distends the blood vessels would be followed by a return of flow to the previous control level by contraction of the smooth muscles of the resistance vessels.

An example of a myogenic response is shown in Fig. 8-4. Arterioles isolated from the hearts of young pigs were cannulated at each end, and the transmural pressure (intravascular pressure minus extravascular pressure) and flow through the arteriole could be adjusted to desired levels. With no flow through the arteri-

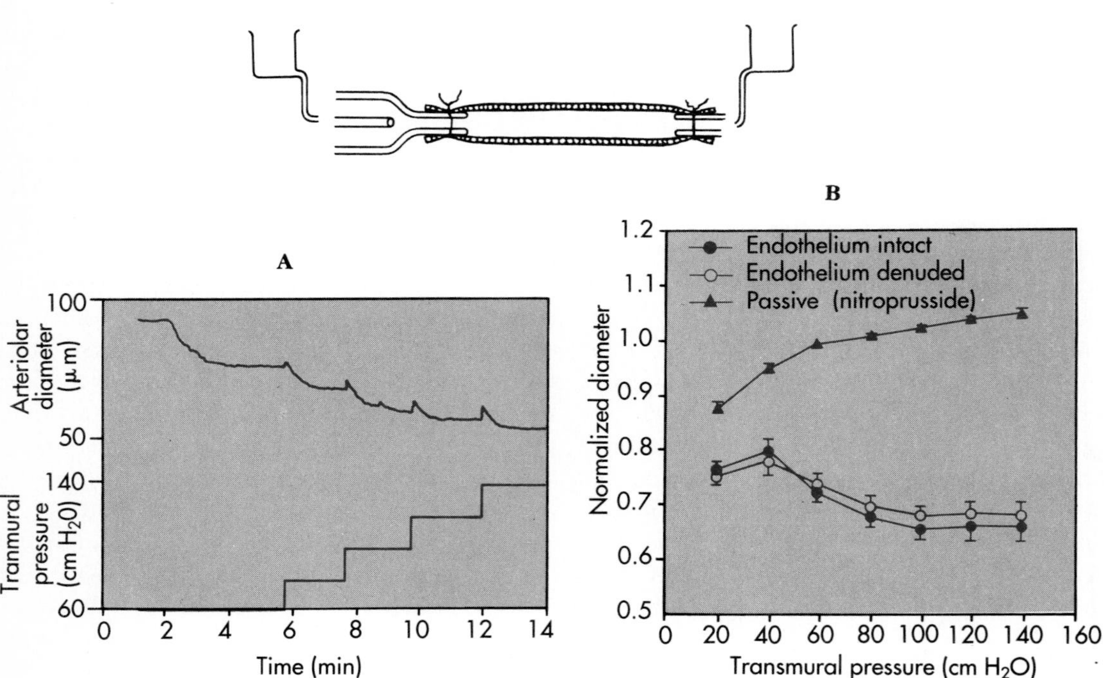

Fig. 8-4 ■ **A,** Constriction of an isolated cardiac arteriole in response to increases in transmural pressure without flow through the blood vessel. **B,** Constrictor response of the arteriole to an increase in transmural pressure is unaffected by removal of its endothelium. When the smooth muscle is relaxed by nitroprusside, the arteriole is passively distended by the increase in transmural pressure. (Redrawn from Kuo, L., Davis, M.J., and Chilian, W.M.: Am. J. Physiol. 259:H1063, 1990).

ole, successive increases of transmural pressure elicited progressive decreases in the vessel diameter (Fig. 8-4, *A*). This response was independent of the endothelium because it was identical in intact vessels and in vessels denuded of endothelium (Fig. 8-4, *B*). Arterioles that were relaxed by direct action of nitroprusside on the vascular smooth muscle showed only a passive increase in diameter when transmural pressure was increased. How vessel distension elicits contraction is unsettled, but because stretch of vascular smooth muscle elevates intracellular Ca^{++}, it has been proposed that an increase in transmural pressure activates membrane calcium channels.

Because blood pressure is reflexly maintained at a fairly constant level under normal conditions, operation of a myogenic mechanism would be expected to be minimized. However, when one changes position (from lying to standing) a large change in transmural pressure occurs in the lower extremities. The precapillary vessels constrict in response to this imposed stretch, which results in cessation of flow in most capillaries. After flow stops, capillary filtration diminishes until the increase in plasma oncotic pressure and the increase in interstitial fluid pressure balance the elevated capillary hydrostatic pressure produced by changing from a horizontal to a vertical position. If arteriolar resistance did not increase with standing, the hydrostatic pressure in the lower parts of the legs would reach such high levels that large volumes of fluid would pass from the capillaries into the interstitial fluid compartment and produce edema.

Endothelial-Mediated Regulation

As discussed on p. 156, stimulation of the endothelium can elicit a vasoactive response of the vascular smooth muscle. Endothelial-mediated dilation, in the same preparation described for Fig. 8-4, is illustrated in Fig. 8-5. Transmural pressure is kept constant and flow through the isolated arteriole is increased by raising the perfusion fluid reservoir connected to one end of the arteriole and simultaneously lowering the reservoir connected to the other

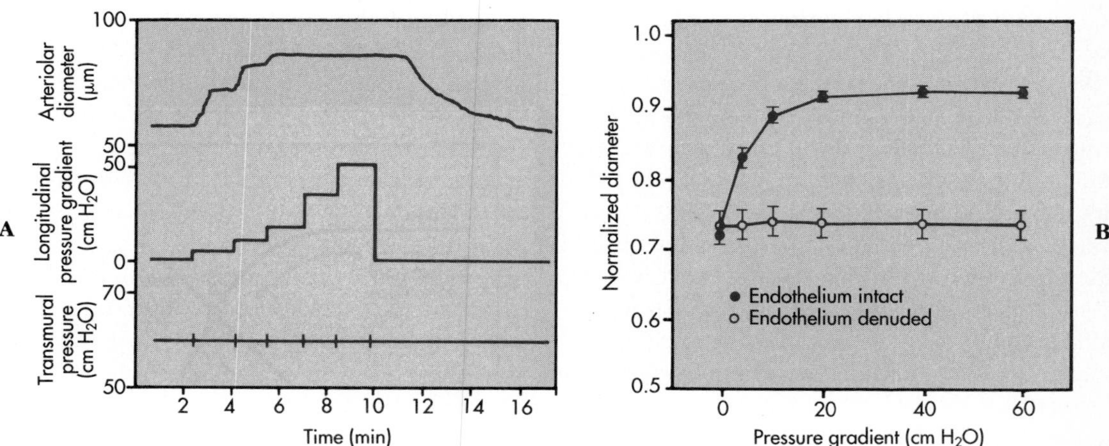

Fig. 8-5 ■ **A,** Flow-induced vasodilation in an isolated cardiac arteriole at constant transmural pressure. Flow was increased progressively by increasing the pressure gradient in the long axis of the arteriole (longitudinal pressure gradient). **B,** Flow-induced vasodilation is abolished by removal of the endothelium of the arteriole. (Redrawn from Kuo, L., Davis, M.J., and Chilian, W.M.: Am. J. Physiol. 259:H1063, 1990).

end of the arteriole by an equal distance. This elevation of pressure gradient along the vessel axis (longitudinal pressure gradient) increases flow and increases vessel diameter (Fig. 8-5, *A*). If the arteriole is denuded of endothelium, the dilation of the vessel in response to increased flow is abolished (Fig. 8-5, *B*). The vasodilation is presumably caused by the endothelial-derived relaxing factor (EDRF) (see p. 156), which is released from the endothelium in response to the shear stress consequent to the increase in velocity of flow.

Metabolic Regulation

According to the metabolic mechanism, blood flow is governed by the metabolic activity of the tissue. Any intervention that results in an O_2 supply that is inadequate for the requirements of the tissue gives rise to the formation of vasodilator metabolites. These metabolites are released from the tissue and act locally to dilate the resistance vessels. When the metabolic rate of the tissue increases or the O_2 delivery to the tissue decreases, more vasodilator substance is released and the metabolite concentration in the tissue increases.

Many substances have been proposed as mediators of metabolic vasodilation. Some of the earliest ones suggested are lactic acid, CO_2, and hydrogen ions. However, the decrease in vascular resistance induced by supernormal concentrations of these dilator agents falls considerably short of the dilation observed under physiological conditions of increased metabolic activity.

Changes in O_2 tension can evoke changes in the contractile state of vascular smooth muscle; an increase in Po_2 elicits contraction, and a decrease in Po_2, relaxation. If significant reductions in the intravascular Po_2 occur before the arterial blood reaches the resistance vessels (diffusion through the arterial and arteriolar walls, p. 162), small changes in O_2 supply or consumption could elicit contraction or relaxation of the resistance vessels. However, direct measurements of Po_2 at the resistance vessels indicate that over a wide range of Po_2 (11 to 343 mm Hg) there is no correlation between O_2 tension and arteriolar diameter. Furthermore, if Po_2 were directly responsible for vascular smooth muscle tension, one would not expect to find a parallelism between the duration of arterial occlusion and the duration of the reactive hyperemia (flow above control level upon release of an arterial occlusion) (Fig. 8-6). With either short occlusions (5 to 10 seconds) or long occlusions (1 to 3 minutes) the venous blood becomes bright red (well oxygenated) within 1 or 2 seconds after release of the arterial occlusion and hence the smooth muscle of the resistance vessels must be exposed to a high Po_2 in each instance. Nevertheless, the longer occlusions result in longer periods of reactive hyperemia. These observations are more compatible with the release of a vasodilator metabolite from the tissue than with a direct effect of Po_2 on the vascular smooth muscle.

Potassium ions, inorganic phosphate, and interstitial fluid osmolarity can also induce vasodilation. Because K^+ and phosphate are released and osmolarity is increased during skeletal muscle contraction, it has been proposed that these factors contribute to **active hyperemia** (increased blood flow caused by enhanced tissue activity). However, significant increases of phosphate concentration and osmolarity are not consistently observed during muscle contraction, and they may produce only transient increases in blood flow. Therefore, they are not likely candidates as mediators of the vasodilation observed with muscular activity. Potassium release occurs with the onset of skeletal muscle contraction or an increase in cardiac activity and could be responsible for the initial decrease in vascular

Bradykinin also has been reported to be formed in other exocrine glands, such as the lacrimal glands and the sweat glands. Its presence in sweat is thought to be partly responsible for the dilation of cutaneous blood vessels that occurs with sweating.

Humoral Factors

Epinephrine and norepinephrine exert a profound effect on the peripheral blood vessels. In skeletal muscle, epinephrine in low concentrations dilates resistance vessels (**beta-adrenergic effect**) and in high concentrations produces constriction (**alpha-adrenergic effect**). In skin only vasoconstriction is obtained with epinephrine, whereas in all vascular beds the primary effect of norepinephrine is vasoconstriction. When stimulated, the adrenal gland can release epinephrine and norepinephrine into the systemic circulation. However, under physiological conditions, the effect of catecholamine release from the adrenal medulla is of lesser importance than norepinephrine release produced by sympathetic nerve activation.

Vascular Reflexes

Areas of the medulla that mediate sympathetic and vagal effects are under the influence of neural impulses arising in the baroreceptors, chemoreceptors, hypothalamus, cerebral cortex, and skin. These areas of the medulla are also affected by changes in the blood concentrations of CO_2 and O_2.

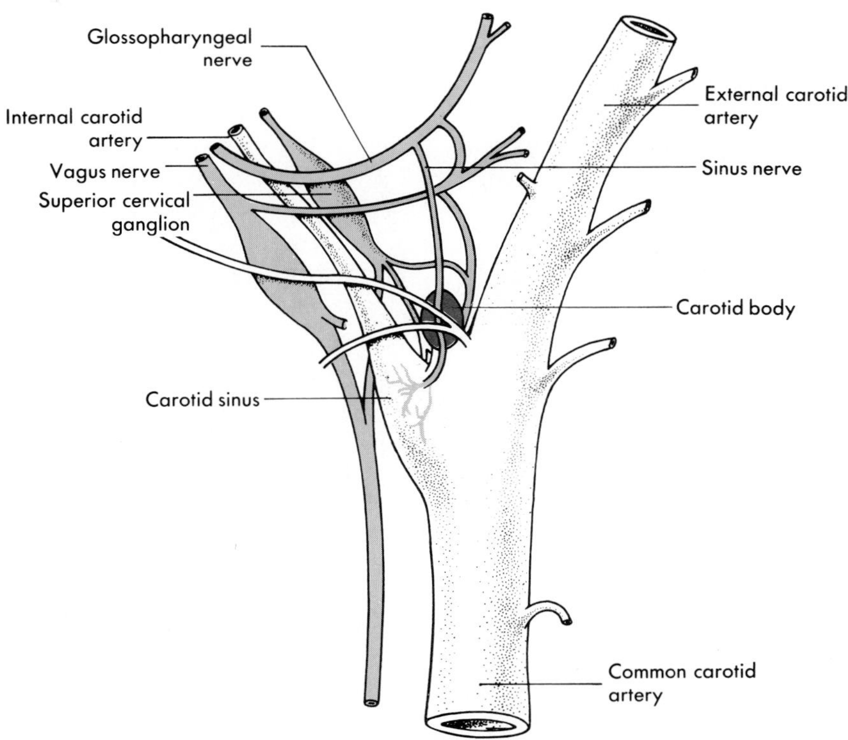

Fig. 8-8 ■ Diagrammatic representation of the carotid sinus and carotid body and their innervation in the dog. (Redrawn from Adams, W.E.: The comparative morphology of the carotid body and carotid sinus, Springfield, Ill., 1958, Charles C Thomas, Publisher.)

Arterial Baroreceptors. The **baroreceptors** (or **pressoreceptors**) are stretch receptors located in the carotid sinuses (slightly widened areas of the internal carotid arteries at their points of origin from the common carotid arteries) and in the aortic arch (Figs. 8-8 and 8-9). Impulses arising in the carotid sinus travel up the sinus nerve (nerve of Hering) to the glossopharyngeal nerve and, via the latter, to the nucleus of the tractus solitarius (NTS) in the medulla. The NTS is the site of central projection of the chemoreceptors and baroreceptors. Stimulation of the NTS inhibits sympathetic nerve impulses to the peripheral blood vessels (depressor), whereas lesions of the NTS produce vasoconstriction (pressor). Impulses arising in the pressoreceptors of the aortic arch reach the NTS via afferent fibers in the vagus nerves. The pressoreceptor nerve terminals in the walls of the carotid sinus and aortic arch respond to the stretch and deformation of the vessel induced by the arterial pressure. The frequency of firing is enhanced by an increase in blood pressure and diminished by a reduction in blood pressure. An increase in impulse frequency, as occurs with a rise in arterial pres-

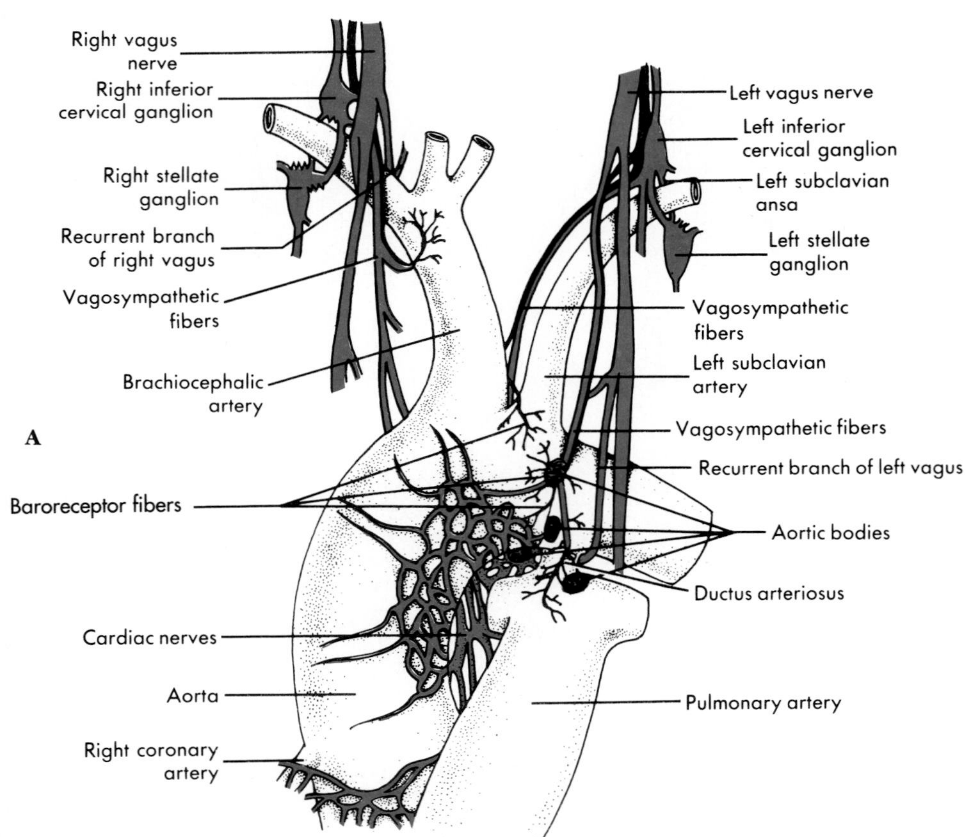

Fig. 8-9 ■ Anterior view of the aortic arch showing the innervation of the aortic bodies and pressoreceptors in the dog. (Modified from Nonidez, J.F.: Anat. Rec. 69:299, 1937.)

sure, inhibits the vasoconstrictor regions, resulting in peripheral vasodilation and a lowering of blood pressure. Contributing to a lowering of the blood pressure is a bradycardia brought about by stimulation of the vagal regions. The carotid sinus and aortic baroreceptors are not equipotent in their effects on peripheral resistance in response to nonpulsatile alterations in blood pressure. The carotid sinus baroreceptors are more sensitive than those in the aortic arch. Changes in pressure in the carotid sinus evoke greater alterations in systemic arterial pressure than do equivalent changes in aortic arch pressure. However, with pulsatile changes in blood pressure the two sets of baroreceptors respond similarly.

The carotid sinus with the sinus nerve intact can be isolated from the rest of the circulation and perfused by either a donor animal or an artificial perfusion system. Under these conditions changes in the pressure within the carotid sinus are associated with reciprocal changes in the blood pressure of the experimental animal. The receptors in the walls of the carotid sinus show some adaptation and therefore are more responsive to constantly

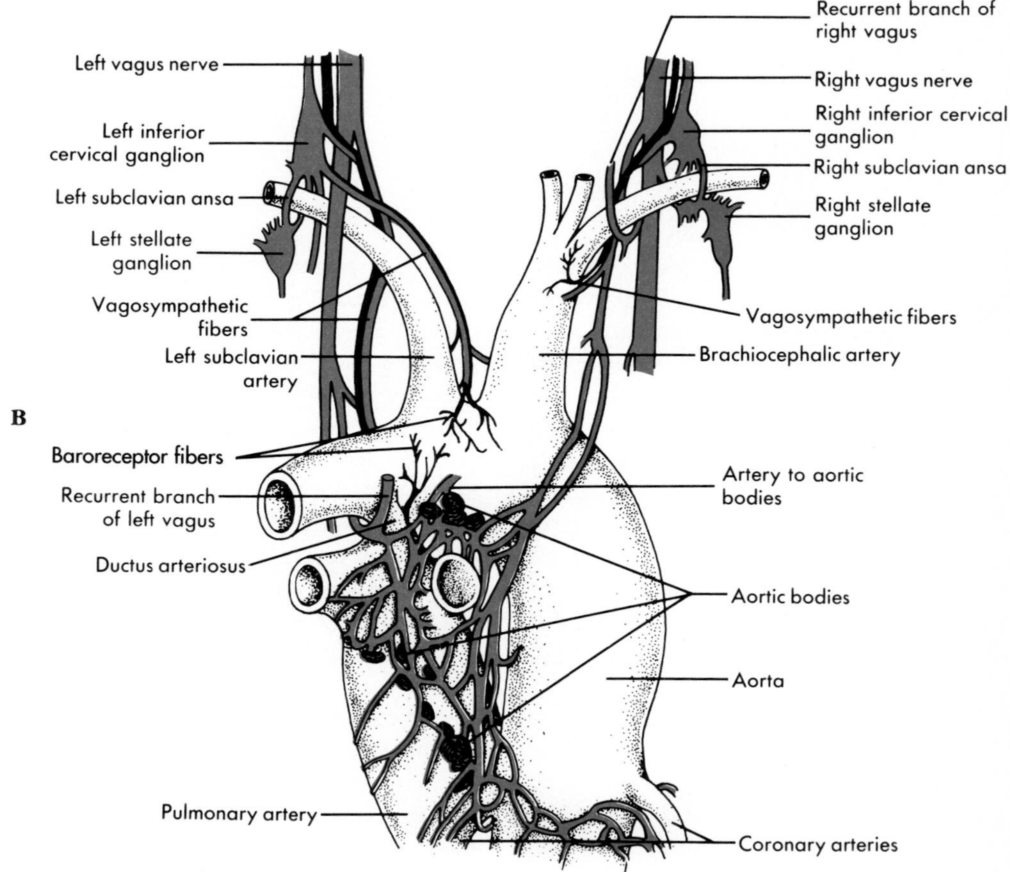

Fig. 8-9, cont'd ■ Posterior view of the aortic arch showing the innervation of the aortic bodies and pressoreceptors in the dog. (Modified from Nonidez, J.F.: Anat. Rec. 69:299, 1937.)

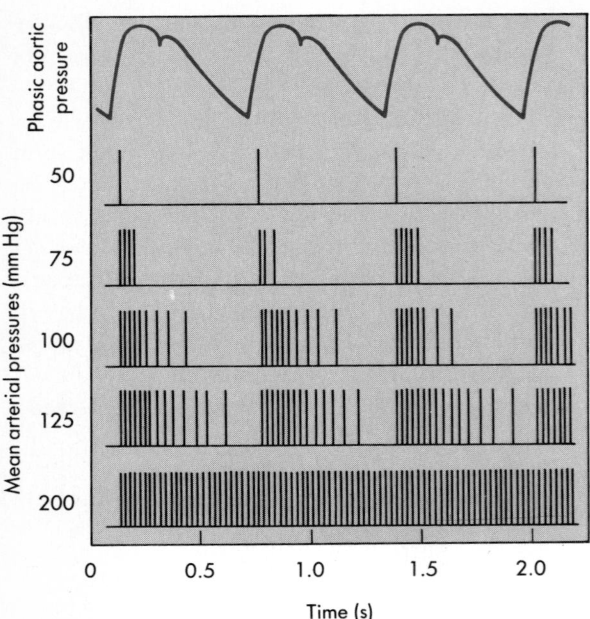

Fig. 8-10 ■ Relationship of phasic aortic blood pressure in the firing of a single afferent nerve fiber from the carotid sinus at different levels of mean arterial pressure.

changing pressures than to sustained constant pressures. This is illustrated in Fig. 8-10, where at normal levels of blood pressure a barrage of impulses from a single fiber of the sinus nerve is initiated in early systole by the pressure rise and only a few spikes are observed during late systole and early diastole. At lower pressures these phasic changes are even more evident, but the overall frequency of discharge is reduced. The blood pressure threshold for eliciting sinus nerve impulses is about 50 mm Hg, and a maximum sustained firing is reached at around 200 mm Hg. Because the pressoreceptors show some degree of adaptation, their response at any level of mean arterial pressure is greater with a large than with a small pulse pressure. This is illustrated in Fig. 8-11, which shows the effects of damping pulsations in the carotid sinus on the frequency of firing in a fiber of the sinus nerve and on the systemic arterial pressure. When the pulse pressure in the carotid sinuses is reduced with an air chamber, but mean pressure remains constant, the rate of electrical impulses recorded from a sinus nerve fiber decreases and the systemic arterial pressure increases. Restoration of the pulse pressure in the carotid sinus restores the frequency of sinus nerve discharge and systemic arterial pressure to control levels (see Fig. 8-11).

The resistance increases that occur in the peripheral vascular beds in response to a reduced pressure in the carotid sinus vary from one vascular bed to another and thereby produce a redistribution of blood flow. For example, in the dog the resistance changes elicited by altering carotid sinus pressure around the normal operating sinus pressure are greatest in the femoral vessels, less in the renal, and least in the mesenteric and celiac vessels. Furthermore, the sensitivity of the carotid sinus reflex can be altered. Local application of norepinephrine or stimulation of sympathetic nerve fibers to the carotid sinuses enhances the sen-

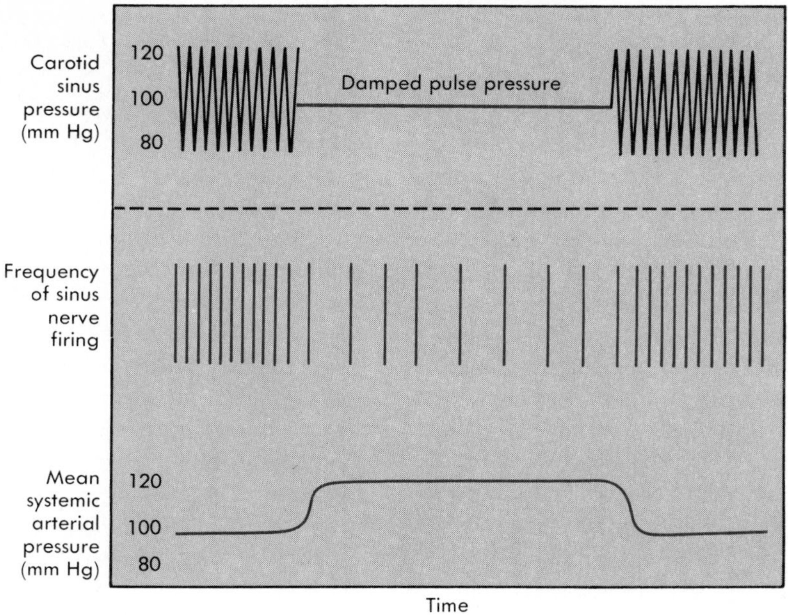

Fig. 8-11 ■ Effect of reducing pulse pressure in the vascularly isolated perfused carotid sinuses *(top record)* on impulses recorded from a fiber of a sinus nerve *(middle record)* and on mean systemic arterial pressure *(bottom record).* Mean pressure in the carotid sinuses *(colored line, top record)* is held constant when pulse pressure is damped.

sitivity of the receptors in the sinus so that a given increase in intrasinus pressure produces a greater depressor response. A decrease in baroreceptor sensitivity occurs in hypertension when the carotid sinus becomes stiffer and less deformable as a result of the high intraarterial pressure. Under these conditions a given increase in carotid sinus pressure elicits a smaller decrement in systemic arterial pressure than it does at normal levels of blood pressure. In other words, the set point of the baroreceptors is raised in hypertension so that the threshold is increased and the receptors are less sensitive to change in transmural pressure.

In some individuals the carotid sinus is quite sensitive to pressure. Hence tight collars or other forms of external pressure over the region of the carotid sinus may elicit marked hypotension and fainting. In some patients with severe coronary artery disease and chest pain **(angina pectoris),** symptoms have been temporarily relieved by stimulation of the sinus nerve by means of a chronically implanted stimulator that can be activated externally. The reduction in blood pressure achieved by sinus nerve stimulation decreases the pressure work of the heart and its oxygen needs. Hence, the myocardial ischemia (oxygen deprivation) that is responsible for the pain is alleviated. As would be expected, denervation of the carotid sinus can produce temporary, and in some instances prolonged, hypertension.

The arterial baroreceptors play a key role in short-term adjustments of blood pressure when relatively abrupt changes in blood vol-

ume, cardiac output, or peripheral resistance (as in exercise) occur. However, long-term control of blood pressure—that is, over days, weeks, and longer—is determined by the fluid balance of the individual, namely, the balance between fluid intake and fluid output. By far the single most important organ in the control of body fluid volume, and hence blood pressure, is the kidney. With overhydration, excessive fluid intake is excreted, whereas with dehydration there is a marked reduction in urine output.

Cardiopulmonary Baroreceptors. In addition to the carotid sinus and aortic baroreceptors, there are also cardiopulmonary receptors with vagal and sympathetic afferent and efferent nerves. These cardiopulmonary reflexes are tonically active and can alter peripheral resistance with changes in intracardiac, venous, or pulmonary vascular pressures. The receptors are located in the atria, ventricles, and pulmonary vessels.

The atria contain two types of receptors, one that is activated by the tension developed during atrial contraction **(A receptors)** and one that is activated by the stretch of the atria during atrial filling **(B receptors).** Stimulation of these atrial receptors sends impulses up vagal fibers to the vagal center in the medulla. Consequently, the sympathetic activity is decreased to the kidney and is increased to the sinus node. These changes in sympathetic activity increase renal blood flow, urine flow, and heart rate.

Activation of the cardiopulmonary receptors can also lower blood pressure reflexly by inhibiting the vasoconstrictor center in the medulla. Stimulation of the receptors inhibits angiotensin, aldosterone, and vasopressin (antidiuretic hormone) release; interruption of the reflex pathway has the opposite effects. Changes in urine volume elicited by changes in cardiopulmonary baroreceptor activation are important in the regulation of blood volume. For example, a decrease in blood volume (hypovolemia), as occurs in hemorrhage, enhances sympathetic vasoconstriction in the kidney and increases secretion of renin, angiotensin, aldosterone, and antidiuretic hormone. The renal vasoconstriction (primarily afferent arteriolar) reduces glomerular filtration and increases renin release from the kidney. Renin acts on a plasma substrate to form angiotensin, which increases aldosterone release from the adrenal cortex. The enhanced release of antidiuretic hormone increases water reabsorption. The net result is retention of salt and water by the kidney and a sensation of thirst. Angiotensin II (formed from angiotensin I bv converting enzyme) also raises systemic arteriolar tone.

Peripheral Chemoreceptors. The chemo receptors consist of small, highly vascular bodies in the region of the aortic arch and just medial to the carotid sinuses (see Figs. 8-8 and 8-9). They are sensitive to changes in the Po_2, Pco_2, and pH of the blood. Although they are primarily concerned with the regulation of respiration, they reflexly influence the vasomotor regions to a minor degree. A reduction in arterial blood O_2 tension (Pao_2) stimulates the chemoreceptors, and the increase in the number of impulses in the afferent nerve fibers from the carotid and aortic bodies stimulates the vasoconstrictor regions, resulting in increased tone of the resistance and capacitance vessels. The chemoreceptors are also stimulated by increased arterial blood CO_2 tension ($Paco_2$) and reduced pH, but the reflex effect induced is quite small compared to the direct effect of hypercapnia (high $Paco_2$) and hydrogen ions on the vasomotor regions in the medulla. When hypoxia and hypercapnia occur at the same time, the stimulation of the chemoreceptors is greater than the sum of the two stimuli when they act alone. When the chemoreceptors are stimulated simultaneously with a reduction in pressure in the baroreceptors, the chemoreceptors potentiate the vasoconstriction observed in the peripheral vessels. However, when the baroreceptors and chemoreceptors are both stimulated (for example, high carotid sinus pressure and low $Pa{O_2}$), the effects of the baroreceptors predominate.

There are also chemoreceptors with sympathetic afferent fibers in the heart. These cardiac chemoreceptors are activated by ischemia and transmit the precordial pain (angina pectoris) associated with an inadequate blood supply to the myocardium.

Hypothalamus. Optimum function of the cardiovascular reflexes requires the integrity of pontine and hypothalamic structures. Furthermore, these structures are responsible for behavioral and emotional control of the cardiovascular system. Stimulation of the anterior hypothalamus produces a fall in blood pressure and bradycardia, whereas stimulation of the posterolateral region of the hypothalamus produces a rise in blood pressure and tachycardia. The hypothalamus also contains a temperature-regulating center that affects the skin vessels. Stimulation by cold applications to the skin or by cooling of the blood perfusing the hypothalamus results in constriction of the skin vessels and heat conservation, whereas warm stimuli result in cutaneous vasodilation and enhanced heat loss (see p. 253).

Cerebrum. The cerebral cortex can also exert a significant effect on blood flow distribution in the body. Stimulation of the motor and premotor areas can affect blood pressure; usually a pressor response is obtained. However, vasodilation and depressor responses may be evoked, as in blushing or fainting, in response to an emotional stimulus.

Skin and Viscera. Painful stimuli can elicit either pressor or depressor responses, depending on the magnitude and location of the stimulus. Distension of the viscera often evokes a depressor response, whereas painful stimuli on the body surface usually evoke a pressor response. In the anesthetized animal, strong electrical stimulation of a sensory nerve will produce a strong pressor response. However, it is sometimes possible to obtain a depressor response with low-intensity and low-frequency stimulation. Furthermore, all vascular beds do not exhibit the same response; in some, resistance increases, whereas in others it decreases. In addition, muscle contractions can elicit reflex changes in the magnitude of vasoactivity in the muscle. For the most part, these reflexes are mediated through the vasomotor areas in the medulla, but there are also spinal areas that can aid in the regulation of peripheral resistance.

Pulmonary Reflexes. Inflation of the lungs reflexly induces systemic vasodilation and a decrease in arterial blood pressure. Conversely, collapse of the lungs evokes systemic vasoconstriction. Afferent fibers mediating this reflex run in the vagus nerves and possibly to a limited extent in the sympathetic nerves. Their stimulation by stretch of the lungs inhibits the vasomotor areas. The magnitude of the depressor response to lung inflation is directly related to the degree of inflation and to the existing level of vasoconstrictor tone.

Central Chemoreceptors. Increases of $Pa{CO_2}$ stimulate chemosensitive regions of the medulla and elicit vasoconstriction and increased peripheral resistance. Reduction in $Pa{CO_2}$ below normal levels (as with hyperventilation) decreases the degree of tonic activity of these areas in the medulla, thereby decreasing peripheral resistance. The chemosensitive regions are also affected by changes in pH. A lowering of blood pH stimulates and a rise in blood pH inhibits these areas. These effects of changes in $Pa{CO_2}$ and blood pH possibly operate through changes in cerebrospinal fluid pH, as appears to be the case for the respiratory center. Whether there are special hydrogen ion chemoreceptors mediating pH-induced vasomotor effects has not been established.

Oxygen tension has relatively little direct effect on the medullary vasomotor region. The primary effect of hypoxia is reflexly mediated via the carotid and aortic chemoreceptors. Moderate reduction of Pa_{O_2} will stimulate the vasomotor region, but severe reduction will depress vasomotor activity in the same manner that other areas of the brain are depressed by very low O_2 tensions.

Cerebral ischemia, which may occur because of excessive pressure exerted by an expanding intracranial tumor, results in a marked increase in peripheral vasoconstriction. The stimulation is probably caused by a local accumulation of CO_2 and reduction of O_2, and possibly by excitation of intracranial baroreceptors. With prolonged, severe ischemia, central depression eventually supervenes, and the blood pressure falls.

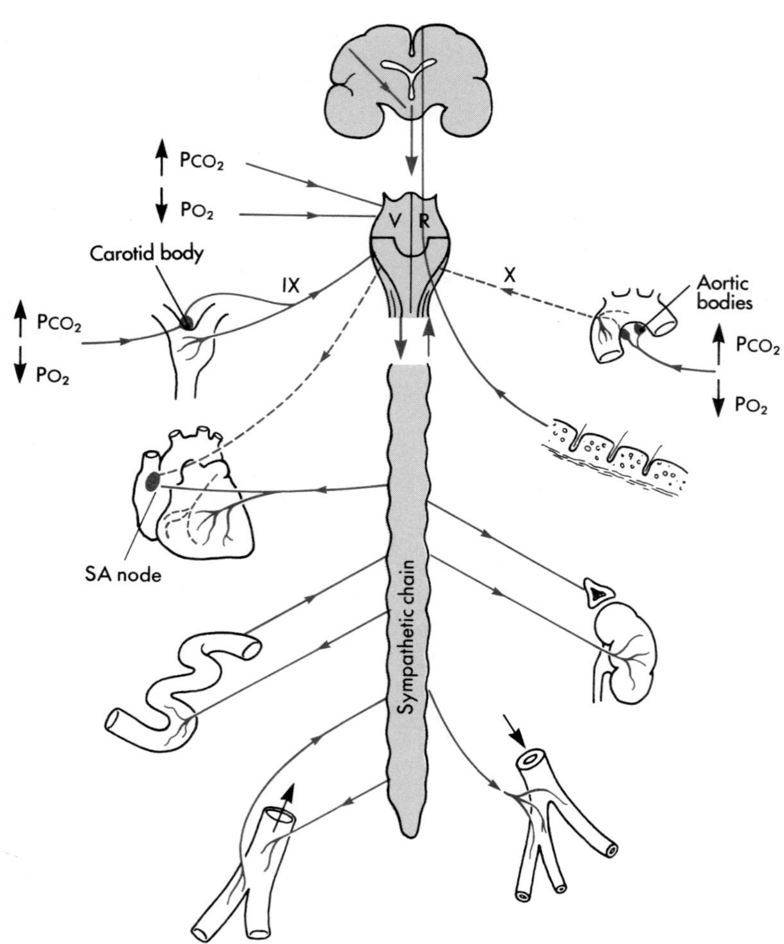

Fig. 8-12 ■ Schematic diagram illustrating the neural input and output of the vasomotor region *(VR). IX,* Glossopharyngeal nerve; *X,* vagus nerve.

■ BALANCE BETWEEN EXTRINSIC AND INTRINSIC FACTORS IN REGULATION OF PERIPHERAL BLOOD FLOW

Dual control of the peripheral vessels by intrinsic and extrinsic mechanisms makes possible a number of vascular adjustments that enable the body to direct blood flow to areas where it is needed in greater supply and away from areas whose immediate requirements are less. In some tissues a more or less fixed relative potency of extrinsic and intrinsic mechanisms exists, and in other tissues the ratio is changeable, depending on the state of activity of that tissue.

In the brain and the heart, both vital structures with very limited tolerance for a reduced blood supply, intrinsic flow-regulating mechanisms are dominant. For instance, massive discharge of the vasoconstrictor region over the sympathetic nerves, which might occur in severe, acute hemorrhage, has negligible effects on the cerebral and cardiac resistance vessels, whereas skin, renal, and splanchnic blood vessels become greatly constricted.

In the skin the extrinsic vascular control is dominant. Not only do the cutaneous vessels participate strongly in a general vasoconstrictor discharge, but they also respond selectively through hypothalamic pathways to subserve the heat loss and heat conservation function required in body temperature regulation. However, intrinsic control can be demonstrated by local changes of temperature that can modify or override the central influence on resistance and capacitance vessels.

In skeletal muscle the interplay and changing balance between extrinsic and intrinsic mechanisms can be clearly seen. In resting skeletal muscle, neural control (vasoconstrictor tone) is dominant, as can be demonstrated by the large increment in blood flow that occurs immediately after section of the sympathetic nerves to the tissue. In anticipation of and at the start of exercise, such as running, blood flow increases in the leg muscles. After the onset of exercise the intrinsic flow-regulating mechanism assumes control, and because of the local increase in metabolites, vasodilation occurs in the active muscles. Vasoconstriction occurs in the inactive tissues as a manifestation of the general sympathetic discharge, but constrictor impulses reaching the resistance vessels of the active muscles are overridden by the local metabolic effect. Operation of this dual control mechanism thus provides increased blood where it is required and shunts it away from relatively inactive areas. Similar effects may be achieved with an increase in Pa_{CO_2}. Normally the hyperventilation associated with exercise keeps Pa_{CO_2} at normal levels. However, were Pa_{CO_2} to increase, a generalized vasoconstriction would occur because of stimulation of the medullary vasoconstrictor region by CO_2. In the active muscles, where the CO_2 concentration is highest, the smooth muscle of the arterioles would relax in response to the local P_{CO_2}. Factors affecting and affected by the vasomotor region are summarized in Fig. 8-12.

■ SUMMARY

1. The arterioles, often referred to as the resistance vessels, are important in the regulation of blood flow through their cognate capillaries. The smooth muscle, which comprises a major fraction of the wall of the arterioles, contracts and relaxes in response to neural and humoral stimuli.
2. Most tissues show autoregulation of blood flow, a phenomenon characterized by a constant blood flow in the face of a change in perfusion pressure. A logical explanation of autoregulation is the myogenic mechanism whereby stretch of the vessel wall by an increase in transmural pressure elicits a contractile response, whereas a decrease in transmural pressure elicits relaxation.

3. The striking parallelism between tissue blood flow and tissue oxygen consumption indicates that *blood flow is largely regulated by a metabolic mechanism.* A decrease in the oxygen supply/oxygen demand ratio of a tissue releases a vasodilator metabolite that dilates arterioles to enhance the oxygen supply.
4. *Neural regulation of blood flow is almost completely accomplished by the sympathetic nervous system.* Sympathetic nerves to blood vessels are tonically active; inhibition of the vasoconstrictor center in the medulla reduces peripheral vascular resistance. Stimulation of the sympathetic nerves constricts resistance and capacitance (veins) vessels. Parasympathetic fibers innervate the head, viscera, and genitalia; they do not innervate skin and muscle.
5. The baroreceptors (pressoreceptors) in the internal carotid arteries and aorta are tonically active and regulate blood pressure on a moment to moment basis. Stretch of these receptors by an increase in arterial pressure reflexly inhibits the vasoconstrictor center in the medulla and induces vasodilation, whereas a decrease in arterial pressure disinhibits the vasoconstrictor center and induces vasoconstriction. The carotid baroreceptors predominate over those in the aorta and respond more vigorously to **changes in pressure** (stretch) than they do to elevated or reduced constant pressures; they adapt to an imposed constant pressure. Baroreceptors are also present in the cardiac chambers and large pulmonary vessels (cardiopulmonary baroreceptors); they have less influence on blood pressure but participate in blood volume regulation.
6. Peripheral chemoreceptors in the carotid bodies and aortic arch and central chemoreceptors in the medulla oblongata are stimulated by a decrease in blood oxygen tension (Pao_2) and an increase in blood carbon dioxide tension ($Paco_2$). Stimulation of these chemoreceptors primarily increases the rate and depth of respiration but also produces peripheral vasoconstriction.
7. Peripheral resistance and hence blood pressure can be affected by stimuli arising in the skin, viscera, lungs, and brain.
8. The combined effect of neural and local metabolic factors is to distribute blood to active tissues and divert it from inactive tissues. In vital structures, such as the heart and brain and in contracting skeletal muscle, the metabolic factors predominate.

■ BIBLIOGRAPHY

Journal articles

Belloni, F.L., and Sparks, H.V.: The peripheral circulation, Ann. Rev. Physiol. 40:67, 1978.

Berne, R.M., Knabb, R.M., Ely, S.W., and Rubio, R.: Adenosine in the local regulation of blood flow: a brief overview, Fed. Proc. 42:3136, 1983.

Brown, A.M.: Receptors under pressure—an update on baroreceptors, Circ. Res. 46:1, 1980.

Coleridge, H.M., and Coleridge, J.C.G.: Cardiovascular afferents involved in regulation of peripheral vessels, Ann. Rev. Physiol. 42:413, 1980.

Donald, D.E., and Shepherd, J.T.: Autonomic regulation of the peripheral circulation, Ann. Rev. Physiol. 42:429, 1980.

Hilton, S.M., and Spyer, K.M.: Central nervous regulation of vascular resistance, Ann. Rev. Physiol. 42:399, 1980.

Kuo, L., Davis, J.J., and Chilian, W.M.: Endothelium-dependent flow-induced dilation of isolated coronary arterioles, Am. J. Physiol. 259:H1063, 1990.

Shen, Y-T, Knight, D.R., Thomas, J.X., Jr., and Vatner, S.F.: Relative roles of cardiac receptors and arterial baroreceptors during hemorrhage in conscious dogs, Circ. Res. 66:397, 1990.

Shepherd, J.T.: Reflex control of arterial blood pressure, Cardiovasc. Res. 16:357, 1982.

Books and monographs

Abboud, F.M., and Thames, M.D.: Interaction of cardiovascular reflexes in circulatory control. In Handbook of physiology; Section 2: The cardiovascular system—peripheral circulation and organ blood flow, vol. III, Bethesda, Md., 1983, American Physiological Society.

Bevan, J.A., Bevan, R.D., and Duckles, S.P.: Adrenergic regulation of vascular smooth muscle. In Handbook of physiology; Section 2: The cardiovascular system—vascular smooth muscle, vol. II, Bethesda, Md., 1980, American Physiological Society.

Bishop, V.S., Malliani, A., and Thoren, P.: Cardiac mechanoreceptors. In Handbook of physiology; Section 2: The cardiovascular system, vol. III, Bethesda, Md., 1983, American Physiological Society.

Brown, A.M.: Cardiac reflexes. In Handbook of physiology; Section 2: The cardiovascular system—the heart, vol. I, Bethesda, Md., 1979, American Physiological Society.

Crass, M.F., and Barnes, D.C., editors: Vascular smooth muscle—metabolic, ionic and contractile mechanisms, New York, 1982, Academic Press, Inc.

Eyzaguirre, C., Fitzgerald, R.S., Lahiri, S., and Zapata, P.: Arterial chemoreceptors. In Handbook of physiology; Section 2: The cardiovascular system—peripheral circulation and organ blood flow, vol. III, Bethesda, Md., 1983, American Physiological Society.

Johnson, P.C.: The myogenic response. In Handbook of physiology; Section 2: The cardiovascular system—vascular smooth muscle, vol. II, Bethesda, Md., 1980, American Physiological Society.

Korner, P.I.: Central nervous control of autonomic cardiovascular function. In Handbook of physiology; Section 2: The cardiovascular system—the heart, vol. I, Bethesda, Md., 1979, American Physiological Society.

Kovach, A.G.B., Sandos, P., and Kollii, M., editors: Cardiovascular physiology: neural control mechanisms, New York, 1981, Academic Press, Inc.

Mancia, G., and Mark, A.L.: Arterial baroreflexes in humans. In Handbook of physiology; Section 2: The cardiovascular system—peripheral circulation and organ blood flow, vol. III, Bethesda, Md., 1983, American Physiological Society.

Mark, A.L., and Mancia, G.: Cardiopulmonary baroreflexes in humans. In Handbook of physiology; Section 2: The cardiovascular system—peripheral circulation and organ blood flow, vol. III, Bethesda, Md., 1983, American Physiological Society.

Mulvany, M.J., Strandgaard, S., and Hammersen, F., editors: Resistance vessels: physiology, pharmacology and hypertensive pathology, Basel, Switzerland, 1985, S. Karger.

Rothe, C.F.: Venous system: physiology of the capacitance vessels. In Handbook of physiology; Section 2: The cardiovascular system—peripheral circulation and organ blood flow, vol. III, Bethesda, Md., 1983, American Physiological Society.

Sagawa, K.: Baroreflex control of systemic arterial pressure and vascular bed. In Handbook of physiology; Section 2: The cardiovascular system—peripheral circulation and organ blood flow, vol. III, Bethesda, Md., 1983, American Physiological Society.

Shepherd, J.T.: Cardiac mechanoreceptors. In Fozzard, H.A. et al. editors: The heart and cardiovascular system, scientific foundations, ed. 2, New York, 1991, Raven Press.

Somlyo, A.P., and Somlyo, A.V. Smooth muscle structure and function. In Fozzard, H.A. et al. editors: The heart and cardiovascular system, scientific foundations, ed. 2, New York, 1991, Raven Press.

Sparks, H.V., Jr.: Effect of local metabolic factors on vascular smooth muscle. In Handbook of physiology; Section 2: The cardiovascular system—vascular smooth muscle, vol. II, Bethesda, Md., 1980, American Physiological Society.

9 Control of Cardiac Output: Coupling of Heart and Blood Vessels

Four factors control cardiac output: heart rate, myocardial contractility, preload, and afterload (Fig. 9-1). Heart rate and myocardial contractility are strictly **cardiac factors.** They are characteristics of the cardiac tissues, although they are modulated by various neural and humoral mechanisms. Preload and afterload, however, depend on the characteristics of both the heart and the vascular system. On the one hand, preload and afterload are important **determinants** of cardiac output. On the other hand, preload and afterload are themselves **determined by** the cardiac output and certain vascular characteristics. Preload and afterload may be designated **coupling factors,** because they constitute a functional coupling between the heart and blood vessels. The heart pumps the blood around the vascular system. Concomitantly, the vessels partly determine the preload and afterload and hence the vessels regulate the quantity of blood that the heart will pump around the circuit per unit time.

To understand the regulation of cardiac output, therefore, it is important to appreciate the nature of the coupling between the heart and the vascular system. Guyton and his colleagues have developed graphic techniques that we have modified to analyze the interactions between the cardiac and vascular components of the circulatory system. The graphic analysis involves two simultaneous functional relationships between the **cardiac output** and the **central venous pressure** (that is, the pressure in the right atrium and thoracic venae cavae).

The curve defining one of these relationships will be called the **cardiac function curve.** It is an expression of the well-known Frank-Starling relationship (p. 94) and reflects the dependence of cardiac output on preload (that is, the central venous, or right atrial, pressure). The cardiac function curve is a characteristic of the heart itself and has been studied in hearts completely isolated from the rest of the circulatory system (see Fig. 4-16).

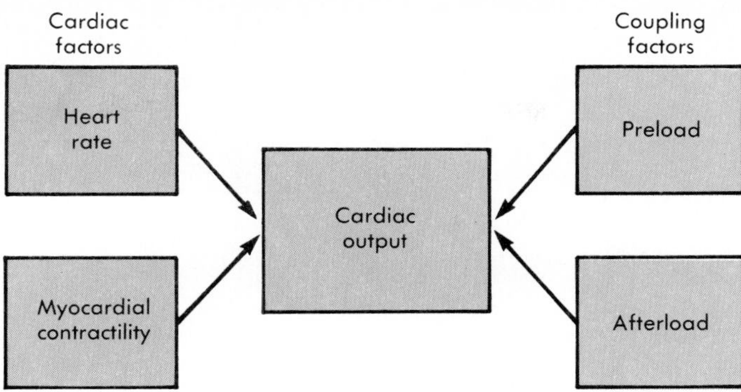

Fig. 9-1 ■ The four factors that determine cardiac output.

The second curve, which we shall call the **vascular function curve,** defines the dependence of central venous pressure on cardiac output. This relationship depends only on certain vascular system characteristics, namely, the peripheral resistance, the arterial and venous compliances, and the blood volume. The vascular function curve is entirely independent of the characteristics of the heart, and it can be studied even if the heart were replaced by a mechanical pump.

■ VASCULAR FUNCTION CURVE

The vascular function curve defines the changes in central venous pressure evoked by changes in cardiac output; that is, central venous pressure is the **dependent variable** (or **response**), and cardiac output is the **independent variable** (or **stimulus**). This contrasts with the cardiac function curve, for which the central venous pressure (or preload) is the **independent variable** and the cardiac output is the **dependent variable.**

The simplified model of the circulation illustrated in Fig. 9-2 will help explain how the cardiac output determines the level of the central venous pressure. The essential components of the cardiovascular system have been lumped into four elements. The right and left sides of the heart, as well as the pulmonary vascular bed, are considered simply as a **pump,** much as that employed during open heart surgery. The high-resistance microcirculation is designated the **peripheral resistance.** Finally, the compliance of the system is subdivided into two components, the **arterial compliance,** C_a, and the **venous compliance,** C_v. As defined on p. 138, compliance (C) is the increment of volume (dV) accommodated per unit change of pressure (dP); that is,

$$C = dV/dP \quad (1)$$

The venous compliance is about twenty times as great as the arterial compliance. In the example to follow, the ratio of C_v to C_a will be set at 19:1 to simplify certain calculations. Thus, if it were necessary to add x ml of blood to the arterial system to produce a 1 mm Hg increment in arterial pressure, then it would be necessary to add 19x ml of blood to the venous system to raise venous pressure by the same amount.

To illustrate why the central venous pressure varies inversely with the cardiac output, let us first give our model the characteristics that resemble those of an average adult person (Fig. 9-2, *A*). Let the flow (Q_h) generated by the heart (i.e., the cardiac output) be 5 L/min,

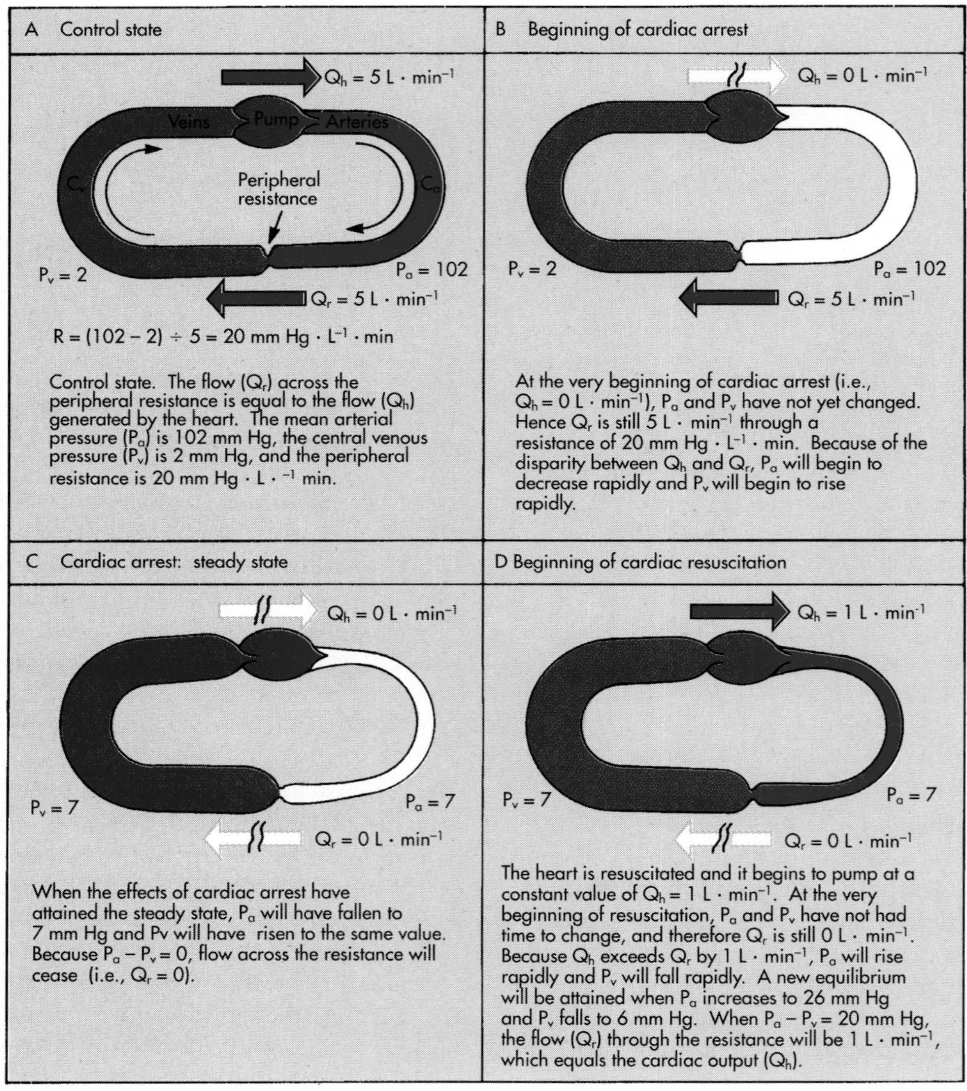

Fig. 9-2 ■ Simplified model of the cardiovascular system, consisting of a pump, arterial compliance *(C_a)*, peripheral resistance, and venous compliance *(C_v)*.

the mean arterial pressure, P_a, be 102 mm Hg, and the central venous pressure, P_v, be 2 mm Hg. The peripheral resistance, R, is the ratio of pressure difference ($P_a - P_v$) to flow (Q_r) through the resistance vessels; this ratio equals 20 mm Hg/L/min. An arteriovenous pressure difference of 100 mm Hg is sufficient to force a flow (Q_r) of 5 L/min through a peripheral resistance of 20 mm Hg/L/min; this flow (Q_r) is precisely equal to the flow (Q_h) generated by the heart. From heartbeat to heartbeat, the volume (V_a) of blood in the arteries and the volume (V_v) of blood in the veins remain constant because the volume of blood transferred from the veins to the arteries by the heart equals the volume of blood that flows from the arteries through the resistance vessels and into the veins.

Fig. 9-2, *B* illustrates the status of the circulation at the very beginning of an episode of cardiac arrest; i.e., $Q_h = 0$. Initially, the volumes of blood in the arteries (V_a) and veins (V_v) have not had time to change. The arterial and venous pressures depend on V_a and V_v, respectively. Therefore, these pressures are identical to the respective pressures in panel *A* (i.e., $P_a = 102$ and $P_v = 2$). The arteriovenous pressure gradient of 100 mm Hg will force a flow of 5 L/min through the peripheral resistance of 20 mm Hg/L/min. Thus, although cardiac output now equals 0 L/min, the flow through the microcirculation equals 5 L/min. In other words, the potential energy stored in the arteries by the previous pumping action of the heart causes blood to be transferred from arteries to veins, initially at the control rate, even though the heart can no longer transfer blood from the veins into the arteries.

As time passes, the blood volume in the arteries progressively decreases and the blood volume in the veins progressively increases. Because the vessels are elastic structures, the arterial pressure falls gradually and the venous pressure rises gradually. This process will continue until the arterial and venous pressures become equal (Fig. 9-2, *C*). Once this condition is reached, the flow (Q_r) from the arteries to the veins through the resistance vessels will be zero, as is the cardiac output (Q_h).

At zero flow equilibrium (Fig. 9-2, *C*), the pressure attained in the arteries and veins depends on the relative compliances of these vessels. Had the arterial (C_a) and venous (C_v) compliances been equal, the decline in P_a would have been equal to the rise in P_v because the decrement in arterial volume equals the increment in venous volume (principle of conservation of mass). P_a and P_v would have both attained the average of P_a and P_v in panels *A* and *B*; i.e., $P_a = P_v = (102 + 2)/2 = 52$ mm Hg.

However, the veins are much more compliant than the arteries; the ratio is approximately equal to the ratio ($C_v:C_a = 19$) that we have assumed for the model. Hence, the transfer of blood from arteries to veins at equilibrium would induce a fall in arterial pressure nineteen times as great as the concomitant rise in venous pressure. As Fig. 9-2, *C* shows, P_v would increase by 5 mm Hg (to 7 mm Hg), whereas P_a would fall by $19 \times 5 = 95$ mm Hg (to 7 mm Hg). This equilibrium pressure that prevails in the circulatory system in the absence of flow is often referred to as the **mean circulatory pressure,** or the **static pressure.** The pressure in the static system reflects the total volume of blood in the system and the overall compliance ($C_a + C_v$) of the system.

The example of cardiac arrest in Fig. 9-2 provides the basis for understanding the vascular function curves. Two important points on the curve have already been derived, as shown in Fig. 9-3. One point *(A)* represents the normal status (depicted in Fig. 9-2, *A*). At that point, when cardiac output was 5 L/min, P_v was 2 mm Hg. Then, when flow stopped (cardiac output = 0), P_v became 7 mm Hg at equilibrium; this pressure is the mean circulatory pressure, P_{mc}.

The inverse relation between P_v and cardiac output simply expresses that when cardiac output is suddenly decreased, the rate at which blood flows from arteries to veins through the capillaries is temporarily greater than the rate at which the heart pumps it from the veins back into the arteries. During that transient period, a net volume of blood is translocated from arteries to veins; hence P_a falls and P_v rises.

An example of a sudden increase in cardiac output will illustrate how a third point *(B)* on the vascular function curve is derived. Consider that the arrested heart is suddenly restarted, and it immediately begins pumping blood from the veins into the arteries at a rate of 1 L/min (Fig. 9-2, *D*). When the heart first begins to beat, the arteriovenous pressure gradient is zero, and hence no blood is being transferred from the arteries through the capillaries and into the veins. Hence, when beating has just resumed, blood is being depleted from the veins at the rate of 1 L/min, and the arterial volume is being repleted at the same rate. Hence, P_v begins to fall, and P_a begins to rise. Because of the difference in compliances, P_a will rise nineteen times more rapidly than P_v will fall.

The resultant pressure gradient will cause blood to flow through the resistance. If the heart maintains a constant output of 1 L/min, P_a will continue to rise and P_v will continue to fall until the pressure gradient becomes 20 mm Hg. This gradient will force a flow of 1 L/min through a resistance of 20 mm Hg/L/min. This gradient will be achieved by a 19 mm Hg rise (to 26 mm Hg) in P_a and a 1 mm Hg fall (to 6 mm Hg) in P_v. This equilibrium value of P_v = 6 mm Hg for a cardiac output of 1 L/min also appears *(B)* on the vascular function curve of Fig. 9-3. It reflects a net transfer of blood from the venous to the arterial side of the circuit and a consequent reduction of P_v.

The reduction of P_v that can be achieved by an increase in cardiac output is limited. At some critical maximum value of cardiac output, sufficient fluid will be translocated from the venous to the arterial side of the circuit to

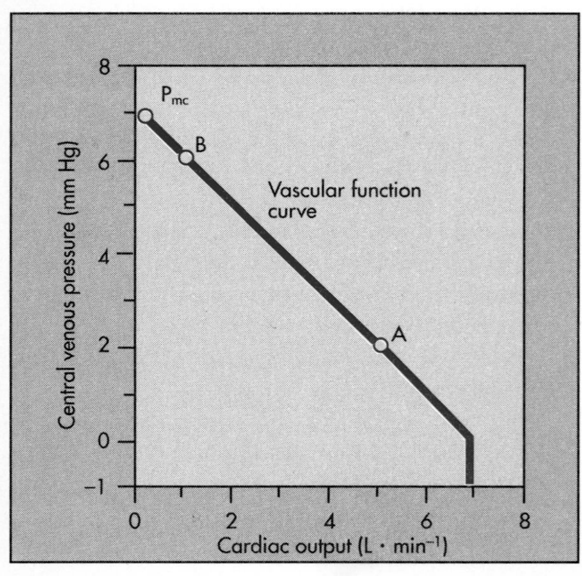

Fig. 9-3 ■ Changes in central venous pressure produced by changes in cardiac output. The mean circulatory pressure (or static pressure), P_{mc}, is the equilibrium pressure throughout the cardiovascular system when cardiac output is 0. Points *B* and *A* represent the values of venous pressure at cardiac outputs of 1 and 5 L/min, respectively.

reduce P_v below the ambient pressure. In a system of very distensible vessels, such as the venous system, the vessels will be collapsed by the greater external pressure. This venous collapse constitutes an impediment to venous return to the heart. Hence, it will limit the maximum value of cardiac output to 7 L/min (see Fig. 9-3), regardless of the capabilities of the pump. For readers interested in the mathematical derivation of these results, the basic equations are presented in the next section.

Mathematical Analysis

From the definition of **peripheral resistance** (p. 122):

$$R = (P_a - P_v) / Q_r, \qquad (2)$$

where R is resistance, P_a is arterial pressure, P_v is venous pressure, and Q_r is blood flow through the resistance vessels.

At equilibrium, Q_r equals cardiac output, Q_h. Assume that R = 20, and that Q_h had been 0, but that it had then been increased to a constant value of 1 L/min (Fig. 9-4, arrow *1*). If we solve equation 2 for P_a at equilibrium (i.e., $Q_r = Q_h$):

$$P_a = P_v + Q_r R = P_v + (1 \times 20) \qquad (3)$$

Thus, P_a will increase to a value 20 mm Hg greater than P_v. It will continue to be 20 mm Hg above P_v, as long as the pump output is maintained at 1 L/min and the peripheral resistance remains at 20 mm Hg/L/min.

We can calculate what the actual changes in P_a and P_v will be when Q_r attains a constant value of 1 L/min. The arterial volume increment needed to achieve the required level of P_a depends entirely on the arterial compliance, C_a. For a rigid arterial system (low compliance) this volume will be small; for a distensible system the volume will be large. Whatever the magnitude, however, the change in volume represents the translocation of some quantity of blood from the venous to the arterial side of the circuit.

For a given total blood volume, any increment in arterial volume (ΔV_a) must equal the decrement in venous volume (ΔV_v); that is

$$\Delta V_a = -\Delta V_v \qquad (4)$$

From the definition of compliance,

$$C_a = \Delta V_a / \Delta P_a \qquad (5)$$

and

$$C_v = \Delta V_v / \Delta P_v \qquad (6)$$

By substitution into equation 4,

$$\frac{\Delta P_v}{\Delta P_a} = -\frac{C_a}{C_v} \qquad (7)$$

Given that C_v is nineteen times as great as C_a, then the increment in P_a will be nineteen times as great as the decrement in P_v; that is

$$\Delta P_a = -19 \Delta P_v \qquad (8)$$

To calculate the absolute values of P_a and P_v, let ΔP_a represent the difference between the prevailing P_a and the mean circulatory pressure (P_{mc}); that is, let

$$\Delta P_a = P_a - P_{mc} \qquad (9)$$

and let ΔP_v represent the difference between the prevailing P_v and the mean circulatory pressure:

$$\Delta P_v = P_v - P_{mc} \qquad (10)$$

Substituting these values for ΔP_a and ΔP_v into equation 8:

$$P_a - P_{mc} = -19 (P_v - P_{mc}) \qquad (11)$$

By solving equations 3 and 11 simultaneously:

$$P_a = P_{mc} + 19 \qquad (12)$$

and

$$P_v = P_{mc} - 1 \qquad (13)$$

Hence for a mean circulatory pressure of 7 mm Hg, P_a increases to 26 mm Hg and P_v decreases to 6 mm Hg when Q_h increases from 0 to 1 L/min (see Fig. 9-4). These pressure

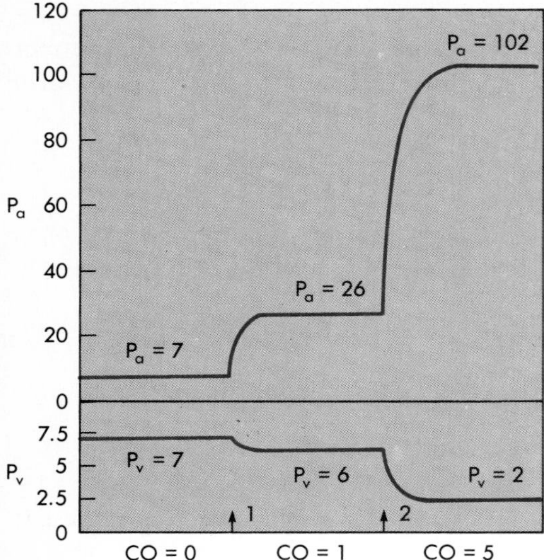

Fig. 9-4 ■ The changes in arterial *(P_a)* and venous *(P_v)* pressures in the circulatory model shown in the preceding figure. The total peripheral resistance is 20 mm Hg/L/min, and the ratio of C_v to C_a is 19:1. The cardiac output *(CO)* is 0 to the left of arrow *1*. It is increased to 1 L/min at arrow *1*, and to 5 L/min at arrow *2*.

changes provide the required arteriovenous pressure gradient of 20 mm Hg.

If the pump output is abruptly increased to a constant level of 5 L/min (see Fig. 9-4, arrow *2*) and peripheral resistance remains constant at 20 mm Hg/L/min, an additional volume of blood again will be translocated from the venous to the arterial side of the circuit. It will progressively accumulate in the arteries until P_a reaches a level of 100 mm Hg above P_v, as shown by substitution into equation 3:

$$P_a = P_v + Q_rR = P_v + (5 \times 20) \tag{14}$$

By solving equations 11 and 14 simultaneously, we find that P_a rises to a value of 95 mm Hg above P_{mc}, and P_v falls to a value 5 mm Hg below P_{mc}. In Fig. 9-4, therefore, P_v declines to 2 mm Hg and P_a rises to 102 mm Hg. The resultant pressure gradient of 100 mm Hg will force a cardiac output of 5 L/min through a constant peripheral resistance of 20 mm Hg/L/min.

Venous Pressure Dependence on Cardiac Output

Experimental and clinical observations have shown that changes in cardiac output do indeed evoke the alterations in P_a and P_v that have been predicted above for our simplified model. In an experiment on an anesthesized dog, a mechanical pump was substituted for the right ventricle (Fig. 9-5). As the cardiac output, Q, was diminished in a series of small steps, P_a fell and P_v rose. Similarly, a major coronary artery may suddenly become occluded in a human patient. The resultant **acute myocardial infarction (death of myocardial tissue)** often diminishes cardiac output, which is attended by a fall in the arterial pressure and a rise in the central venous pressure.

The changes in P_v evoked by the alterations in blood flow (Q_r) in the experiment illustrated in Fig. 9-5 resemble those derived from our simplified model (see Fig. 9-3). The following equation for P_v as a function of Q_r in the model is derived from equations 2, 7, 9, and 10 above.

$$P_v = -\frac{RC_a}{C_a + C_v} Q_r + P_{mc} \tag{15}$$

Note that the slope depends only on R, C_a; and C_v. Note also that when $Q_r = 0$, then $P_v = P_{mc}$; that is, at zero flow, P_v equals the mean circulatory pressure.

Blood Volume

The vascular function curve is affected by variations in total blood volume. During circulatory standstill (zero cardiac output), the mean circulatory pressure depends only on total vascular compliance and blood volume, as stated previously. Thus for a given vascular

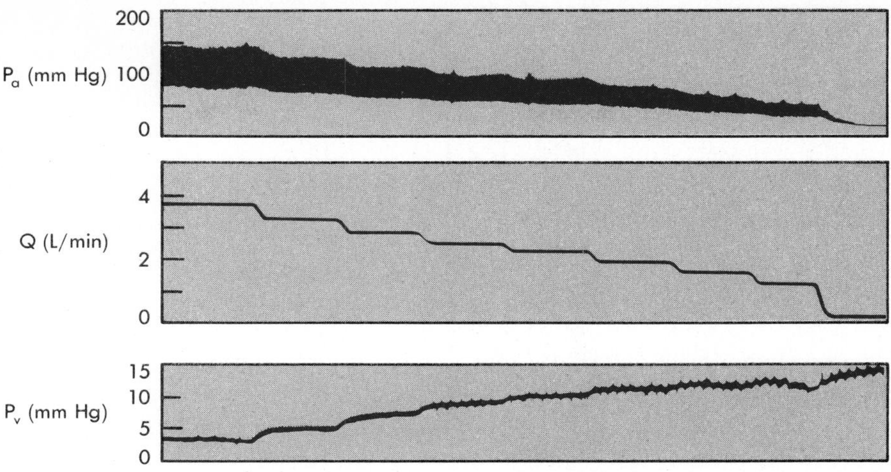

Fig. 9-5 ■ The changes in arterial *(P_a)* and central venous *(P_v)* pressures produced by changes in systemic blood flow *(Q_r)* in a canine right-heart bypass preparation. Stepwise changes in Q_r were produced by altering the rate of a mechanical pump. (From Levy, M.N.: Circ. Res. 44:739, 1979. By permission of the American Heart Association, Inc.)

compliance the mean circulatory pressure will be increased when the blood volume is expanded **(hypervolemia)** and decreased when the blood volume is diminished **(hypovolemia).** This is illustrated by the Y-axis intercepts in Fig. 9-6, where the mean circulatory pressure is 5 mm Hg after hemorrhage and 9 mm Hg after transfusion, as compared with the value of 7 mm Hg at the normal blood volume **(normovolemia).**

Furthermore, the differences in P_v during hypervolemia, normovolemia, and hypovolemia in the static system are preserved at each level of cardiac output such that the vascular function curves parallel each other (Fig. 9-6). To illustrate, consider the example of hypervolemia, in which the mean circulatory pressure is 9 mm Hg. In Fig. 9-6 both P_a and P_v would be 9 mm Hg, instead of 7 mm Hg, when the cardiac output is zero. With a sudden increase in cardiac output to 1 L/min (at arrow *1,* Fig. 9-4), if the peripheral resistance were still 20 mm Hg/L/min, an arteriovenous pressure gradient of 20 mm Hg would still be necessary for 1 L/min to flow through the resistance vessels. This does not differ from the example for normovolemia. Assuming the same ratio of C_v to C_a of 19:1, the pressure gradient would be achieved by a 1 mm Hg decline in P_v and a 19 mm Hg rise in P_a. Hence, a change in cardiac output from 0 to 1 L/min would evoke the same 1 mm Hg reduction in P_v irrespective of the blood volume, as long as C_a, C_v, and the peripheral resistance were independent of blood volume. Equation 15 also discloses that the slope of the vascular function curve remains constant as long as R, C_v, and C_a do not change.

From Fig. 9-6 it is also apparent that the cardiac output at which P_v = 0 varies directly with the blood volume. Therefore, the maximum value of cardiac output becomes progressively more limited as the total blood volume is reduced. However, the pressure at which the veins collapse (sharp change in slope of the vascular function curve) is not altered ap-

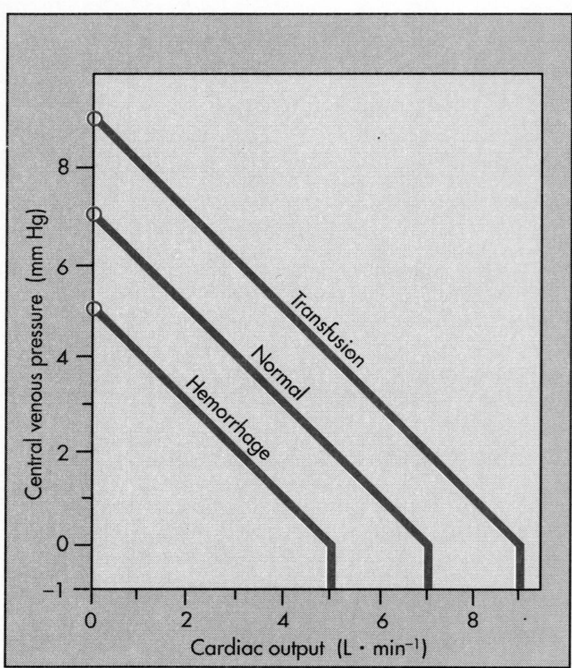

Fig. 9-6 ■ Effects of increased blood volume *(transfusion curve)* and of decreased blood volume *(hemorrhage curve)* on the vascular function curve. Similar shifts in the vascular function curve are produced by increases and decreases, respectively, in venomotor tone.

preciably by changes in blood volume. This pressure depends only on the pressure surrounding the central veins.

Venomotor Tone

The effects of changes in venomotor tone on the vascular function curve closely resemble those for changes in blood volume. In Fig. 9-6, for example, the transfusion curve could just as well represent increased venomotor tone, whereas the hemorrhage curve could represent decreased tone. During circulatory standstill, for a given blood volume, the pressure within the vascular system will rise as the tension exerted by the smooth muscle within the vascular walls increases. It is principally the arteriolar and venous smooth muscle that is under any notable nervous or humoral control. The fraction of the blood volume located within the arterioles is very small, whereas the blood volume in the veins is large (see Fig. 1-2). Therefore, only changes in venous tone can alter the mean circulatory pressure appreciably. Hence, mean circulatory pressure rises with increased venomotor tone and falls with diminished tone.

Experimentally, the pressure attained shortly after abrupt circulatory standstill is usually above 7 mm Hg, even when blood volume is normal. This is attributable to the generalized venoconstriction elicited by cerebral ischemia, activation of the chemoreceptors, and reduced excitation of the baroreceptors. If resuscitation is not successful, this reflex response subsides as central nervous activity ceases. At normal blood volume the mean circulatory pressure usually approaches a value close to 7 mm Hg.

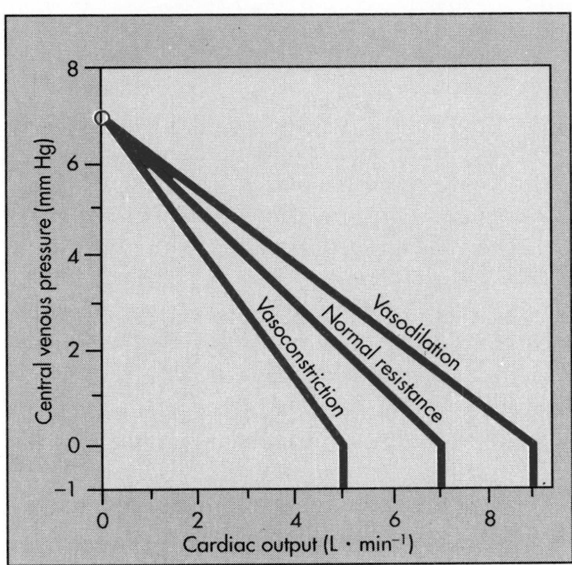

Fig. 9-7 ■ Effects of arteriolar vasodilation and vasoconstriction on the vascular function curve.

Blood Reservoirs

Venoconstriction is considerably greater in certain regions of the body than in others. In effect, vascular beds that undergo appreciable venoconstriction constitute blood reservoirs. The vascular bed of the skin is one of the major blood reservoirs in people. Blood loss evokes profound subcutaneous venoconstriction, giving rise to the characteristic pale appearance of the skin. The resultant diversion of blood away from the skin liberates several hundred milliliters of blood to be perfused through more vital regions. The vascular beds of the liver, lungs, and spleen are important blood reservoirs. In the dog the spleen is packed with red blood cells and can constrict to a small fraction of its normal size. During hemorrhage this mechanism autotransfuses blood of high erythrocyte content into the general circulation. However, in humans the volume changes of the spleen are considerably less extensive.

Peripheral Resistance

The changes in the vascular function curve induced by changes in arteriolar tone are shown in Fig. 9-7. The arterioles contain only about 3% of the total blood volume (see Fig. 1-2). Hence, changes in the contractile state of these vessels do not significantly alter the mean circulatory pressure, as stated previously. Thus the family of vascular function curves representing different peripheral resistances converges at a common point on the abscissa.

At any given cardiac output, P_v varies inversely with the arteriolar tone, all other factors remaining constant. Arteriolar constriction sufficient to double the peripheral resistance will cause a twofold rise in P_a (p. 144). In the example shown in Fig. 9-4, a change in the cardiac output from 0 to 1 L/min (arrow *1*) caused P_a to rise from 7 to 26 mm Hg, an increment of 19 mm Hg. If peripheral resistance had been twice as great, the same change in cardiac output would have evoked twice as great an increment in P_a.

To achieve this greater rise in P_a, twice as great an increment in blood volume would be required on the arterial side of the circulation, assuming a constant arterial compliance. Given a constant total blood volume, this larger arterial volume signifies a corresponding reduction in venous volume. Hence the decrement in venous volume would be twice as great when the peripheral resistance is doubled. If venous compliance remained constant, a twofold reduction in venous volume would be reflected by a twofold decline in P_v. Therefore, in Fig. 9-4, an increase in cardiac output from 0 L / min to 1 L / min (arrow *1*) would have caused a 2 mm Hg decrement in P_v, to a level of 5 mm Hg, instead of the 1 mm Hg decrement that occurred with the normal peripheral resistance. Similarly, greater increases in cardiac output would have evoked proportionately greater decrements in P_v under conditions of increased peripheral resistance than with normal levels of resistance.

This relationship between the peripheral resistance and the decrement in P_v, together with the failure of peripheral resistance to affect the mean circulatory pressure, accounts for the clockwise rotation of the vascular function curves with increased peripheral resistance (Fig. 9-7). Conversely, arteriolar vasodilation produces a counterclockwise rotation from the same vertical axis intercept. A higher maximum level of cardiac output is attainable with vasodilation than with normal or increased arteriolar tone (Fig. 9-7).

■ INTERRELATIONSHIPS BETWEEN CARDIAC OUTPUT AND VENOUS RETURN

Cardiac output and venous return are inextricably interdependent. Clearly, except for small, transient disparities, the heart is unable to pump any more blood than is delivered to it through the venous system. Similarly, because the circulatory system is a closed circuit, the venous return must equal the cardiac output over any appreciable time interval. The flow around the entire closed circuit depends on the capability of the pump, the characteristics of the circuit, and the total volume of fluid in the system. Cardiac output and venous return are simply two terms for the flow around the closed circuit. Cardiac output is the volume of blood being pumped by the heart per unit time. Venous return is the volume of blood returning to the heart per unit time. At equilibrium, these two flows are equal.

The techniques of circuit analysis will be applied in an effort to gain some insight into the control of flow around the circuit. Acute changes in cardiac contractility, peripheral resistance, or blood volume may transiently affect cardiac output and venous return disparately. Except for such brief disparities, however, such factors simply alter flow around the entire circuit. Whether one thinks of that flow as "cardiac output" or "venous return" is irrelevant. Commonly, authors have ascribed the reduction in cardiac output during hemorrhage, for example, to a decrease in venous return. It will become clear that such an explanation is a blatant example of circular reasoning. Hemorrhage reduces flow around the entire circuit, for reasons to be elucidated. To attribute the reduction in cardiac output to a curtailment of venous return is equivalent to ascribing the decrease in total flow to a decrease in total flow!

■ COUPLING BETWEEN THE HEART AND THE VASCULATURE

In accordance with Starling's law of the heart, cardiac output is intimately dependent on the right atrial or central venous pressure. Furthermore, the right atrial pressure is approximately equal to the right ventricular end-diastolic pressure, because the normal tricuspid valve constitutes a low resistance junction between the right atrium and ventricle. In the

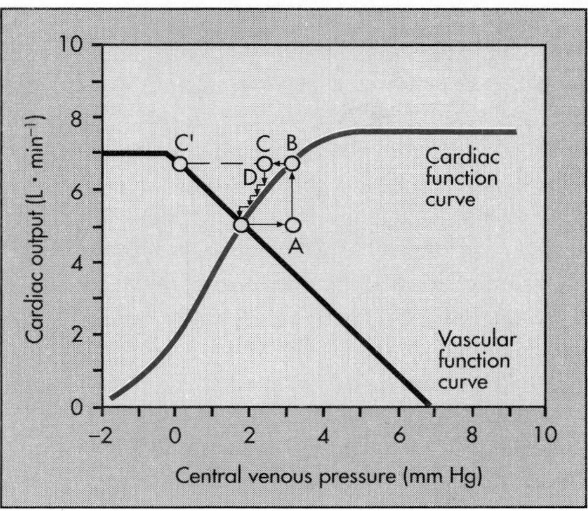

Fig. 9-8 ■ Typical vascular and cardiac function curves plotted on the same coordinate axes. Note that to plot both curves on the same graph, it is necessary to reverse the X and Y axes for the vascular function curves shown in Figs. 9-3, 9-6, and 9-7. The coordinates of the equilibrium point, at the intersection of the cardiac and vascular function curves, represent the stable values of cardiac output and central venous pressure at which the system tends to operate. Any perturbation (e.g., when venous pressure is suddenly increased to point *A*) institutes a sequence of changes in cardiac output and venous pressure that restore these variables to their equilibrium values.

discussion to follow, graphs of cardiac output as a function of central venous pressure (P_v) will be called **cardiac function curves.** Extrinsic regulatory influences may be expressed as shifts in such curves, as indicated previously (p. 99).

A typical cardiac function curve is plotted on the same coordinates as a normal vascular function curve in Fig. 9-8. The cardiac function curve is plotted according to the usual convention; that is, the variable (P_v) plotted along the abscissa is the independent variable (stimulus), and the variable (cardiac output) plotted along the ordinate is the dependent variable (response). In accordance with the Frank-Starling mechanism, the cardiac function curve reveals that a rise in P_v causes an increase in cardiac output.

Conversely, the vascular function curve describes an inverse relationship between cardiac output and P_v, that is, a rise in cardiac output causes a reduction in P_v. P_v is the dependent variable (or response) and cardiac output is the independent variable (or stimulus) for the vascular function curve. By convention, P_v should be scaled along the Y-axis and cardiac output should be scaled along the X-axis. Note that this convention is observed for the vascular function curves displayed in Figs. 9-5 to 9-7.

However, to include the vascular function curve on the same set of coordinate axes with the cardiac function curve (see Fig. 9-8), it is necessary to violate the plotting convention for one of these curves. We have arbitrarily **violated the convention** for the vascular function curve. Note that the vascular function curve in Fig. 9-8 reflects how P_v (scaled along the X-axis) varies in response to a change of cardiac output (scaled along the Y-axis).

The **equilibrium point** of a system represented by a given pair of cardiac and vascular function curves is defined by the intersection of these two curves. The coordinates of this equilibrium point represent the values of cardiac output and P_v at which such a system tends to operate. Only transient deviations from such values for cardiac output and P_v are possible, as long as the given cardiac and vascular function curves accurately describe the system.

The tendency for the cardiovascular system to operate about such an equilibrium point may best be illustrated by examining its response to a sudden perturbation. Consider the changes elicited by a sudden rise in P_v from the equilibrium point to point *A* in Fig. 9-8. Such a change might be induced by the rapid injection, during ventricular diastole, of a given volume of blood on the venous side of the circuit, accompanied by the withdrawal of an equal volume from the arterial side so that total blood volume would remain constant.

As defined by the cardiac function curve, this elevated P_v would increase cardiac output *(A* to *B)* during the very next ventricular systole. The increased cardiac output, in turn, would result in the net transfer of blood from the venous to the arterial side of the circuit, with a consequent reduction in P_v.

In one heart beat, the reduction in P_v would be small *(B* to *C)* because the heart would transfer only a tiny fraction of the total venous blood volume over to the arterial side. Because of this reduction in P_v, the cardiac output during the very next beat diminishes *(C* to *D)* by an amount dictated by the cardiac function curve. Because *D* is still above the intersection point, the heart will pump blood from the veins to the arteries at a rate greater than that at which the blood will flow across the peripheral resistance from arteries to veins. Hence, P_v will continue to fall. This process will continue in diminishing steps until the point of intersection is reached. Only one specific combination of cardiac output and venous pressure (denoted by the coordinates of the point of intersection) will satisfy simultaneously the requirements of the cardiac and vascular function curves.

Myocardial Contractility

Combinations of cardiac and vascular function curves help explain the effects of alterations in ventricular contractility. In Fig. 9-9 the lower cardiac function curve represents the control state, whereas the upper curve reflects an improved contractility. This pair of curves is analogous to the family of ventricular

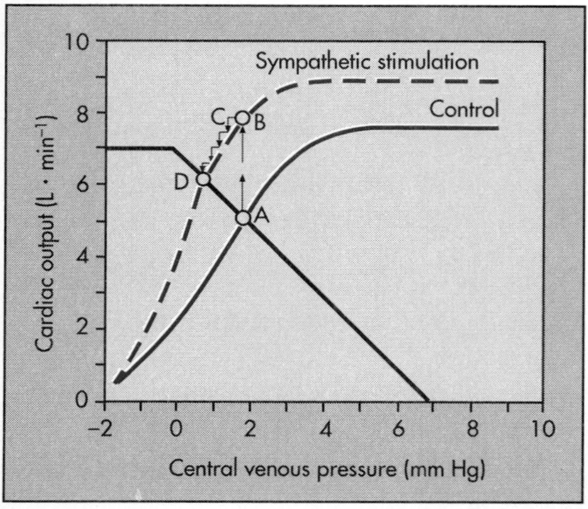

Fig. 9-9 ■ Enhancement of myocardial contractility, as by cardiac sympathetic nerve stimulation, causes the equilibrium values of cardiac output and P_v to shift from the intersection (point *A*) of the control vascular and cardiac function curves *(continuous lines)* to the intersection (point *D*) of the same vascular function curve with the cardiac function curve *(dashed line)* that represents enhanced myocardial contractility.

function curves described on p. 99. The enhancement of ventricular contractility might be achieved by electrical stimulation of the cardiac sympathetic nerves. If the effects of such stimulation are restricted to the heart, the vascular function curve would be unaffected. Therefore, one vascular function curve would suffice, as shown in Fig. 9-9.

During the control state the equilibrium values for cardiac output and P_v are designated by point *A*. Cardiac sympathetic nerve stimulation would abruptly raise cardiac output to point *B* because of the enhanced contractility before P_v would change appreciably. However, this high cardiac output would increase the net transfer of blood from the venous to the arterial side of the circuit, and consequently, P_v would then begin to fall (point *C*). Cardiac output would continue to fall until a new equilibrium point (D) is reached, which is located at the intersection of the vascular function curve with the new cardiac function curve. The new equilibrium point *(D)* lies above and to the left of the control equilibrium point *(A)*, revealing that sympathetic stimulation evokes a greater cardiac output at a lower level of P_v.

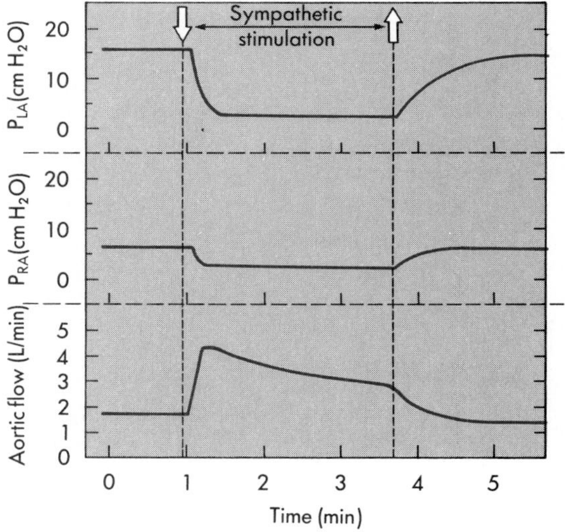

Fig. 9-10 ■ During electrical stimulation of the left stellate ganglion (containing cardiac sympathetic nerve fibers), aortic blood flow increased while pressures in the left atrium *(P_{LA})* and right atrium *(P_{RA})* diminished. These data conform with the conclusions derived from Fig. 9-9, in which the equilibrium values of cardiac output and venous pressure are observed to shift from point *A* to point *D* during cardiac sympathetic nerve stimulation. (Redrawn from Sarnoff, S.J., Brockman, S.K., Gilmore, J.P., Linden, R.J., and Mitchell, J.H.: Circ. Res. 8:1108, 1960.)

Such a change accurately describes the true response. In the experiment depicted in Fig. 9-10, the left stellate ganglion was stimulated between the two arrows. During stimulation aortic flow (cardiac output) rose quickly to a peak value, and then fell gradually to a steady state value that was significantly greater than the control level. The increased aortic flow was accompanied by reductions in right and left atrial pressures (P_{RA} and P_{LA}).

Blood Volume

Changes in blood volume do not directly affect myocardial contractility but they do influence the vascular function curve in the manner shown in Fig. 9-6. Therefore, to understand the circulatory alterations evoked by a given change in blood volume, it is necessary to plot the appropriate cardiac function curve along with the vascular function curves that represent the control and experimental states.

Fig. 9-11 illustrates the response to a blood transfusion. Equilibrium point *B*, which denotes the values for cardiac output and P_v after transfusion, lies above and to the right of the control equilibrium point *A*. Thus transfusion increases both cardiac output and P_v. Hemorrhage has the opposite effect. Pure increases or decreases in venomotor tone elicit responses that are analogous to those evoked by augmentations or reductions, respectively, of the total blood volume, for reasons that were discussed on p. 202.

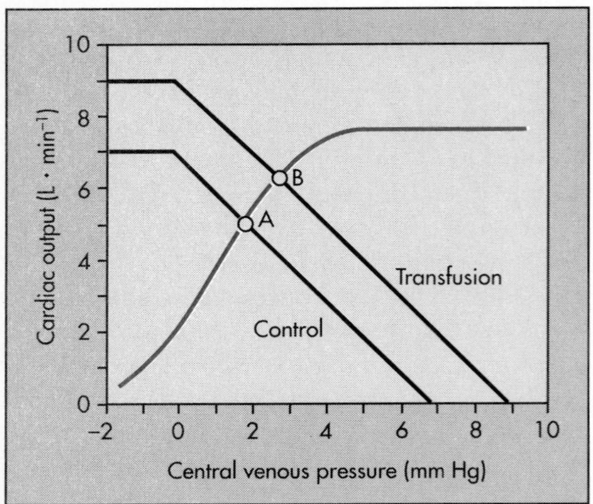

Fig. 9-11 ■ After a blood transfusion the vascular function curve is shifted to the right. Therefore, cardiac output and venous pressure are both increased, as denoted by the translocation of the equilibrium point from *A* to *B*.

Heart Failure

Heart failure may be acute or chronic. Acute heart failure may be caused by toxic quantities of drugs and anesthetics or by certain pathological conditions, such as a sudden coronary artery occlusion. Chronic heart failure may occur in such conditions as essential hypertension or ischemic heart disease. In these various forms of heart failure, myocardial contractility is impaired. Consequently, the cardiac function curve is shifted downward and to the right, as depicted in Fig. 9-12.

In acute heart failure blood volume does not change immediately. Therefore the equilibrium point will shift from the intersection of the normal curves (Fig. 9-12, point *A*) to the intersection of the normal vascular function curve with a depressed cardiac function curve (point *B* or *C*).

In chronic heart failure both the cardiac function and the vascular function curves shift. The vascular function curve shifts because of an increase in blood volume caused in part by fluid retention by the kidneys. The fluid retention is related to the concomitant reduction in

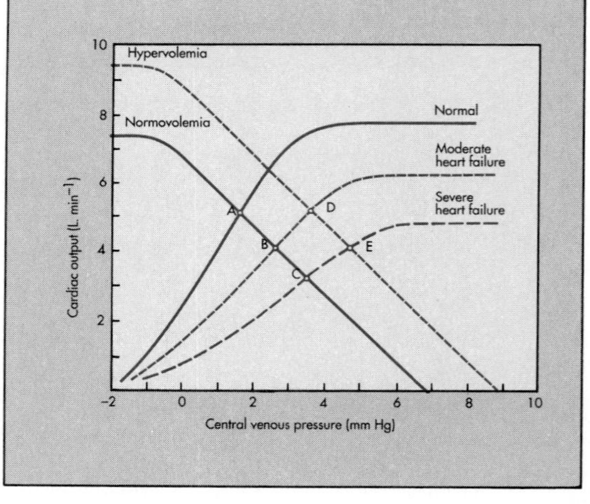

Fig. 9-12 ■ With moderate or severe heart failure, the cardiac function curves are shifted to the right. Before any change in blood volume, cardiac output decreases and central venous pressure rises (from control equilibrium point *A* to point *B* or point *C*). After the increase in blood volume that usually occurs in heart failure, the vascular function curve is shifted to the right. Hence central venous pressure may be elevated with no reduction in cardiac output (point *D*) or (in severe heart failure) with some diminution in cardiac output (point *E*).

glomerular filtration rate and to the increased secretion of aldosterone by the adrenal cortex. The resultant hypervolemia is reflected by a rightward shift of the vascular function curve, as shown in Fig. 9-12. Hence, with moderate degrees of heart failure, P_v will be elevated but cardiac output will be approximately normal (point *D*). With more severe degrees of heart failure, P_v will be still higher but cardiac output will be subnormal (point *E*).

Peripheral Resistance

Predictions concerning the effects of changes in peripheral resistance are also complex because both the cardiac and vascular function curves shift. With increased peripheral resistance (Fig. 9-13) the vascular function curve is rotated counterclockwise but it converges to the same P_v-axis intercept as the control curve (see Fig. 9-7); the direction of rotation differs in Figs. 9-7 and 9-13 because the axes were switched for the vascular function curves in the two figures. The cardiac function curve is also shifted downward because at any given P_v the heart is able to pump less blood against a greater afterload. Because both curves are displaced downward, the new equilibrium point, *B,* will fall below the control point, *A.*

Whether point *B* will fall directly below point *A* or will lie to the right or left of it depends on the magnitude of the shift in each curve. For example, if a given increase in peripheral resistance shifts the vascular function curve more than the cardiac function curve, equilibrium point *B* would fall below and to the left of *A;* that is, both cardiac output and P_v would diminish. Conversely, if the cardiac function curve is displaced more than the vascular function curve, point *B* will fall below and to the right of point *A;* that is, cardiac output would decrease but P_v would rise.

■ ROLE OF HEART RATE

Cardiac output is the product of stroke volume and heart rate. The preceding analysis of the control of cardiac output was, in reality, restricted to the control of stroke volume, and the role of heart rate was neglected.

The effect of changes in heart rate on cardiac output will now be considered. The analysis is complex, because a change in heart rate

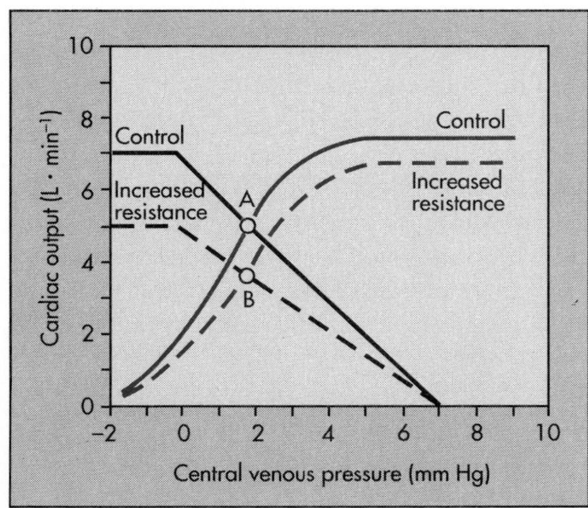

Fig. 9-13 ■ An increase in peripheral resistance shifts the cardiac and the vascular function curves downward. At equilibrium the cardiac output is less *(B)* when the peripheral resistance is high than when it is normal *(A).*

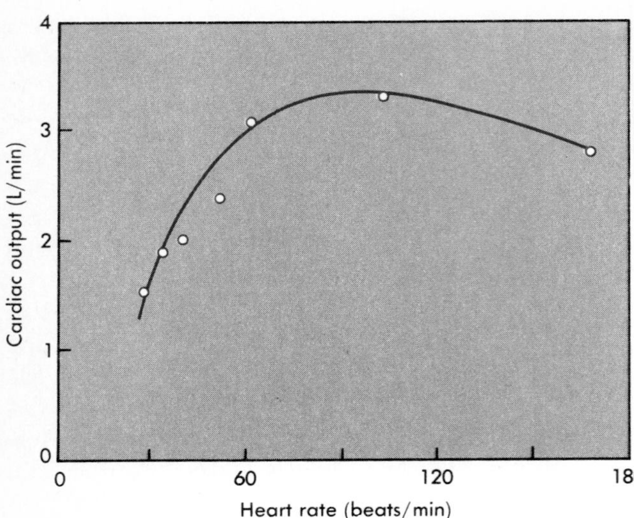

Fig. 9-14 ■ The changes in cardiac output induced by changing the rate of ventricular pacing in a dog with complete heart block. (Redrawn from Miller, D.E., Gleason, W.L., Whalen, R.E., Morris, J.J., and McIntosh, H.D.: Circ. Res. 10:658, 1962. By permission of the American Heart Association, Inc.)

alters the other three factors (preload, afterload, and contractility) that determine stroke volume (see Fig. 9-1). An increase in heart rate, for example, would decrease the duration of diastole. Hence, ventricular filling would be diminished; that is, preload would be reduced. If the proposed increase in heart rate did alter cardiac output, the arterial pressure would change; that is, afterload would be altered. Finally, the rise in heart rate would increase the net influx of Ca^{++} per minute into the myocardial cells, and this would enhance myocardial contractility (p. 100).

Heart rate has been varied by artificial pacing in many types of experimental preparations and in humans. The effects on cardiac output have usually resembled the experimental results shown in Fig. 9-14. In that experiment on a dog with third-degree heart block, contraction frequency was varied by ventricular pacing. As the ventricular rate was increased from 30 to 60 beats per minute, the cardiac output increased substantially. Presumably, at the slowest heart rates within this range, the greater filling per cardiac cycle is not adequate to compensate for the decreased number of contractions per minute.

Over the frequency range from 60 to 170 beats per minute, however, cardiac output did not change very much (Fig. 9-14). Hence, as heart rate was increased, the stroke volume was proportionately reduced. The decreased time for filling at the faster rates partly accounts for the observed proportionality between heart rate increase and stroke volume decrease. Also, vascular autoregulation tends to hold tissue blood flow constant. This adaptation leads to changes in preload and afterload that maintain cardiac output nearly constant. As the heart rate is increased to levels in excess of about 150 to 170 beats per minute, the filling time is so severely restricted that compensation is inadequate and cardiac output decreases precipitously (not shown in Fig. 9-14).

During certain activities, such as physical exercise, the cardiac output increases (see Chapter 12). This change in output is attended predominantly by an increase in heart rate and a slight increase in stroke volume. The temptation is great to conclude that the increase in cardiac output must be caused by the observed increase in heart rate, because of the striking correlation between cardiac output and heart rate. Yet Fig. 9-14 emphasizes that, over a wide range of heart rates, a change in heart rate has little influence on cardiac output. Several studies on exercising subjects have confirmed that, even during exercise, changes in pacing frequency do not alter cardiac output very much.

The principal increase in cardiac output during exercise must therefore be ascribed to the pronounced reduction in peripheral vascular resistance. The attendant changes in heart rate are not inconsequential, however. If the heart rate cannot increase normally during exercise, the augmentation of cardiac output and the capacity for exercise may be severely limited. The increase in heart rate does play a **permissive role** in augmenting cardiac output, even if it is not proper to assign it a primary, causative role. The mechanisms responsible for raising heart rate in precise proportion to the increase in cardiac output are undoubtedly neural in origin, but the specific components of the reflex arcs remain to be elucidated.

■ ANCILLARY FACTORS THAT AFFECT THE VENOUS SYSTEM AND CARDIAC OUTPUT

We have oversimplified the interrelationships between central venous pressure and cardiac output. We have described effects evoked by changes in single variables. However, because many feedback control loops regulate the cardiovascular system, an isolated change in a single response rarely occurs. A change in blood volume, for example, reflexly alters cardiac function, peripheral resistance, and venomotor tone. Several auxiliary factors also regulate cardiac output. Such ancillary factors may be considered to modulate the more basic factors that have been considered above.

Gravity

Gravitational forces may affect cardiac output profoundly. It is not unusual for some soldiers standing at attention to faint because of reduced cardiac output. Gravitational effects are exaggerated in airplane pilots during pullouts from dives. The centrifugal force in the footward direction may be several times greater than the force of gravity. Such individuals characteristically black out momentarily during the maneuver, as blood is drained from the cephalic regions and pooled in the lower parts of the body.

The explanation for the reduction in cardiac output under such conditions is often specious. It is argued that when an individual is standing, the forces of gravity impede venous return from the dependent regions of the body. This statement is incomplete, however, because it ignores the facilitative counterforce on the arterial side of the same circuit.

In this sense the vascular system resembles a U tube. To comprehend the action of gravity on flow through such a system, the models depicted in Figs. 9-15 and 9-16 will be analyzed. In Fig. 9-15 all the U tubes represent rigid cylinders of constant diameter. With both limbs of the U tube oriented horizontally *(A)* the flow depends only on the pressures at the inflow and outflow ends of the tube (P_i and P_o, respectively), the viscosity of the fluid, and the length and radius of the tube, in accordance with Poiseuille's equation (p. 120). With a constant cross section the pressure gradient will be uniform; hence the pressure midway down the tube (P_m) will equal the average of the inflow and outflow pressures.

When the U tube is oriented vertically *(B to D),* hydrostatic forces must be taken into consideration. In tube *B* both limbs are open to atmospheric pressure and both ends are located at the same hydrostatic level; hence there is no flow. The pressure at the midpoint of the tube will simply be ρhg. It will depend on the den-

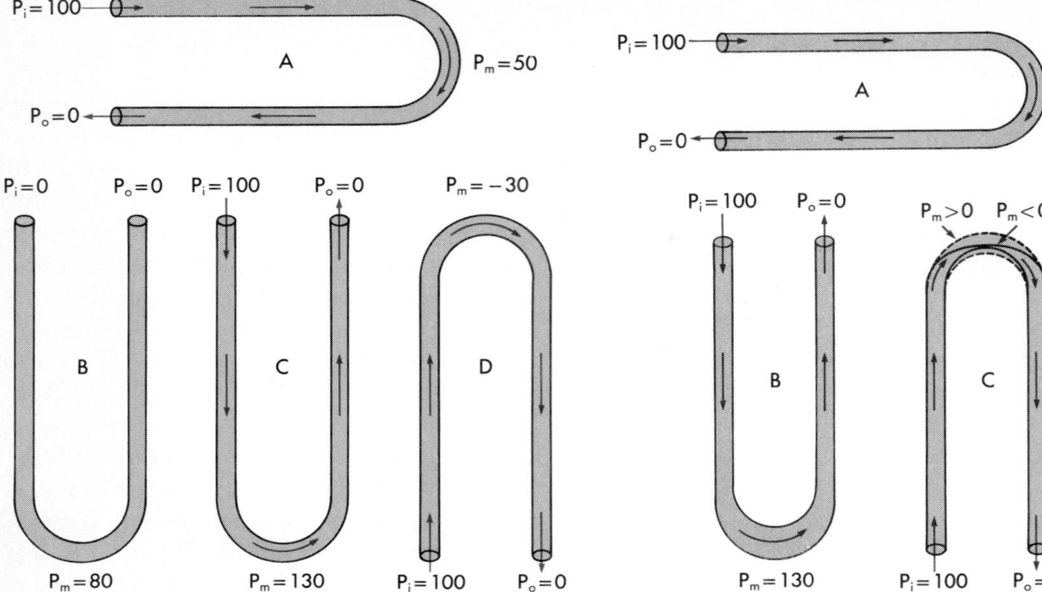

Fig. 9-15 ■ Pressure distributions in **rigid** U tubes with constant internal diameters, all with the same dimensions. For a given inflow pressure ($P_i = 100$) and outflow pressure ($P_o = 0$), the pressure at the midpoint (P_m) depends on the orientation of the U tube, but the flow through the tube is independent of the orientation.

Fig. 9-16 ■ In U tubes with a **distensible** section at the bend, even when inflow (P_i) and outflow (P_o) pressures are the same, the resistance to flow, and the fluid volume contained within each tube vary with the orientation of the tube. P_m, Pressure at the midpoint of the tube.

sity of the fluid, ρ; the height of the U tube, h; and the acceleration of gravity, g. In the example, the length of the U tube is such that the midpoint pressure is 80 mm Hg.

Now consider tube *C*, where the tube is oriented the same as tube *B*, but where a 100 mm Hg pressure difference is applied across the two ends. The flow will precisely equal that in *A*, because the pressure gradient, tube dimensions, and fluid viscosity are all the same. Gravitational forces are precisely equal in magnitude but opposite in direction in the two limbs of the U tube. Because the flow will be the same as that in *A*, there will be a pressure drop of 50 mm Hg at the midpoint because of the viscous losses resulting from flow. Furthermore, gravity will tend to increase pressure by 80 mm Hg at the midpoint, just as in tube *B*. The actual pressure at the midpoint of tube *C* will be the resultant of the viscous loss and hydrostatic gain, or 130 mm Hg in this example.

In *D* a pressure gradient of 100 mm Hg is applied to the same U tube, but the tube is oriented in the opposite direction. Gravitational forces will be so directed that the pressure at the midpoint will tend to be 80 mm Hg less than that at the end of the U tube. Viscous losses will still produce a 50 mm Hg pressure drop at the midpoint relative to P_i. Hence, with this orientation, pressure at the midpoint of the U tube will be 30 mm Hg below ambient pressure. Flow will, of course, be the same as in tubes *A* and *C*, for the reasons stated in relation to *C*.

In a system of rigid U tubes gravitational effects will not alter the rate of fluid flow. However, experience shows that gravity does affect the cardiovascular system. The reason is that the vessels are distensible rather than rigid. To explain the gravitational effects, the pressures in a set of U tubes with distensible components (at the bends in the tubes of Fig. 9-16) will be examined. In tubes *A* and *B* the pressure distributions will resemble those in tubes *A* and *C*, respectively, of Fig. 9-15. Because the pressure is higher at the bend of tube *B* than at the bend of tube *A* in Fig. 9-16 and because the segments are distensible in this region, the distension at bend *B* will exceed that at bend *A*. The extent of the distension will depend on the compliance of these tube segments. Because flow varies directly with the tube diameter, the flow through *B* will exceed the flow through *A* for a given pressure difference applied at the ends.

Because orienting a U tube with its bend downward actually increases rather than diminishes flow, how then is the observed impairment of cardiovascular function explained when the body is similarly oriented? The explanation is that the cardiovascular system is a closed circuit of constant fluid (blood) volume, whereas the U tube is an open conduit supplied by a fluid source of unlimited volume. In the dependent regions of the cardiovascular system, the distension will occur more on the venous than on the arterial side of the circuit, because the venous compliance is so much greater than the arterial compliance. Such venous distension is readily observed on the back of the hands when the arms are allowed to hang down. The hemodynamic effects of such venous distension **(venous pooling)** resemble those caused by the hemorrhage of an equivalent volume of blood from the body. When an adult person shifts from a supine position to a relaxed standing position, from 300 to 800 ml of blood are pooled in the legs. This may reduce cardiac output by about 2 L/min.

The compensatory adjustments to the erect position are similar to the adjustments to blood loss. For example, the diminished baroreceptor excitation reflexly speeds the heart, strengthens the cardiac contraction, and constricts the arterioles and veins. The baroreceptor reflex has a greater effect on the resistance than on the capacitance vessels.

Warm ambient temperatures interfere with the compensatory vasomotor reactions, and the absence of muscular activity exaggerates the effects. Many of the drugs used to treat hypertension also interfere with the reflex adaptation to standing. Similarly, astronauts exposed to weightlessness lose their adaptations after a few days in space, and they experience difficulties when they first return to earth. When individuals with impaired reflex adaptations stand, their blood pressures may drop substantially. This response is called **orthostatic hypotension,** which may cause lightheadedness or fainting.

When the U tube is rotated so that the bend is directed upward (Fig. 9-16, tube *C*), the effects are opposite to those that take place in tube *B*. The pressure at the bend of tube *C* would tend to be −30 mm Hg, just as in tube *D* of Fig. 9-15. Because the ambient pressure exceeds the internal pressure, however, the distensible segment of tube *C* will collapse. Flow will then cease, and therefore, the decline of pressure associated with viscous flow will cease. In U tube *C*, when flow stops, the pressure at the top of each limb will be 80 mm Hg less than at the bottom (the hydrostatic pressure difference). Hence, in the left, or inflow, limb the pressure will approach 20 mm Hg. As soon as this pressure exceeds ambient pressure (0 mm Hg), the collapsed tubing will be forced open and flow will begin. With the onset of flow, however, pressure at the bend will again drop below the ambient pressure. Thus the tubing at the bend will flutter; that is, it will fluctuate between the open and closed states.

When an arm is raised, the cutaneous veins in the hand and forearm collapse, for the reasons described previously. Fluttering does not occur here because the deeper veins are protected from collapse by being tethered to surrounding structures. This protection allows these deeper veins to accommodate the flow ordinarily carried by the collapsed superficial veins. The analogy would be to add a rigid tube (representing the deeper veins) in parallel with the collapsible tube (representing the superficial veins) at the bend of tube *C* in Fig. 9-16. The collapsible tube would no longer flutter, but would remain closed. All flow would occur through the rigid tube, just as in tube *D* in Fig. 9-15.

The superficial veins in the neck are ordinarily partially collapsed when a normal individual is upright. Venous return from the head is conducted largely through the deeper cervical veins. However, when **central venous pressure** is abnormally elevated, the superficial neck veins are distended and they do not collapse even when the subject sits or stands. Such cervical venous distension is an important clinical sign of congestive heart failure.

Muscular Activity and Venous Valves

When a recumbent person stands but remains at rest, the pressure rises in the veins in the dependent regions of the body. The venous pressure in the legs increases gradually and does not reach an equilibrium value until almost 1 minute after standing. The slowness of this rise in P_v is attributable to the venous valves, which permit flow only toward the heart. When the person stands, the valves prevent blood in the veins from actually falling toward the feet. Hence the column of venous blood is supported at numerous levels by these valves; temporarily the venous column consists of many discontinuous segments. However, blood continues to enter the column from many venules and small tributary veins, and the pressure continues to rise. As soon as the pressure in one segment exceeds that in the segment just above it, the intervening valve is forced open. Ultimately, all the valves are open, and the column is continuous, similar to the state in the outflow limbs of the U tubes shown in Figs. 9-15 and 9-16.

Precise measurement reveals that the final level of P_v in the feet during quiet standing is only slightly greater than that in a static column of blood extending from the right atrium to the feet. This indicates that the pressure drop caused by blood flow from the foot veins to the right atrium is very small. This very low resistance justifies lumping all the veins as a common venous compliance in the circulatory system model illustrated in Fig. 9-2.

When an individual who has been standing quietly begins to walk, the venous pressure in the legs decreases appreciably. Because of the intermittent venous compression exerted by the contracting leg muscles and because of the presence of the venous valves, blood is forced from the veins toward the heart. Hence, muscular contraction lowers the mean venous pressure in the legs and serves as an **auxiliary pump.** Furthermore, it prevents venous pooling and lowers capillary hydrostatic pressure. Thereby, it reduces the tendency for edema fluid to collect in the feet during standing.

Respiratory Activity

The normal, periodic activity of the respiratory muscles causes rhythmic variations in vena caval flow. Thus, respiration constitutes an auxiliary pump to promote venous return. Coughing, straining at stool, and other activities that require respiratory muscle exertion may affect cardiac output substantially.

The changes in blood flow in the superior

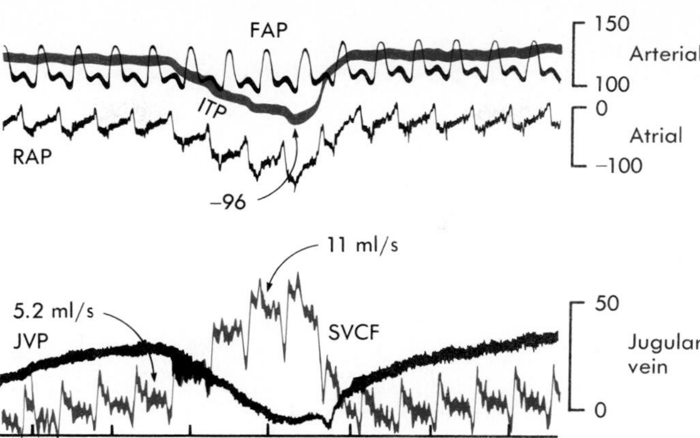

Fig. 9-17 ■ During a normal inspiration, intrathoracic *(ITP)*, right atrial *(RAP)*, and jugular venous *(JVP)* pressures decrease, and flow in the superior vena cava *(SVCF)* increases (from 5.2 to 11 ml/s). All pressures are in millimeters of water, except for femoral arterial pressure *(FAP)*, which is in millimeters of mercury. (Modified from Brecher, G.A.: Venous return, New York, 1956, Grune & Stratton, Inc.)

vena cava during the normal respiratory cycle are shown in Fig. 9-17. During respiration the reduction in intrathoracic pressure is transmitted to the lumina of the thoracic blood vessels. The reduction in central venous pressure during inspiration increases the pressure gradient between extrathoracic and intrathoracic veins. The consequent acceleration of venous return to the right atrium is displayed in Fig. 9-17 as an increase in superior vena caval blood flow from 5.2 ml/s during expiration to 11 ml/s during inspiration.

An exaggerated reduction in intrathoracic pressure achieved by a strong inspiratory effort against a closed glottis (called **Müller's maneuver**) does not increase venous return proportionately. The extrathoracic veins collapse near their entry into the chest when their internal pressures fall below the ambient level. As the veins collapse, flow into the chest momentarily stops. The cessation of flow raises pressure upstream, forcing the collapsed segment to open again. The process is repetitive; the venous segments adjacent to the chest alternately open and close.

During normal expiration, flow into the central veins decelerates. However, the mean rate of venous return during normal respiration exceeds the flow during a brief period of **apnea** (cessation of respiration). Hence normal inspiration apparently facilitates venous return more than normal expiration impedes it. In part, this must be attributable to the valves in the veins of the extremities and neck. These valves prevent any reversal of flow during expiration. Thus the respiratory muscles and venous valves constitute an **auxiliary pump** for venous return.

Sustained expiratory efforts increase intrathoracic pressure and thereby impede venous return. Straining against a closed glottis (termed **Valsalva's maneuver**) regularly occurs during coughing, defecation, and heavy lifting. Intrathoracic pressures in excess of 100 mm Hg have been recorded in trumpet players and pressures over 400 mm Hg have been observed during paroxysms of coughing. Such pressure increases are transmitted directly to the lumina of the intrathoracic arteries. After cessation of coughing the arterial

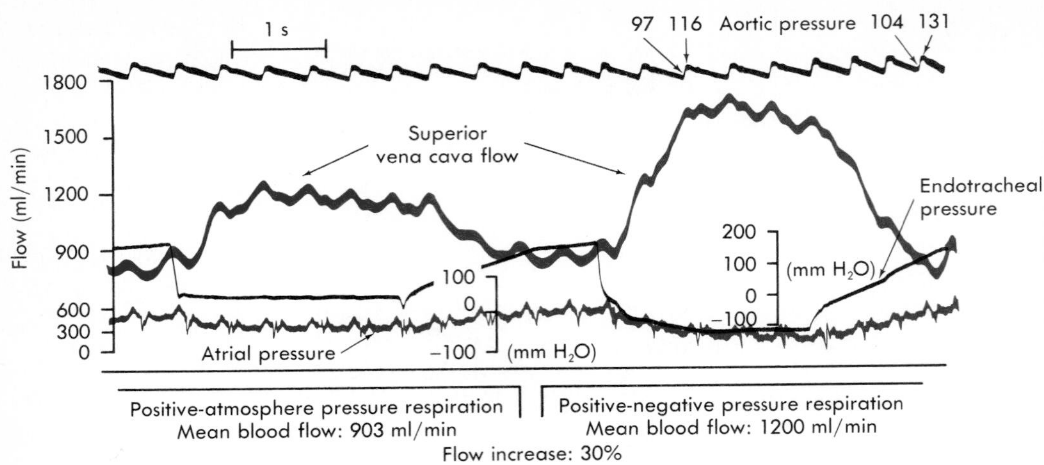

Fig. 9-18 ■ During intermittent positive-pressure respiration, the flow in the superior vena cava is approximately 30% greater when the lungs are deflated actively by applying negative endotracheal pressure *(right side)* than when they are allowed to deflate passively against atmospheric pressure *(left side)*. (Modified from Brecher, G.A.: Venous return, New York, 1956, Grune & Stratton, Inc.)

blood pressure may fall precipitously because of the preceding impediment to venous return.

The dramatic increase in intrathoracic pressure induced by coughing constitutes an **auxiliary pumping mechanism** for the blood, despite its concurrent tendency to impede venous return. During certain diagnostic procedures, such as coronary angiography or electrophysiological testing, patients are at increased risk for ventricular fibrillation. Such patients have been trained to cough rhythmically on command. If ventricular fibrillation does occur, substantial arterial blood pressure increments are generated by each cough, and enough cerebral blood flow may be promoted to sustain consciousness. The cough raises the intravascular pressure equally in intrathoracic arteries and veins. Blood is propelled through the extrathoracic tissues, however, because the increased pressure is transmitted to the extrathoracic arteries but not to the extrathoracic veins, because of the valves in the extrathoracic veins.

Artificial Respiration

In most forms of artificial respiration (mouth-to-mouth resuscitation, mechanical respiration), lung inflation is achieved by applying endotracheal pressures above atmospheric pressure, and expiration occurs by passive recoil of the thoracic cage. Thus lung inflation is attended by an appreciable rise in intrathoracic pressure. Vena cava flow decreases sharply during the phase of positive-pressure lung inflation (indicated by the progressive rise in endotracheal pressure in the central portion of Fig. 9-18). When negative endotracheal pressure (indicated by the abrupt decrease in endotracheal pressure in the right half of Fig. 9-18) is used to facilitate deflation, vena cava flow accelerates more than when the lungs are allowed to deflate passively (near the left border of Fig. 9-18).

■ SUMMARY

1. Two important relationships between cardiac output (CO) and central venous pressure (P_v) prevail in the cardiovascular system. One applies to the heart and the other to the vascular system.
2. With respect to the heart, CO varies **directly** with P_v (or preload) over a very wide range of P_v. This relationship is represented by the **cardiac function curve,** and it expresses the Frank-Starling mechanism.
3. With respect to the vascular system, P_v varies **inversely** with CO. This relationship is represented by the **vascular function curve,** and it reflects the fact that as CO increases, for example, a greater fraction of the total blood volume resides in the arteries and a smaller volume resides in the veins.
4. The principal mechanisms that govern the cardiac function curve are the changes in numbers of crossbridges that interact and in the affinity of the contractile proteins for calcium. These mechanisms are evoked by changes in the cardiac filling pressure (preload).
5. The principal factors that govern the vascular function curve are the arterial and venous compliances, the peripheral vascular resistance, and the total blood volume.
6. The equilibrium values of CO and P_v that prevail under a given set of conditions are determined by the **intersection** of the cardiac and vascular function curves.
7. At very low and very high **heart rates,** the heart is unable to pump adequate CO. At the very low rates, the increment in filling during diastole cannot compensate for the small number of cardiac contractions per minute. At the very high rates, the large number of contractions per minute cannot compensate for the inadequate filling time.
8. Gravity influences CO because the veins are so compliant, and substantial quantities of blood tend to pool in the veins of the dependent portions of the body.
9. Respiration changes the pressure gradient between the intrathoracic and extrathoracic veins. Hence, respiration serves as an **auxiliary pump,** which may affect the mean level of CO and the transitory changes in stroke volume during the various phases of the respiratory cycle.

■ BIBLIOGRAPHY

Journal articles

Bedford, T.G., and Dormer, K.J.: Arterial hemodynamics during head-up tilt in conscious dogs, J. Appl. Physiol. 65:1556, 1988.

Bromberger-Barnea, B.: Mechanical effects of inspiration on heart functions: a review, Fed. Proc. 40:2172, 1981.

Carneiro, J.J., and Donald, D.E.: Blood reservoir function of dog spleen, liver, and intestine, Am. J. Physiol. 232:H67, 1977.

Freeman, G.L., Little, W.C., and O'Rourke, R.A.: Influence of heart rate on left ventricular performance in conscious dogs, Circ. Res., 61:455, 1987.

Greenway, C.V.: Mechanisms and quantitative assessment of drug effects on cardiac output with a new model of the circulation, Pharmacol. Rev. 33:213, 1982.

Johnston, W.E., Vinten-Johansen, J., Santamore, W.P., Case, L.D., and Little, W.C.: Mechanism of reduced cardiac output during positive end-expiratory pressure in the dog, Am. Rev. Respir. Dis. 140:1257, 1989.

Levy, M.N.: The cardiac and vascular factors that determine systemic blood flow, Circ. Res. 44:739, 1979.

Miller, R.R., Fennell, W.H., Young, J.B., Palomo, A.R., and Quinones, M.A.: Differential systemic arterial and venous actions and consequent cardiac effects of vasodilator drugs, Prog. Cardiovasc. Dis. 24:353, 1982.

Narahara, K.A., and Blettel, M.L.: Effect of rate on left ventricular volumes and ejection fraction during chronic ventricular pacing, Circulation 67:323, 1983.

Peters, J., Fraser, C., Stuart, R.S., Baumgartner, W., and Robotham, J.L.: Negative intrathoracic pressure decreases independently left ventricular filling and emptying, Am. J. Physiol. 257:H120, 1989.

Rothe, C.F.: Physiology of venous return. An unappreciated boost to the heart, Arch. Intern. Med., 146:977, 1986.

Rothe, C.F., and Gaddis, M.L.: Autoregulation of cardiac output by passive elastic characteristics of the vascular capacitance system, Circ. 81:360, 1990.

Shoukas, A.A., and Bohlen, H.G.: Rat venular pressure-diameter relationships are regulated by sympathetic activity, Am. J. Physiol. 259:H674, 1990.

Shoukas, A.A., and Sagawa, K.: Control of total systemic vascular capacity by the carotid sinus baroreceptor reflex, Circ. Res. 33:22, 1973.

Books and monographs

Green, J.F.: Determinants of systemic blood flow. International Review of Physiology III: Cardiovascular Physiology, vol. 18, Baltimore, 1979, University Park Press.

Guyton, A.C., Jones, C.E., and Coleman, T.G.: Circulatory physiology: cardiac output and its regulation, ed. 2, Philadelphia, 1973, W.B. Saunders Co.

Rothe, C.F.: Venous system: physiology of the capacitance vessels. In Handbook of physiology; Section 2: The cardiovascular system—peripheral circulation and organ blood flow, vol. III, Bethesda, Md., 1983, American Physiological Society.

Yin, F.C.P., editor: Ventricular/vascular coupling, New York, 1987, Springer-Verlag.

10 Coronary Circulation

■ FUNCTIONAL ANATOMY OF CORONARY VESSELS

The right and left coronary arteries, which arise at the root of the aorta behind the right and left cusps of the aortic valve, respectively, provide the entire blood supply to the myocardium. The right coronary artery supplies principally the right ventricle and atrium; the left coronary artery, which divides near its origin into the anterior descendens and the circumflex branches, supplies principally the left ventricle and atrium, but there is some overlap. In the dog the left coronary artery supplies about 85% of the myocardium, whereas in humans the right coronary artery is dominant in 50% of individuals, the left coronary artery is dominant in another 20%, and the flow delivered by each main artery is about equal in the remaining 30%.

Coronary blood flow is most commonly measured in humans by thermodilution. Thermodilution is the same procedure used for the measurement of cardiac output (p. 78), except that the indicator (cold saline) is ejected at the tip of a catheter inserted into the coronary sinus via a peripheral vein. The thermal sensor (thermistor) is located on the catheter a few centimeters from the catheter tip. The greater the coronary sinus outflow, the less the temperature decrease produced by the cold saline injection. This method does not measure total coronary blood flow because only about two thirds of coronary arterial inflow returns to the venous circulation through the coronary sinus. However, almost all of the blood flow that does empty into the coronary sinus comes from the left ventricle. Hence the thermodilution method provides a good estimate of left ventricular coronary blood flow. Right and left coronary artery inflow, as well as inflow of the major branches of the left coronary artery, can be measured with reasonable accuracy by injection of a radioactive tracer (for example, ^{133}Xe) through a catheter threaded into the coronary artery via a peripheral artery. Myocardial clearance of the isotope is monitored with a detector appropriately placed over the precordium.

Recently, newer methods for measurement of coronary blood flow have been developed. In the major coronary arteries, blood flow can be measured by the pulsed Doppler technique. An ultrasound signal is emitted from a crystal at the tip of a cardiac catheter that is inserted into the origin of the artery to be studied. The sound is reflected by the flowing blood, and the frequency shift of the reflected sound is proportional to the velocity of the blood flow. From an estimate of the cross-sectional area of the coronary artery and the measured flow velocity, the blood flow can be calculated. Coronary blood flow can also be estimated by videodensitometry where the movement a bolus of a radioopaque substance injected into the coronary artery can be monitored by rapid sequential radiographs. Similarly, intracoronary injection of microbubbles and tracking their movement by echocardiography is used to measure coronary blood flow. Also, ciné computed tomography and magnetic resonance imaging are being developed for determination of total and regional myocardial blood flow.

After passage through the capillary beds, most of the venous blood returns to the right atrium through the coronary sinus, but some reaches the right atrium by way of the anterior coronary veins. There are also vascular communications directly between the vessels of the myocardium and the cardiac chambers; these comprise the **arteriosinusoidal,** the **arterioluminal,** and the **thebesian vessels.** The arteriosinusoidal channels consist of small arteries or arterioles that lose their arterial structure as they penetrate the chamber walls and divide into irregular, endothelium-lined sinuses (50 to 250 μm). These sinuses anastomose with other sinuses and with capillaries and communicate with the cardiac chambers. The arterioluminal vessels are small arteries or arterioles that open directly into the atria and ventricles. The thebesian vessels are small veins that connect capillary beds directly with the cardiac chambers and also communicate with cardiac veins and other thebesian veins. On the basis of anatomical studies, intercommunication appears to exist among all the minute vessels of the myocardium in the form of an extensive plexus of subendocardial vessels. It has been suggested that some myocardial nutrition can be derived from the cardiac cavities through those channels. Isotope-labeled blood in the cardiac chambers does penetrate a short distance into the endocardium, but does not constitute a significant source of oxygen and nutrients to the myocardium. In the dog a major fraction of the left coronary inflow returns to the right atrium via the coronary sinus, and a small fraction that supplies the interventricular septum returns directly to the right ventricular cavity. Right coronary artery drainage is mainly via the anterior cardiac veins to the right atrium. The epicardial distribution of the coronary arteries and veins is illustrated in Fig. 10-1.

■ FACTORS THAT INFLUENCE CORONARY BLOOD FLOW

Physical factors

The primary factor responsible for perfusion of the myocardium is the aortic pressure, which is, of course, generated by the heart itself. Changes in aortic pressure generally evoke parallel directional changes in coronary blood flow. However, alterations of cardiac work, produced by an increase or decrease in aortic pressure, have a considerable effect on coronary resistance. Increased metabolic activity of the heart results in a decrease in coronary resistance, and a reduction in cardiac metabolism produces an increase in coronary resistance. If a cannulated coronary artery is perfused by blood from a pressure-controlled reservoir, perfusion pressure can be altered without changing aortic pressure and cardiac work. Under these conditions abrupt variations in perfusion pressure produce equally abrupt changes in coronary blood flow in the same direction. However, maintenance of the perfusion pressure at the new level is associated with a return of blood flow toward the level observed before the induced change in perfusion pressure (Fig. 10-2). This phenomenon is an example of autoregulation of blood flow and is discussed in Chapter 8. Under normal

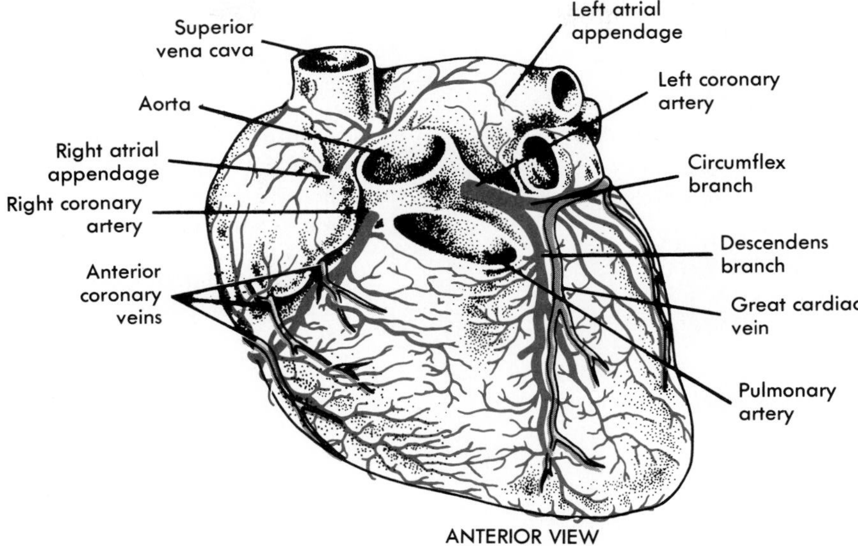

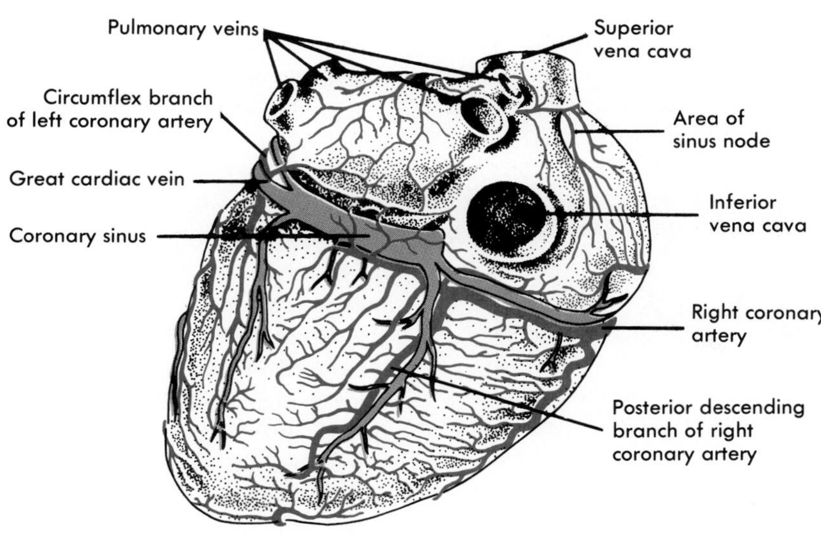

Fig. 10-1 ■ Anterior and posterior surfaces of the heart, illustrating the location and distribution of the principal coronary vessels.

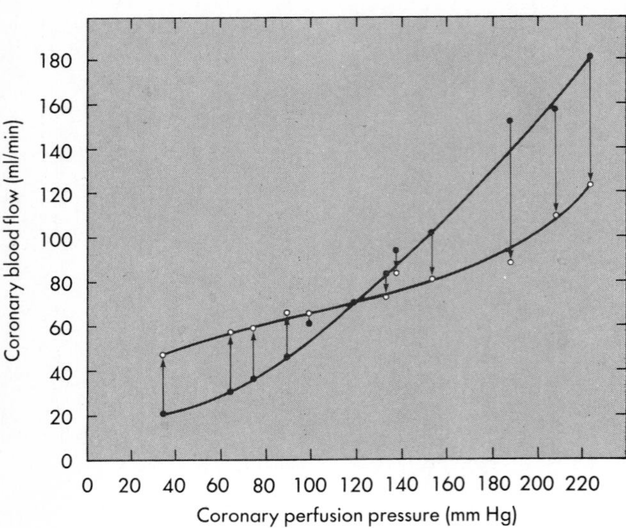

Fig. 10-2 ■ Pressure-flow relationships in the coronary vascular bed. At constant aortic pressure, cardiac output, and heart rate, coronary artery perfusion pressure was abruptly increased or decreased from the control level indicated by the point where the two lines cross. The closed circles represent the flows that were obtained immediately after the change in perfusion pressure, and the open circles represent the steady-state flows at the new pressures. There is a tendency for flow to return toward the control level (autoregulation of blood flow), and this is most prominent over the intermediate pressure range (about 60 to 180 mm Hg).

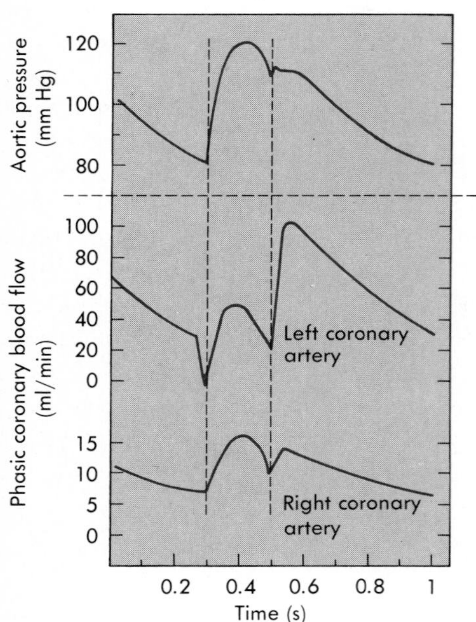

Fig. 10-3 ■ Comparison of phasic coronary blood flow in the left and right coronary arteries.

conditions blood pressure is kept within relatively narrow limits by the baroreceptor reflex mechanisms so that changes in coronary blood flow are primarily caused by caliber changes of the coronary resistance vessels in response to metabolic demands of the heart.

In addition to providing the head of pressure to drive blood through the coronary vessels, the heart also influences its blood supply by the squeezing effect of the contracting myocardium on the blood vessels that course through it (**extravascular compression** or **extracoronary resistance**). This force is so great during early ventricular systole that blood flow, as measured in a large coronary artery that supplies the left ventricle, is briefly reversed. Maximum left coronary inflow occurs in early diastole, when the ventricles have relaxed and extravascular compression of the coronary vessels is virtually absent. This flow pattern is seen in the phasic coronary flow curve for the left coronary artery (Fig. 10-3). After an initial reversal in early systole, left coronary blood flow follows the aortic pressure until early diastole, when it rises abruptly and then declines slowly as aortic pressure falls during the remainder of diastole.

The minimum extravascular resistance and absence of left ventricular work during diastole, are used to advantage clinically to improve myocardial perfusion in patients with damaged myocardium and low blood pressure. The method is called **counterpulsation** and consists of the insertion of an inflatable balloon into the thoracic aorta through a femoral artery. The balloon is inflated during ventricular diastole and deflated during systole. This procedure enhances coronary blood flow during diastole by raising diastolic pressure at a time when coronary extravascular resistance is lowest. Furthermore, it reduces cardiac energy requirements by lowering aortic pressure during ventricular ejection.

Left ventricular myocardial pressure (pressure within the wall of the left ventricle) is greatest near the endocardium and lowest near the epicardium. However, under normal conditions this pressure gradient does not impair endocardial blood flow, because a greater blood flow to the endocardium during diastole compensates for the greater blood flow to the epicardium during systole. In fact, when 10 μm diameter radioactive spheres are injected into the coronary arteries, their distribution indicates that the blood flow to the epicardial and endocardial halves of the left ventricle are approximately equal (slightly higher in the endocardium) under normal conditions. Because extravascular compression is greatest at the endocardial surface of the ventricle, equality of epicardial and endocardial blood flow must mean that the tone of the endocardial resistance vessels is less than that of the epicardial vessels.

Under abnormal conditions, when diastolic pressure in the coronary arteries is low, such as in severe hypotension, partial coronary artery occlusion, or severe aortic stenosis, the ratio of endocardial to epicardial blood flow falls below a value of 1. This indicates that the blood flow to the endocardial regions is more severely impaired than that to the epicardial regions of the ventricle. The redistribution of coronary blood flow is also reflected in an increase in the gradient of myocardial lactic acid and adenosine concentrations from epicardium to endocardium. For this reason, the myocardial damage observed in arteriosclerotic heart disease (for example, following coronary occlusion) is greatest in the inner wall of the left ventricle.

Flow in the right coronary artery shows a similar pattern (see Fig. 10-3), but because of the lower pressure developed during systole by the thin right ventricle, reversal of blood flow does not occur in early systole and systolic blood flow constitutes a much greater proportion of total coronary inflow than it does in the left coronary artery. The extent to which extravascular compression restricts coronary inflow can be readily seen when the heart is suddenly arrested in diastole or with the induction of ventricular fibrillation. Fig. 10-4 depicts mean left coronary flow when the vessel was perfused with blood at a constant pressure from a reservoir. At the arrow in record *A*, ventricular fibrillation was electrically induced and an immediate and substantial increase in blood flow occurred. Subsequent increase in coronary resistance over a period of many minutes reduced myocardial blood flow to below the level existing before induction of ventricular fibrillation (record *B*, before stellate ganglion stimulation).

Tachycardia and bradycardia have dual effects on coronary blood flow. A change in heart rate is accomplished chiefly by shortening or lengthening of diastole. With tachycardia the proportion of time spent in systole, and consequently the period of restricted inflow, increases. However, this mechanical reduction in mean coronary flow is overridden by the coronary dilation associated with the increased

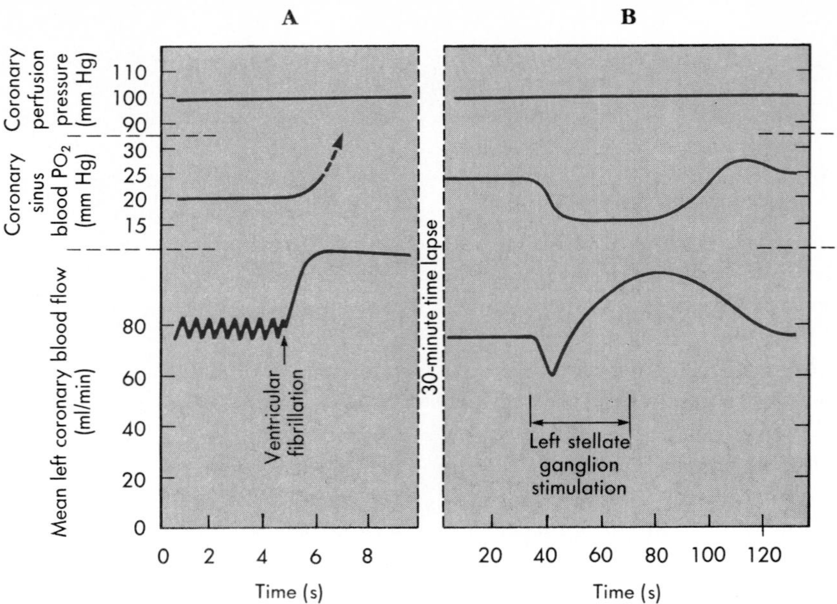

Fig. 10-4 ■ **A,** Unmasking of the restricting effect of ventricular systole on mean coronary blood flow by induction of ventricular fibrillation during constant pressure perfusion of the left coronary artery. **B,** Effect of cardiac sympathetic nerve stimulation on coronary blood flow and coronary sinus blood O_2 tension in the fibrillating heart during constant pressure perfusion of the left coronary artery.

metabolic activity of the more rapidly beating heart. With bradycardia the opposite is true; restriction of coronary inflow is less (more time in diastole) but so are the metabolic (O_2) requirements of the myocardium.

Neural and Neurohumoral Factors

Stimulation of the sympathetic nerves to the heart elicits a marked increase in coronary blood flow. However, the increase in flow is associated with cardiac acceleration and a more forceful systole. The stronger myocardial contractions and the tachycardia (with the consequence that a greater proportion of time is spent in systole) tend to restrict coronary flow, whereas the increase in myocardial metabolic activity, as evidenced by the rate and contractility changes, tends to evoke dilation of the coronary resistance vessels. The increase in coronary blood flow observed with cardiac sympathetic nerve stimulation is the algebraic sum of these factors. In perfused hearts in which the mechanical effect of extravascular compression is eliminated by cardiac arrest or ventricular fibrillation, an initial coronary vasoconstriction is often observed with cardiac sympathetic nerve stimulation before the vasodilation attributable to the metabolic effect comes into play (Fig. 10-4, *B*).

Furthermore, after the beta receptors are blocked to eliminate the chronotropic and inotropic effects, direct reflex activation of the sympathetic nerves to the heart increases coronary resistance. These observations indicate that *the primary action of the sympathetic nerve fibers on the coronary resistance vessels is vasoconstriction.*

Alpha- and beta-adrenergic drugs and their respective blocking agents reveal the presence of alpha-receptors (constrictors) and beta-receptors (dilators) on the coronary vessels. Furthermore, the coronary resistance vessels participate in the baroreceptor and chemoreceptor reflexes and there is sympathetic constrictor tone of the coronary arterioles that can be reflexly modulated. Nevertheless, coronary resistance is predominantly under local nonneural control.

Vagus nerve stimulation slightly dilates the coronary resistance vessels, and activation of the carotid and aortic chemoreceptors can elicit a small decrease in coronary resistance via the vagus nerves to the heart. The failure of strong vagal stimulation to evoke a large increase in coronary blood flow is not because of insensitivity of the coronary resistance vessels to acetylcholine, because intracoronary administration of this agent elicits marked vasodilation.

Reflexes originating in the myocardium and altering vascular resistance in peripheral systemic vessels, including the coronary vessels, have been conclusively demonstrated. However, the existence of extracardiac reflexes, with the coronary resistance vessels as the effector sites, has not been established.

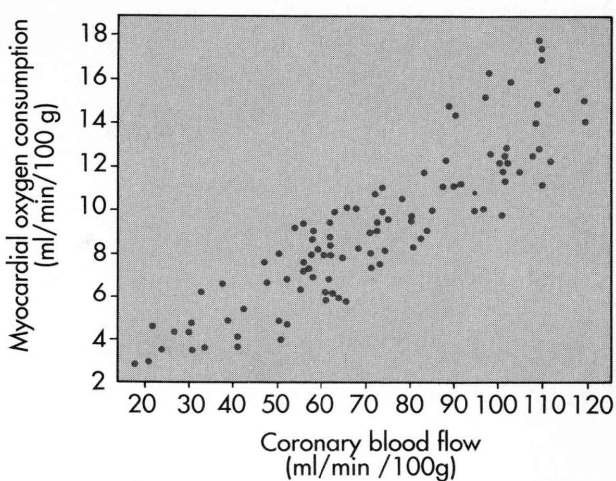

Fig. 10-5 ■ Relationship between myocardial oxygen consumption and coronary blood flow during a variety of interventions that increased or decreased myocardial metabolic rate. (Redrawn from Berne, R.M. and Rubio, R.: Coronary circulation. In Handbook of physiology, the cardiovascular system—the heart, vol. 1, Bethesda, Md., 1979, American Physiological Society.

Metabolic Factors

One of the most striking characteristics of the coronary circulation is the close parallelism between the level of myocardial metabolic activity and the magnitude of the coronary blood flow (Fig. 10-5). This relationship is also found in the denervated heart or the completely isolated heart, whether in the beating or the fibrillating state. The ventricles will continue to fibrillate for many hours when the coronary arteries are perfused with arterial blood from some external source. With the onset of ventricular fibrillation, an abrupt increase in coronary blood flow occurs because of the removal of extravascular compression (see Fig. 10-4). Flow then gradually returns toward, and often falls below, the prefibrillation level. The increase in coronary resistance that occurs despite the elimination of extravascular compression is a manifestation of the heart's ability to adjust its blood flow to meet its energy requirements. The fibrillating heart utilizes less O_2 than the pumping heart, and blood flow to the myocardium is reduced accordingly.

The link between cardiac metabolic rate and coronary blood flow remains unsettled. However, it appears that a decrease in the ratio of oxygen supply to oxygen demand (whether produced by a reduction in oxygen supply or

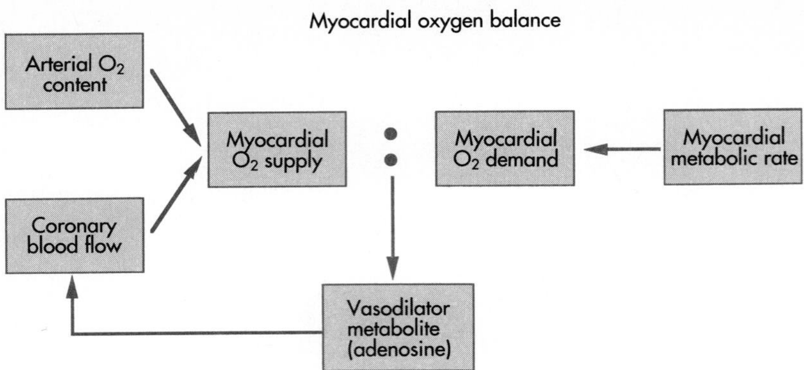

Fig. 10-6 ■ Imbalance in the oxygen supply/oxygen demand ratio alters coronary blood flow by the rate of release of a vasodilator metabolite from the cardiomyocytes. A decrease in the ratio elicits an increase in vasodilator release, whereas an increase in the ratio has the opposite effect.

by an increment in oxygen demand) releases a vasodilator substance from the myocardium into the interstitial fluid, where it can relax the coronary resistance vessels. As diagrammed in Fig. 10-6 a decrease in arterial blood oxygen content, coronary blood flow or both, or an increase in metabolic rate decreases the oxygen supply/demand ratio. This causes the release of a vasodilator substance such as adenosine, which dilates the arterioles, thereby adjusting oxygen supply to demand. A decrease in oxygen demand would reduce the vasodilator release and permit greater expression of basal tone. Numerous agents, generally referred to as metabolites, have been suggested as mediators of the vasodilation observed with increased cardiac work. Accumulation of vasoactive metabolites also may be responsible for reactive hyperemia, because the duration of coronary flow after release of the briefly occluded vessel is, within certain limits, proportional to the duration of the period of occlusion. Among the substances implicated are CO_2, O_2 (reduced O_2 tension), hydrogen ions (lactic acid), potassium ions, and adenosine. Of these agents adenosine comes closest to satisfying criteria for the physiologic mediator. According to the adenosine hypothesis, a reduction in myocardial O_2 tension produced by low coronary blood flow, hypoxemia, or increased metabolic activity of the heart leads to the myocardial formation of adenosine. This nucleoside crosses the interstitial fluid space to reach the coronary resistance vessels and induces vasodilation by activating an adenosine receptor.

Although potassium release from the myocardium can account for about half of the initial decrease in coronary resistance, it cannot be responsible for the increased coronary flow observed with prolonged enhancement of cardiac metabolic activity, because its release from the cardiac muscle is transitory. There is little evidence that CO_2, hydrogen ions, or O_2 play a significant **direct** role in the regulation of coronary blood flow. Factors that alter coronary vascular resistance are schematized in Fig. 10-7.

■ CORONARY COLLATERAL CIRCULATION AND VASODILATORS

In the normal human heart there are virtually no functional intercoronary channels, whereas in the dog there are a few small vessels that link branches of the major coronary

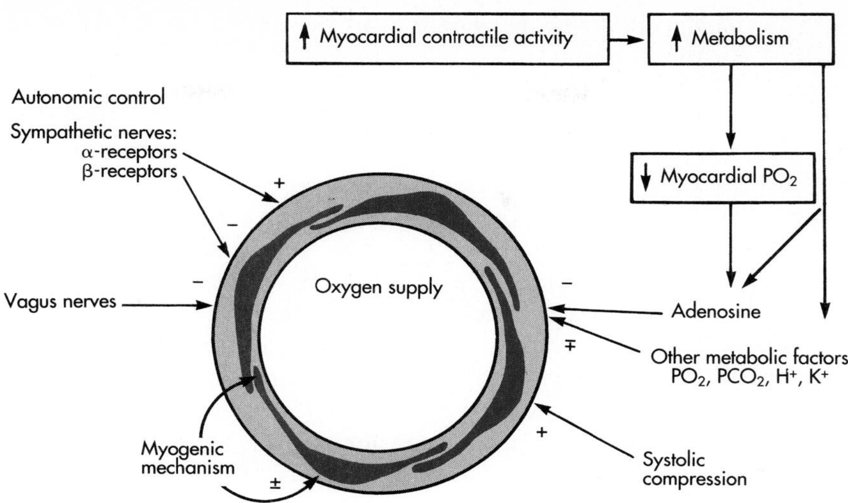

Fig. 10-7 ■ Schematic representation of factors that increase (+) or decrease (−) coronary vascular resistance. The intravascular pressure (arterial blood pressure) stretches the vessel wall.

arteries. Abrupt occlusion of a coronary artery or one of its branches in a human or dog leads to ischemic necrosis and eventual fibrosis of the areas of myocardium supplied by the occluded vessel. However, if narrowing of a coronary artery occurs slowly and progressively over a period of days, weeks, or longer, collateral vessels develop and may furnish sufficient blood to the ischemic myocardium to prevent or reduce the extent of necrosis. The development of collateral coronary vessels has been extensively studied in dogs, and the clinical picture of coronary atherosclerosis, as it occurs in humans, can be simulated by gradual narrowing of the normal dog's coronary arteries. Collateral vessels develop between branches of occluded and nonoccluded arteries. They originate from preexisting small vessels that undergo proliferative changes of the endothelium and smooth muscle, possibly in response to wall stress and chemical agents released by the ischemic tissue.

Numerous surgical attempts have been made to enhance the development of coronary collateral vessels. However, the techniques used do not increase the collateral circulation over and above that produced by coronary artery narrowing alone. When discrete occlusions or severe narrowing occur in coronary arteries (even vessels as small as 1 mm in diameter), the lesions can be bypassed with a vein graft or the narrow segment can be dilated by inserting a balloon-tipped catheter into the diseased vessel via a peripheral artery and inflating the balloon. Distension of the vessel by balloon inflation **(angioplasty)** can produce a lasting dilation of a narrowed coronary artery.

A number of drugs are available that induce coronary vasodilation, and they are used in patients with coronary artery disease to relieve **angina pectoris,** the chest pain associated with myocardial ischemia. Many of these compounds are nitrites. They are not selective dilators of the coronary vessels, and the mechanism whereby they accomplish their beneficial effects has not been established. The arterioles that would dilate in response to the drugs are undoubtedly already maximally dilated by the ischemia responsible for the symptoms.

In fact, in a patient with marked narrowing of a coronary artery, administration of a vasodilator can fully dilate normal vessel branches proximal to the narrowed segment and reduce the head of pressure to the partially occluded vessel. This will further compromise blood flow to the ischemic myocardium and elicit pain and electrocardiographic changes indicative of tissue injury. This phenomenon is known as **coronary steal,** and it can be observed with vasodilator drugs such as dipyridamole, which acts by blocking cellular uptake and metabolism of endogenous adenosine. Nitrites alleviate angina pectoris, at least partly, by reducing cardiac work and myocardial oxygen requirements by relaxing the great veins (decreased preload) and by decreasing blood pressure (decreased afterload).

In short, the reduction in pressure work and O_2 requirement must be greater than the reduction in coronary blood flow and O_2 supply consequent to the lowered coronary perfusion pressure. It has also been demonstrated that nitrites dilate large coronary arteries and coronary collateral vessels, thus increasing blood flow to ischemic myocardium and alleviating precordial pain.

■ CARDIAC OXYGEN CONSUMPTION AND WORK

The volume of O_2 consumed by the heart is determined by the amount and the type of activity the heart performs. Under basal conditions, myocardial O_2 consumption is about 8 to 10 ml/min/100 g of heart. It can increase severalfold with exercise and decrease moderately under conditions such as hypotension and hypothermia. The cardiac venous blood is normally quite low in O_2 (about 5 ml/dl), and the myocardium can receive little additional O_2 by further O_2 extraction from the coronary blood. Therefore, increased O_2 demands of the heart must be met primarily by an increase in coronary blood flow. When the heartbeat is arrested, as with administration of potassium, but coronary perfusion is maintained experimentally, the O_2 consumption falls to 2 ml/min/100 g or less, which is still six to seven times greater than that for resting skeletal muscle.

Left ventricular work per beat (**stroke work,** p. 99) is generally considered to be equal to the product of the stroke volume and the mean aortic pressure against which the blood is ejected by the left ventricle. At resting levels of cardiac output the kinetic energy component is negligible (p. 114). However, at high cardiac outputs as in severe exercise, the kinetic component can account for up to 50% of total cardiac work. One can simultaneously halve the aortic pressure and double the cardiac output, or vice versa, and still arrive at the same value for cardiac work. However, the O_2 requirements are greater for any given amount of cardiac work when a major fraction is pressure work as opposed to volume work. An increase in cardiac output at a constant aortic pressure (volume work) is accomplished with a small increase in left ventricular O_2 consumption, whereas increased arterial pressure at constant cardiac output (pressure work) is accompanied by a large increment in myocardial O_2 consumption. Thus myocardial O_2 consumption may not correlate well with overall cardiac work. The magnitude and duration of left ventricular pressure do correlate with left ventricular O_2 consumption.

The greater energy demand of pressure work over volume work is of great clinical importance, especially in aortic stenosis, in which left ventricular O_2 consumption is increased because of the high intraventricular pressures developed during systole, but coronary perfusion pressure is normal or reduced because of the pressure drop across the narrowed orifice of the diseased aortic valve. Work of the right ventricle is one seventh that of the left ventricle because pulmonary vascular resistance is much less than systemic vascular resistance.

■ CARDIAC EFFICIENCY

As with an engine, the efficiency of the heart is the ratio of the work accomplished to the total energy utilized. Assuming an average O_2 consumption of 9 ml/min/100 g for the two ventricles, a 300 g heart consumes 27 ml O_2/ min, which is equivalent to 130 small calories at a respiratory quotient of 0.82. Together the two ventricles do about 8 kg-m of work per minute, which is equivalent to 18.7 small calories. Therefore, the gross efficiency is 14%.

$$\frac{18.7}{130} \times 100 = 14\%$$

The net efficiency is slightly higher (18%) and is obtained by subtracting the O_2 consumption of the nonbeating (asystolic) heart (about 2 ml/min/100 g) from the total cardiac O_2 consumption in the calculation of efficiency. It is thus evident that the efficiency of the heart as a pump is relatively low and is comparable to the efficiency of many mechanical devices used in everyday life. With exercise, efficiency improves, because mean blood pressure shows little change, whereas cardiac output and work increase considerably without a proportional increase in myocardial O_2 consumption. The energy expended in cardiac metabolism that does not contribute to the propulsion of blood through the body appears in the form of heat. The energy of the flowing blood is also dissipated as heat, chiefly in passage through the arterioles.

■ SUBSTRATE UTILIZATION

The heart is quite versatile in its use of substrates, and within certain limits the uptake of a particular substrate is directly proportional to its arterial concentration. The utilization of one substrate is also influenced by the presence or absence of other substrates. For example, the addition of lactate to the blood perfusing a heart metabolizing glucose leads to a reduction in glucose uptake, and vice versa. At normal blood concentrations, glucose and lactate are consumed at about equal rates, whereas pyruvate uptake is very low, but so is its arterial concentration. For glucose the threshold concentration is about 4 mM and below this blood level no myocardial glucose uptake occurs. Insulin reduces this threshold and increases the rate of glucose uptake by the heart. A very low threshold exists for cardiac utilization of lactate; insulin does not affect its uptake by the myocardium. With hypoxia, glucose utilization is facilitated by an increase in the rate of transport across the myocardial cell wall, whereas lactate cannot be metabolized by the hypoxic heart and is in fact produced by the heart under anaerobic conditions. Associated with lactate production by the hypoxic heart is the breakdown of cardiac glycogen.

Of the total cardiac O_2 consumption, only 35% to 40% can be accounted for by the oxidation of carbohydrate. Thus the heart derives the major part of its energy from oxidation of noncarbohydrate sources. The chief noncarbohydrate fuel used by the heart is esterified and nonesterified fatty acid, which accounts for about 60% of myocardial O_2 consumption in the postabsorptive state. The various fatty acids show different thresholds for myocardial uptake but are generally utilized in direct proportion to their arterial concentration. Ketone bodies, especially acetoacetate, are readily oxidized by the heart and contribute a major source of energy in diabetic acidosis. As is true of carbohydrate substrates, utilization of a specific noncarbohydrate substrate is influenced by the presence of other substrates, both noncarbohydrate and carbohydrate. Therefore, within certain limits, the heart uses preferentially that substrate which is available in the largest concentration. Most evidence indicates that the contribution to myocardial energy expenditure provided by the oxidation of amino acids is small.

Normally the heart derives its energy by oxidative phosphorylation, in which each mole of glucose yields 36 moles of ATP. However, during hypoxia, glycolysis supervenes and 2 moles of ATP are provided by each mole of glucose. Beta-oxidation of fatty acids is also curtailed. If hypoxia is prolonged, cellular creatine phosphate and eventually ATP are depleted.

In ischemia, lactic acid accumulates (lack of washout) and causes a decrease in intracellular pH. This condition inhibits glycolysis, fatty acid use, and protein synthesis, which results in, cellular damage and eventually in necrosis of myocardial cells.

■ SUMMARY

1. The physical factors that influence coronary blood flow are the viscosity of the blood, the frictional resistance of the vessel walls, the aortic pressure, and the extravascular compression of the vessels within the walls of the left ventricle. Left coronary blood flow is restricted during ventricular systole as a result of extravascular compression, and it is greatest during diastole when the intramyocardial vessels are not compressed.
2. Neural regulation of coronary blood flow is much less important than is metabolic regulation. Activation of the cardiac sympathetic nerves directly constricts the coronary resistance vessels. However, the enhanced myocardial metabolism caused by the associated increase in heart rate and contractile force produces vasodilation, which overrides the direct constrictor effect of sympathetic nerve stimulation. Stimulation of the cardiac branches of the vagus nerves slightly dilates the coronary arterioles.
3. A striking parallelism exists between metabolic activity of the heart and coronary blood flow. A decrease in oxygen supply or an increase in oxygen demand apparently releases a vasodilator that decreases coronary resistance. Of the known factors (CO_2, O_2, H^+, K^+, adenosine) that can mediate this response, adenosine appears to be the most likely candidate.
4. In response to gradual occlusion of a coronary artery, collateral vessels from adjacent unoccluded arteries develop and supply blood to the compromised myocardium distal to the point of occlusion.
5. The myocardium functions only aerobically and in general utilizes substrates in proportion to their arterial concentration.

■ BIBLIOGRAPHY

Journal articles

Baron, J.F., Vicaut, E., Hou, X., and Duvelleroy, M: Independent role of arterial O_2 tension in local control of coronary blood flow, Am. J. Physiol. 258:H1388, 1990.

Belardinelli, L., Linden, J., and Berne, R.M: The cardiac effects of adenosine, Prog. Cardiovasc. Dis. 32:73, 1989.

Belloni, F.L.: The local control of coronary blood flow, Cardiovasc. Res. 13:63, 1979.

Berne, R.M.: Role of adenosine in the regulation of coronary blood flow, Circ. Res. 47:807, 1980.

Buckberg, G.D., Fixler, D.E., Archie, J.P., Henney, R.P., and Hoffman, J.I.E.: Variable effects of heart rate on phasic and regional left ventricular muscle blood flow in anesthetized dogs, Cardiovasc. Res. 9:1, 1975.

Feigl, E.O.: Sympathetic control of coronary circulation, Circ. Res. 20:262, 1967.

Feigl, E.O.: Parasympathetic control of coronary blood flow in dogs, Circ. Res. 25:509, 1969.

Feigl, E.O.: Coronary physiology, Physiol. Rev. 63:1, 1983.

Gregg, D.E.: The natural history of coronary collateral development, Circ. Res. 35:335, 1974.

Klocke, F.J., and Ellis, A.K.: Control of coronary blood flow, Ann. Rev. Med. 31:489, 1980.

Klocke, F.J., Mates, R.E., Canty, J.M., Jr., and Ellis, A.K.: Coronary pressure-flow relationships—controversial issues and probable implications, Circ. Res. 56:310, 1985.

Murray, P.A., Belloni, F.L., and Sparks, H.V.: The role of potassium in the metabolic control of coronary vascular resistance in the dog, Circ. Res. 44:767, 1979.

Olsson, R.A., and Bunger, R: Metabolic control of coronary blood flow, Prog. Cardiovasc. Dis. 29:369, 1987.

Olsson, R.A., and Pearson, J.D.: Cardiovascular purinoceptors, Physiol. Rev. 70:761, 1990.

Rubio, R., and Berne, R.M.: Regulation of coronary blood flow, Prog. Cardiovasc. Dis. 18:105, 1975.

Wearn, J.T., Mettier, S.R., Klumpp, T.G., and Zschiesche, L.J.: The nature of the vascular communications between the coronary arteries and the chambers of the heart, Am. Heart J. 9:143, 1933.

White, C.W., Wilson, R.F., and Marcus, M.L: Methods of measuring myocardial blood flow in humans, Prog. Cardiovasc. Dis. 31:79, 1988.

Books and monographs

Berne, R.M., and Rubio, R.: Coronary circulation. In Handbook of physiology; Section 2: The cardiovascular system—the heart, vol. I, Bethesda, Md., 1979, American Physiological Society.

Gregg, D.E.: Coronary circulation in health and disease, Philadelphia, 1950, Lea & Febiger.

Marcus, M.L.: The coronary circulation in health and disease, New York, 1983, McGraw-Hill Book Co.

Morgan, H.E., Rannels, D.E., and McKee, E.E.: Protein metabolism of the heart. In Handbook of physiology; Section 2: The cardiovascular system—the heart, vol. I, Bethesda, Md., 1979, American Physiological Society.

Olsson, R.A., Bunger, R., and Spaan, J.A.E. The coronary circulation. In Fozzard, H.A. et al., editors: The heart and cardiovascular system, ed 2, New York, 1991, Raven Press.

Randle, P.J., and Tubbs, P.K.: Carbohydrate and fatty acid metabolism. In Handbook of physiology; Section 2: The cardiovascular system—the heart, vol. I., Bethesda, Md., 1979, American Physiological Society.

Schaper, W.: The collateral circulation of the heart, New York, 1971, North-Holland Publishing Co.

Sparks H.V., Jr., Wangler R.D., and Gorman M.W.: Control of the coronary circulation. In Sperelakis N, editor: Physiology and pathophysiology of the heart, ed. 2, Boston, 1989, Wolters-Kluwer Publishers.

11 Special Circulations

■ CUTANEOUS CIRCULATION

The oxygen and nutrient requirements of the skin are relatively small and, in contrast to most other body tissues, the supply of these essential materials is not the chief governing factor in the regulation of cutaneous blood flow. The primary function of the cutaneous circulation is maintenance of a constant body temperature. Consequently, the skin shows wide fluctuations in blood flow, depending on the need for loss or conservation of body heat. Mechanisms responsible for alterations in skin blood flow are primarily activated by changes in ambient and internal body temperatures.

Regulation of Skin Blood Flow

There are essentially two types of resistance vessels in skin: arterioles and **arteriovenous (AV) anastomoses.** The arterioles are similar to those found elsewhere in the body. AV anastomoses shunt blood from arterioles to venules and venous plexuses; hence they bypass the capillary bed. They are found primarily in the fingertips, palms of the hands, toes, soles of the feet, ears, nose, and lips. AV anastomoses differ morphologically from the arterioles in that they are either short, straight, or long, coiled vessels about 20 to 40 μm in lumen diameter, with thick muscular walls richly supplied with nerve fibers. These vessels are almost exclusively under sympathetic neural control and become maximally dilated when their nerve supply is interrupted. Conversely, reflex stimulation of the sympathetic fibers to these vessels may produce constriction to the point of complete obliteration of the vascular lumen. Although AV anastomoses do not exhibit **basal tone** (tonic activity of the vascular smooth muscle independent of innervation), they are highly sensitive to vasoconstrictor agents like epinephrine and norepinephrine. Furthermore, AV anastomoses do not appear to be under metabolic control, and they fail to show reactive hyperemia or autoregulation of blood flow. *Thus the regulation of blood flow through these **anastomotic channels** is governed principally by the nervous system in response to reflex activation by temperature receptors or from higher centers of the central nervous system.*

The bulk of the skin resistance vessels exhibits some basal tone and is under dual control of the sympathetic nervous system and local regulatory factors, in much the same manner as are other vascular beds. However, in the case of skin, neural control plays a more important role than local factors. Stimulation of sympathetic nerve fibers to skin blood vessels (arteries and veins, as well as arterioles) induces vasoconstriction, and severance of the sympathetic nerves induces vasodilation. With chronic denervation of the cutaneous blood vessels, the degree of tone that existed before denervation is gradually regained over a period of several weeks. This is accomplished by an enhancement of basal tone that compensates for the degree of tone previously contributed by sympathetic nerve fiber activity. Epinephrine and norepinephrine elicit only vasoconstriction in cutaneous vessels. Whether the increased basal tone following denervation of the skin vessels is the result of their enhanced sensitivity to circulating catecholamines **(denervation hypersensitivity)** has not been established.

Parasympathetic vasodilator nerve fibers do not supply the cutaneous blood vessels. However, stimulation of the sweat glands, which are innervated by cholinergic fibers of the sympathetic nervous system, results in dilation of the skin resistance vessels. Sweat contains an enzyme that acts on a protein moiety in the tissue fluid to produce **bradykinin,** a polypeptide with potent vasodilator properties. Bradykinin formed in the tissue can act locally to dilate the arterioles and increase blood flow to the skin. The skin vessels of certain regions, particularly the head, neck, shoulders, and upper chest, are under the influence of the higher centers of the central nervous system. Blushing, as with embarrassment or anger, and blanching, as with fear or anxiety, are examples of cerebral inhibition and stimulation, respectively, of the sympathetic nerve fibers to the affected regions.

In contrast to AV anastomoses in the skin, the cutaneous resistance vessels show autoregulation of blood flow and reactive hyperemia. If the arterial inflow to a limb is stopped with an inflated blood pressure cuff for a brief period of time, the skin shows a marked reddening below the point of vascular occlusion when the cuff is deflated. This increased cutaneous blood flow (reactive hyperemia) is also manifested by the distension of the superficial veins in the erythematous extremity. Autoregulation of blood flow in the skin is best explained by a myogenic mechanism (see p. 176).

Ambient and Body Temperature in Regulation of Skin Blood Flow. *Because the primary function of the skin is to preserve the internal milieu and protect it from adverse changes in the environment, and because ambient temperature is one of the most important external variables the body must contend with, it is not surprising that the vasculature of the skin is chiefly influenced by environmental temperature.* Exposure to cold elicits a generalized cutaneous vasoconstriction that is most pronounced in the hands and feet. This response is chiefly mediated by the nervous system, because arrest of the circulation to a hand with a pressure cuff and immersion of that hand in cold water results in vasoconstriction in the skin of the other extremities that are exposed to room temperature. With the circulation to the chilled hand unoccluded, the reflex vasoconstriction is caused in part by the cooled blood returning to the general circulation and stimulating the temperature-regulating center in the anterior hypothalamus. Direct application of cold to this region of the brain produces cutaneous vasoconstriction.

The skin vessels of the cooled hand also show a direct response to cold. Moderate cooling or exposure for brief periods to severe cold (0° to 15° C) results in constriction of the resistance and capacitance vessels, including AV anastomoses. However, prolonged exposure of the hand to severe cold has a secondary vasodilator effect. Prompt vasoconstriction and severe pain are elicited by immersion of the hand in water near 0° C, but are soon followed by dilation of the skin vessels with reddening of the immersed part and alleviation of the pain. With continued immersion of the hand, alternating periods of constriction and dilation occur, but the skin temperature rarely drops to as low a degree as it did with the initial vasoconstriction. Prolonged severe cold, of course, results in tissue damage. The rosy faces of people working or playing in a cold environment are examples of cold vasodilation. However, the blood flow through the skin of the face may be greatly reduced despite the flushed appearance. The red color of the slowly flowing blood is in large measure the result of the reduced oxygen uptake by the cold skin and the cold-induced shift to the left of the oxyhemoglobin dissociation curve.

Direct application of heat produces not only local vasodilation of resistance and capacitance vessels and AV anastomoses but also reflex dilation in other parts of the body. The local effect is independent of the vascular nerve supply, whereas the reflex vasodilation is a combination of anterior hypothalamic stimulation by the returning warmed blood and of stimulation of receptors in the heated part. However, evidence for a reflex from peripheral temperature receptors is not as definitive for warm stimulation as it is for cold stimulation.

The close proximity of the major arteries and veins to each other permits considerable heat exchange (countercurrent) between artery and vein. Cold blood that flows in veins from a cooled hand toward the heart takes up heat from adjacent arteries, resulting in warming of the venous blood and cooling of the arterial blood. Heat exchange is of course in the opposite direction with exposure of the extremity to heat. Thus heat conservation is enhanced and heat gain is minimized during exposure of extremities to cold and warm environments, respectively.

Skin Color and Special Reactions of the Skin Vessels

The color of the skin is of course caused in large part by pigment; however, in all but very dark skin, the degree of pallor or ruddiness is mainly a function of the amount of blood in the skin. With little blood in the venous plexus the skin appears pale, whereas with moderate to large quantities of blood in the venous plexus, the skin shows color. Whether this color is bright red, blue, or some shade between is determined by the degree of oxygenation of the blood in the subcutaneous vessels. For example, a combination of vasoconstriction and reduced hemoglobin can produce an ashen gray color of the skin, whereas a combination of venous engorgement and reduced hemoglobin can result in a dark purple hue. Skin color provides little information about the rate of cutaneous blood flow. There may coexist rapid blood flow and pale skin when the AV anastomoses are open, and slow blood flow and red skin when the extremity is exposed to cold.

White Reaction and Triple Response. If the skin of the forearm of many individuals is lightly stroked with a blunt instrument, a white line appears at the site of the stroke within 20 seconds. The blanching becomes maximum in about 30 to 40 seconds and then gradually disappears within 3 to 5 minutes. This response is known as a **white reaction** and has been attributed to capillary contraction, because it occurs in the denervated limb and is unaffected by arrest of the limb circulation. Because all direct evidence indicates that capillaries do not contract and because skin color is primarily a result of blood content of venous plexuses, venules, and small veins, it seems logical to attribute the white reaction to venous constriction induced by mechanical stimulation.

If the skin is stroked more strongly with a sharp pointed instrument, a **triple response** is elicited. Within 3 to 15 seconds a thin **red line** appears at the site of the stroke, followed in about 15 to 30 seconds by a red blush, or **flare,** extending out 1 to 2 cm from either side of the red line. This in turn is followed in 3 to 5 minutes by an elevation of the skin along the red line, with gradual fading of the red line as the elevation, a **wheal,** becomes

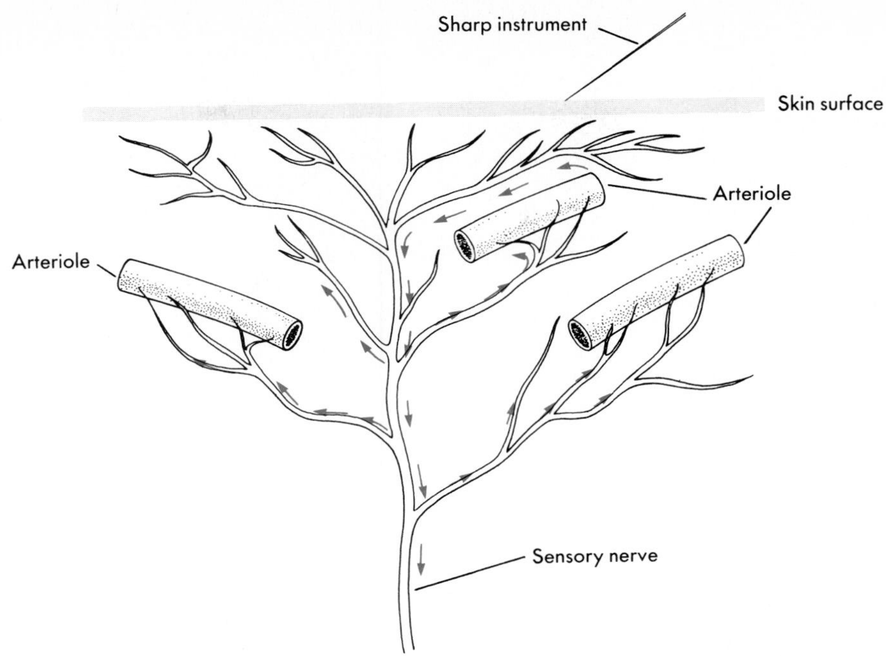

Fig. 11-1 ■ Schematic representation of the axon reflex in response to a scratch on the skin surface with a sharp instrument. Arrows indicate the pathways of impulses in a sensory nerve from the site of stimulation to adjacent arterioles to produce local vasodilation (flare).

more prominent. The red line is probably caused by dilation of the vessels because of mechanical stimulation. The flare, however, is the result of dilation of neighboring arterioles caused to relax by an **axon reflex** originating at the site of mechanical stimulation. In an axon reflex, the nerve impulse travels centripetally in the cutaneous sensory nerve fiber and then antidromically down the small branches of the afferent nerve to adjacent arterioles to elicit vasodilation (Fig. 11-1). The flare is not affected by acute section or anesthetic block of the sensory nerve central to the point of branching, whereas it is abolished when the nerve degenerates after section. The wheal is caused by increased capillary permeability induced by the trauma. Fluid containing protein leaks out of the capillaries locally and produces edema at the site of injury. Because the triple response can be elicited by an intradermal injection of histamine, it has been attributed to histamine or a histamine-like substance **(H-substance).** Whether it is histamine, ATP, a vasoactive polypeptide like bradykinin, or some yet unidentified substance is unknown.

■ SKELETAL MUSCLE CIRCULATION

The rate of blood flow in skeletal muscle varies directly with the contractile activity of the tissue and the type of muscle. Blood flow and capillary density in red (slow-twitch, high-oxidative) muscle are greater than in white (fast-twitch, low-oxidative) muscle. In resting muscle the precapillary arterioles exhibit asynchronous intermittent contractions and relaxations, so that at any given moment, a very large percentage of the capillary bed is not perfused. Consequently, total blood flow through quiescent skeletal muscle is low (1.4 to 4.5 ml/min/100 g). With exercise the resis-

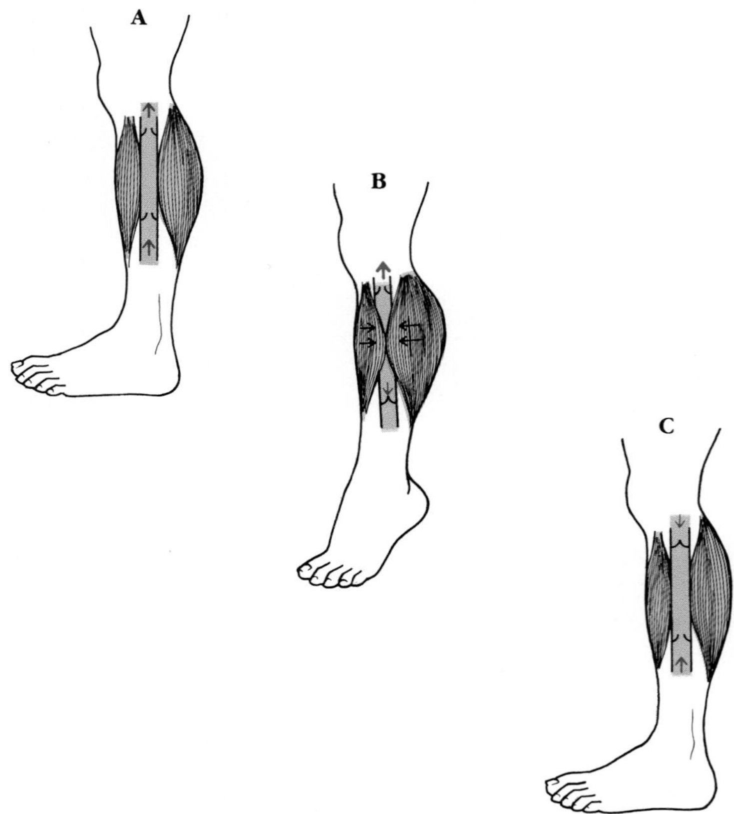

Fig. 11-2 ■ Action of the muscle pump in venous return from the legs. **A,** Standing at rest the venous valves are open and blood flows upward toward the heart by virtue of the pressure generated by the heart and transmitted through the capillaries to the veins from the arterial side of the vascular system **(vis a tergo). B,** Contraction of the muscle compresses the vein so that the increased pressure in the vein drives blood toward the thorax through the upper valve and closes the lower valve in the uncompressed segment of the vein just below the point of muscular compression. **C,** Immediately after muscle relaxation the pressure in the previously compressed venous segment falls, and the reversed pressure gradient causes the upper valve to close. The valve below the previously compressed segment opens because pressure below it exceeds that above it and the segment fills with blood from the foot. As blood flow continues from the foot, the pressure in the previously compressed segment rises. When it exceeds the pressure above the upper valve, this valve opens and continuous flow occurs as in part *A.*

tance vessels relax and the muscle blood flow may increase manyfold (up to fifteen to twenty times the resting level), the magnitude of the increase depending largely on the severity of the exercise.

Regulation of Skeletal Muscle Blood Flow

Control of muscle circulation is achieved by neural and local factors. As with all tissues, physical factors such as arterial pressure, tissue pressure, and blood viscosity influence muscle blood flow. However, another physical factor comes into play during exercise—the squeezing effect of the active muscle on the vessels. With intermittent contractions, inflow is restricted and venous outflow is enhanced during each brief contraction. The presence of the venous valves prevents backflow of blood in the veins between contractions, thereby aiding in the forward propulsion of the blood (Fig. 11-2). With strong sustained contractions the vascular bed can be compressed to the point where blood flow actually ceases temporarily.

Neural Factors. Although the resistance vessels of muscle possess a high degree of basal tone, they also display tone attributable to continuous low frequency activity in the sympathetic vasoconstrictor nerve fibers. The basal frequency of firing in the sympathetic vasoconstrictor fibers is quite low (about 1 to 2 per second), and maximum vasoconstriction is observed at frequencies as low as 8 to 10 per second. Stimulation of the sympathetic nerve fibers to skeletal muscle elicits vasoconstriction that is caused by the release of norepinephrine at the fiber endings. Intraarterial injection of norepinephrine elicits only vasoconstriction, whereas low doses of epinephrine

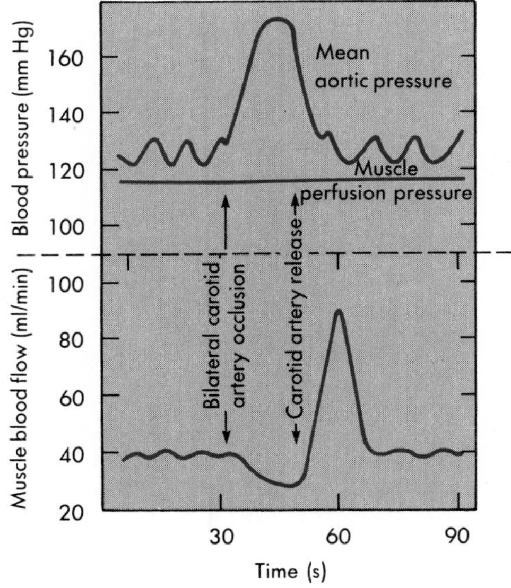

Fig. 11-3 ■ Evidence for participation of the muscle vascular bed in vasoconstriction and vasodilation mediated by the carotid sinus baroreceptors after common carotid artery occlusion and release. In this preparation the sciatic and femoral nerves constituted the only direct connection between the hind leg muscle mass and the rest of the dog. The muscle was perfused by blood at a constant pressure that was completely independent of the animal's arterial pressure. (Redrawn from Jones, R.D., and Berne, R.M.: Am. J. Physiol. 204:461, 1963.)

produce vasodilation in muscle and large doses cause vasoconstriction.

The tonic activity of the sympathetic nerves is greatly influenced by reflexes from the baroreceptors. An increase in carotid sinus pressure results in dilation of the vascular bed of the muscle, and a decrease in carotid sinus pressure elicits vasoconstriction (Fig. 11-3). When the existing sympathetic constrictor tone is high, as in the experiment illustrated in Fig. 11-3, the decrease in blood flow associated with common carotid artery occlusion is small, but the increase following the release of occlusion is large. The vasodilation produced by baroreceptor stimulation is caused by inhibition of sympathetic vasoconstrictor activity. Because muscle is the major body component on the basis of mass and thereby represents the largest vascular bed, the participation of its resistance vessels in vascular reflexes plays an important role in maintaining a constant arterial blood pressure.

A comparison of the vasoconstrictor and vasodilator effects of the sympathetic nerves to blood vessels of muscle and skin is summarized in Fig. 11-4. Note the lower basal tone of the skin vessels, their greater constrictor response, and the absence of active cutaneous vasodilation.

Local Factors. Whether neural or local factors predominate in the regulation of skeletal muscle blood flow depends on the activity of the muscle. In resting muscle the neural factors predominate and superimpose neurogenic

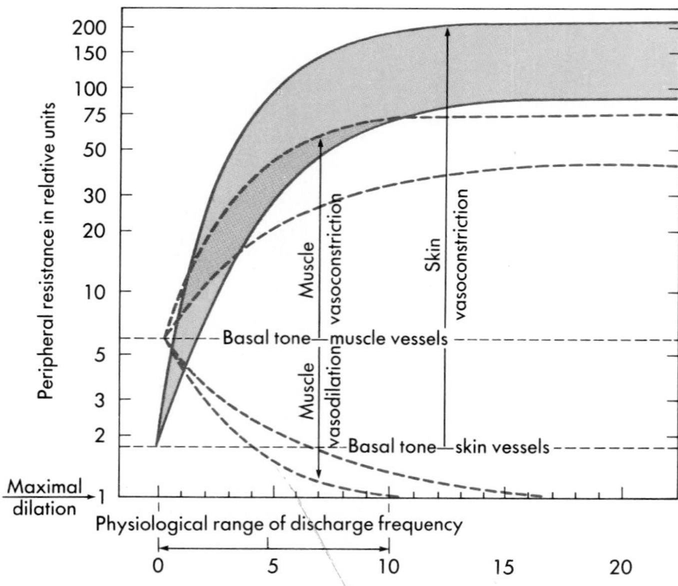

Fig. 11-4 ■ Basal tone and the range of response of the resistance vessels in muscle and skin to sympathetic nerve stimulation. Peripheral resistance plotted on a logarithmic scale. (Redrawn from Celander, O., and Folkow, B.: Acta Physiol. Scand. 29:241, 1953.)

tone on the nonneural basal tone (see Fig. 11-4). Section of the sympathetic nerves to muscle abolishes the neural component of vascular tone and unmasks the intrinsic basal tone of the blood vessels. *Neural and local blood flow regulating mechanisms oppose each other, and during muscle contraction the local vasodilator mechanism supervenes.* However, during exercise, strong sympathetic nerve stimulation slightly reduces the vasodilation induced by locally released metabolites. The identity of the local mediator(s) of the vasodilation that occurs with exercise has not been determined; several mediators are probably involved. Adenosine is released from ischemic muscle and in some cases from contracting muscle during unimpaired blood flow, but the nucleoside accounts for part of the exercise-induced vasodilation only in fast oxidative muscles. Skeletal muscle effectively autoregulates blood flow, particularly during active contractions. As in other cases of autoregulation the mechanism is probably myogenic (see p. 176).

■ CEREBRAL CIRCULATION

Blood reaches the brain through the internal carotid and vertebral arteries. The latter join to form the basilar artery, which, in conjunction with branches of the internal carotid arteries, forms the **circle of Willis.** A unique feature of the cerebral circulation is that it all lies within a rigid structure, the cranium. Because intracranial contents are incompressible, any increase in arterial inflow, as with arteriolar dilation, must be associated with a comparable increase in venous outflow. The volume of blood and of extravascular fluid can vary considerably in most tissues. In brain the volume of blood and extravascular fluid is relatively constant; changes in either of these fluid volumes must be accompanied by a reciprocal change in the other. In contrast to most other organs, the rate of total cerebral blood flow is held within a relatively narrow range and in humans averages 55 ml/min/100 g of brain.

Estimation of Cerebral Blood Flow

Total cerebral blood flow can be measured in humans by the nitrous oxide (N_2O) method, which is based on the Fick principle (p. 75). The subject breathes a gas mixture of 15% N_2O, 21% O_2, and 64% N_2 for 10 minutes, which is sufficient time to permit equilibration of the N_2O between the brain tissue and the blood leaving the brain. Simultaneous samples of arterial (any artery) blood and mixed cerebral venous (internal jugular vein) blood are taken at the start of N_2O inhalation and at 1-minute intervals throughout the 10-minute period of N_2O administration. From these data, the cerebral blood flow can be calculated by the Fick equation:

$$\text{Cerebral blood flow} = \frac{\text{Amount of } N_2O \text{ taken up by brain during time } (t_2 - t_1)}{\text{AV difference of } N_2O \text{ across brain during time } (t_2 - t_1)}$$

Because the arterial and venous concentrations are continuously changing with time, it is necessary to get the true AV difference during the period of N_2O inhalation by integration of the AV difference over the 10-minute period. This is represented in Fig. 11-5, *A,* by the shaded area between the arterial and venous N_2O concentration curves constructed from the blood concentrations observed at successive 1-minute intervals during N_2O administration. The amount of N_2O removed by the brain, as well as the concentration of N_2O in the brain tissue, are unknown. Because the partition coefficient between brain and blood is about 1 and because equilibrium of N_2O between the brain and the blood leaving the brain is reached by the end of 10 minutes, the concentration of N_2O in the brain tissue closely approximates that of the cerebral venous blood in the 10-minute sample. The total weight of the brain is not known, and so for convenience the con-

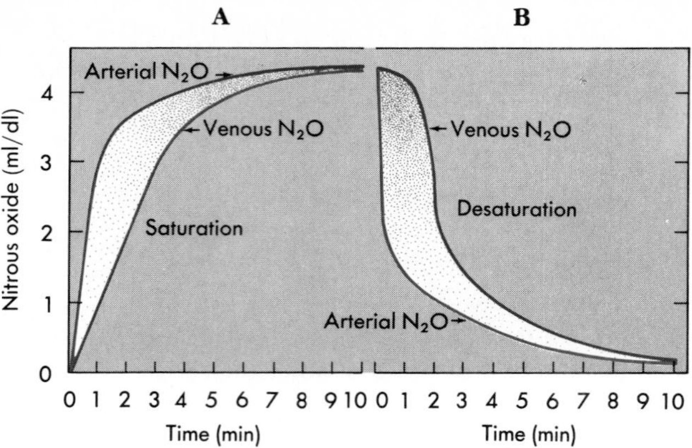

Fig. 11-5 ■ Concentrations of N_2O in arterial and cerebral venous blood during saturation, **A,** and desaturation, **B.** The shaded areas represent the arteriovenous differences of N_2O during the 10-minute period of N_2O inhalation and the 10 minutes after discontinuing the N_2O administration.

centration in brain tissue is multiplied by 100 to express the cerebral blood flow (CBF) in ml/min/100 g of brain tissue. The equation is:

$$CBF = \frac{V_{10} \cdot S \cdot 100}{\int_0^{10} (A - V)dt}$$

V_{10} = Venous concentration of N_2O at equilibrium (at 10 minutes)

S = Partition coefficient of N_2O between brain and blood = 1

A − V = Arteriovenous difference of N_2O

Cerebral blood flow also can be calculated from the desaturation A − V curves, which are constructed from N_2O concentrations of simultaneously drawn arterial and venous blood samples taken each minute for 10 minutes, starting when equilibrium is reached between brain tissue and cerebral venous blood (Fig. 11-5, *B*). In this procedure the subject breathes the N_2O mixture for 10 minutes, and sampling starts at the moment N_2O inhalation is stopped. The only difference from the preceding equation is that the denominator becomes

$$\int_{10}^{20} (V - A)dt$$

Cerebral blood flow and its distribution to different areas of the brain can be measured in animals by injection into the internal carotid artery of microspheres (about 15 μm) labeled with radioactive substances. The microspheres become lodged in the arterioles and capillaries, the brain tissue is sampled, and the radioactivity of the tissue is determined. Blood flow to each tissue sample is proportional to the radioactivity in that sample. By the use of microspheres labeled with different radioactive isotopes, several measurements of cerebral blood flow can be made. A gamma counter is used to measure each isotope independently of the other isotopes in the sample. This method is also used for measurements of blood flow in other tissues, such as the myocardium and is the standard technique for **regional blood flow** measurements. One can also measure cerebral blood flow in animals with the use of ^{14}C-antipyrine, which is taken up by the brain in proportion to the blood flow. The brain is then sliced, and the radioactivity of the slice is determined by radioautography. The advantage of these methods over the N_2O method or the direct measurement of venous outflow from the brain is that blood flow to different regions of the brain can be determined. The obvious disadvantage is that the animals must be sacrificed to obtain the necessary samples of brain tissue.

Recently, the development of multiple collimated scintillation detectors built into a helmet that fits over the cranium has made possible the measurement of regional blood flow (cortical blood flow) in animals and humans. An inert radioactive gas (such as ^{133}Xe) is injected into an internal carotid artery, and from its rate of washout from the brain, regional cerebral blood flow can be determined. The radioactive gas also may be given by inhalation, but more sophisticated techniques are required to eliminate noncerebral blood flow and to distinguish between blood flow to cortical (gray matter) and deep cerebral (white matter) tissue.

Regulation of Cerebral Blood Flow

Of the various body tissues, the brain is the least tolerant of ischemia. Interruption of cerebral blood flow for as little as 5 seconds results in loss of consciousness, and ischemia lasting just a few minutes results in irreversible tissue damage. Fortunately, regulation of the cerebral circulation is primarily under direction of the brain itself. Local regulatory mechanisms and reflexes originating in the brain tend to maintain cerebral circulation relatively constant in the presence of possible adverse extrinsic effects such as sympathetic vasomotor nerve activity, circulating humoral vasoactive agents, and changes in arterial blood pressure. Under certain conditions the brain also regulates its blood flow by initiating changes in systemic blood pressure. For example, elevation of intracranial pressure results in an increase in systemic blood pressure. This response, called **Cushing's phenomenon** is apparently caused by ischemic stimulation of vasomotor regions of the medulla. It aids in maintaining cerebral blood flow in such conditions as expanding intracranial tumors.

Neural Factors. The cerebral vessels receive innervation from the cervical sympathetic nerve fibers that accompany the internal carotid and vertebral arteries into the cranial cavity. The importance of neural regulation of the cerebral circulation is controversial, but the prevalent belief is that relative to other vascular beds sympathetic control of the cerebral vessels is weak and that the contractile state of the cerebral vascular smooth muscle depends primarily on local metabolic factors. There are no known sympathetic vasodilator nerves to the cerebral vessels, but the vessels do receive parasympathetic fibers from the facial nerve, which produce a slight vasodilation on stimulation.

Local Factors. *Generally total cerebral blood flow is constant. However, regional cortical blood flow is associated with regional neural activity.* For example, movement of one hand results in increased blood flow only in the hand area of the contralateral sensorymotor and premotor cortex. Also, talking, reading, and other stimuli to the cerebral center are associated with increased blood flow in the appropriate regions of the contralateral cortex

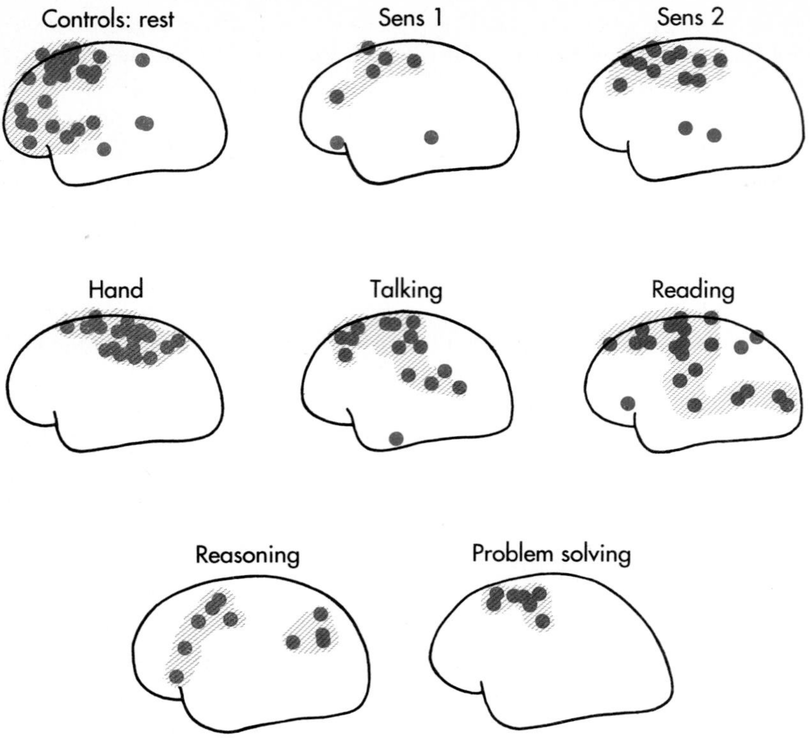

Fig. 11-6 ■ Effects of different stimuli on regional blood flow in the contralateral human cerebral cortex. Sens 1, low intensity electrical stimulation of the hand; Sens 2, high intensity electrical stimulation of the hand (pain). (Redrawn from Ingvar, D.H.: Brain Res. 107:181, 1976).

(Fig. 11-6). Stimulation of the retina with flashes of light increases blood flow only in the visual cortex. Glucose uptake also corresponds with regional cortical neuronal activity. For example, when the retina is stimulated by light, uptake of ^{14}C-2-deoxyglucose is enhanced in the visual cortex. This analogue of glucose is taken up and phosphorylated by cerebral neurons but cannot be metabolized further. The magnitude of its uptake is determined from radioautographs of slices of the brain. The mediator of the link between cerebral activity and blood flow has not been established, but three possible candidates are pH, potassium, and adenosine.

It is well known that the cerebral vessels are very sensitive to carbon dioxide tension. Increases in arterial blood CO_2 tension (Pa_{CO_2}) elicit marked cerebral vasodilation; inhalation of 7% CO_2 results in a twofold increment in cerebral blood flow. By the same token decreases in Pa_{CO_2}, such as elicited by hyperventilation, produce a decrease in cerebral blood flow. CO_2 produces changes in arteriolar resistance by altering perivascular (and probably intracellular vascular smooth muscle) pH. By independently changing P_{CO_2} and bicarbonate concentration, it has been demonstrated that pial vessel diameter (and presumably blood flow) and pH are inversely related, regardless of the level of the P_{CO_2}.

Carbon dioxide can diffuse to the vascular smooth muscle from the brain tissue or from the lumen of the vessels, whereas hydrogen ions in the blood are prevented from reaching the arteriolar smooth muscle by the **blood-brain barrier.** Hence, the cerebral vessels dilate when the hydrogen ion concentration of the cerebrospinal fluid is increased but show only minimal dilation in response to an increase in the hydrogen ion concentration of the arterial blood. Despite the responsiveness of the cerebral vessels to pH changes, the precise role of hydrogen ions in the regulation of cerebral blood flow remains obscure. The initiation of increases in cerebral blood flow produced by seizures has been reported to be associated with transient increases rather than decreases in perivascular pH. Also, the intracellular and extracellular decreases in pH that occur with electrical stimulation of the brain or hypoxia often occur after cerebral blood flow has increased in response to the stimulus. Furthermore, with prolonged hypocapnia, cerebrospinal fluid pH may return to control levels in the face of a persistent reduction in cerebral blood flow. Therefore, pH probably plays no significant role in the normal regulation of cerebral blood flow.

With respect to K^+, such stimuli as hypoxia, electrical stimulation of the brain, and seizures elicit rapid increases in cerebral blood flow and are associated with increases in perivascular K^+. The increments in K^+ are similar to those which produce pial arteriolar dilation when K^+ is applied topically to these vessels. However, the increase in K^+ is not sustained throughout the period of stimulation. Hence, only the initial increment in cerebral blood flow can be attributed to the release of K^+.

Adenosine levels of the brain increase with ischemia, hypoxemia, hypotension, hypocapnia, electrical stimulation of the brain, or induced seizures. When it is applied topically, adenosine is a potent dilator of the pial arterioles. In short, any intervention that either reduces the O_2 supply to the brain or increases the O_2 need of the brain results in rapid (within 5 seconds) formation of adenosine in the cerebral tissue. Unlike pH or K^+, the adenosine concentration of the brain increases with initiation of the stimulus and remains elevated throughout the period of O_2 imbalance. The adenosine released into the cerebrospinal fluid during conditions associated with inadequate brain O_2 supply is available to the brain tissue for reincorporation into cerebral tissue adenine nucleotides.

All three factors, pH, K^+, and adenosine may act in concert to adjust the cerebral blood flow to the metabolic activity of the brain, but how these factors interact to accomplish this regulation of cerebral blood flow remains to be elucidated.

The cerebral circulation shows reactive hyperemia and excellent autoregulation between pressures of about 60 and 160 mm Hg. Mean arterial pressures below 60 mm Hg result in reduced cerebral blood flow and syncope, whereas mean pressures above 160 may lead to increased permeability of the blood-brain barrier and cerebral edema. Autoregulation of cerebral blood flow is abolished by hypercapnia or any other potent vasodilator, and none of the candidates for metabolic regulation of cerebral blood flow has been shown to be responsible for this phenomenon. Hence, autoregulation of cerebral blood flow is probably attributable to a myogenic mechanism, although experimental proof is still lacking.

■ PULMONARY CIRCULATION

The pulmonary and systemic vascular beds are in series with each other. Therefore, under steady-state conditions, the total pulmonary and systemic blood flows are virtually identical. Despite this similarity in the rate of blood flow, the anatomical, hemodynamic, and physiological characteristics of these two sections of the cardiovascular system differ substantially.

Functional Anatomy

Pulmonary vasculature. The pulmonary vascular system is a low-resistance network of

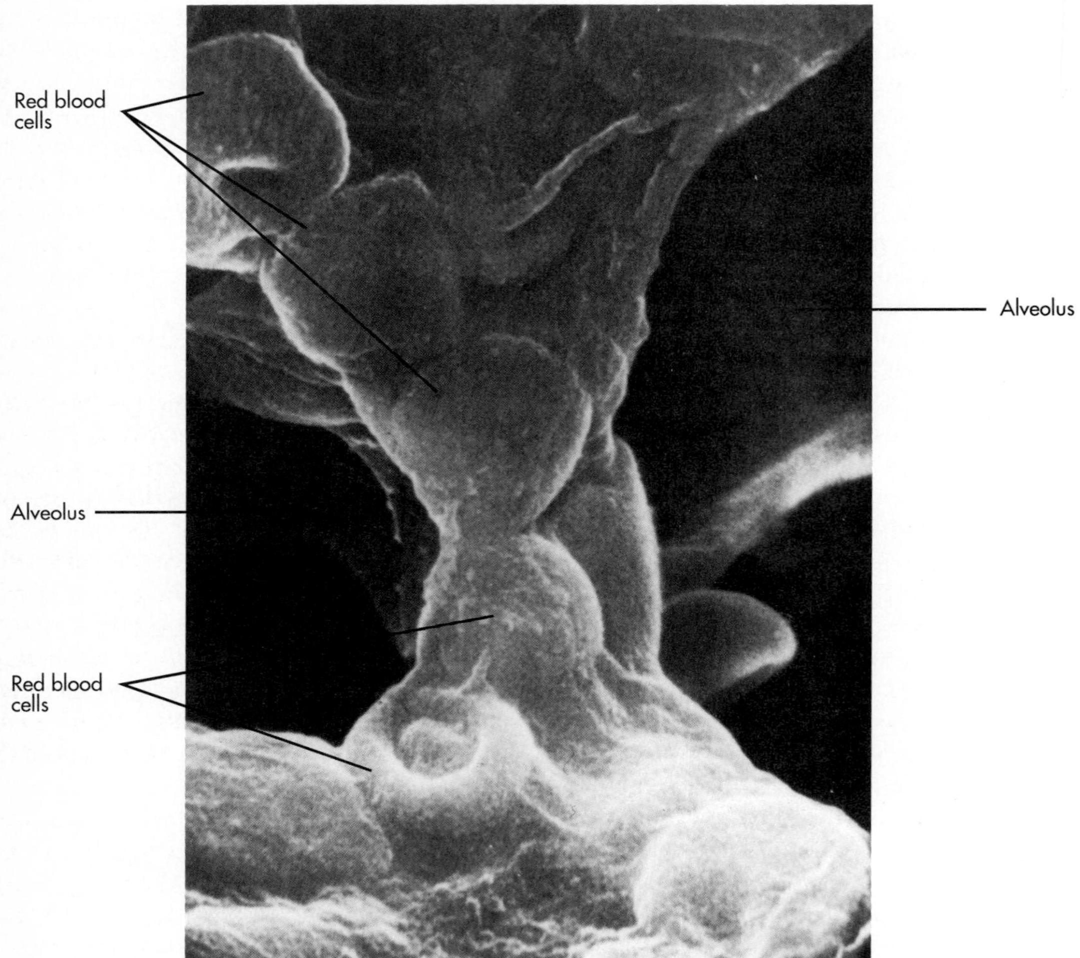

Fig. 11-7 ■ Scanning electron micrograph of mouse lung to show an interalveolar septum. Note that the membranes that separate an alveolus from a capillary are so thin that the shapes of the erythrocytes in the capillary can easily be discerned. (From Greenwood, M.F. and Holland, P.: Lab. Invest. 27:296, 1972.)

highly distensible vessels. The main pulmonary artery is much shorter than the aorta. The walls of the pulmonary artery and its branches are much thinner than the walls of the aorta, and they contain less smooth muscle and elastin. Contrary to systemic arterioles, which have very thick walls comprised mainly of circularly arranged smooth muscle, the pulmonary arterioles are thin and contain little smooth muscle. The pulmonary arterioles do not have the same capacity for vasoconstriction as do their counterparts in the systemic circulation. The pulmonary venules and veins are also very thin and possess little smooth muscle.

The pulmonary capillaries differ markedly from the systemic capillaries. Whereas the systemic capillaries constitute a network of tubular vessels with some interconnections, the pulmonary capillaries are aligned so that the blood flows in thin sheets between adjacent alveoli (Fig. 11-7). Hence, the capillary blood is exposed optimally to the alveolar gases. The total surface area for exchange between alveoli and blood is about 50 to 70 m^2. Only thin layers of vascular and alveolar endothelium separate the blood and alveolar gas. The thickness of the sheets of blood between adjacent alveoli depends on the intravascular pressure and the intraalveolar pressure. Ordinarily, the width of an interalveolar sheet of blood is about equal to the diameter of a red blood cell (Fig. 11-7). During pulmonary vascular congestion, as when the left atrial pressure is elevated, the width of the sheet may increase severalfold. Conversely, when the local alveolar pressure exceeds the adjacent capillary pressure, the capillaries may collapse and blood will not flow to those alveoli. Hydrostatic factors participate in this phenomenon, particularly with respect to the regional distribution of blood flow to the lungs, as described below.

Bronchial Vasculature. The bronchial arteries are branches of the thoracic aorta. These arteries and their branches, down to the arterioles, have the structural characteristics of most systemic arteries; that is, they have much thicker walls and more smooth muscles than do the pulmonary arterial vessels of equivalent caliber. The bronchial vessels supply blood to the tracheobronchial tree down to the terminal bronchioles.

The bronchial veins drain partly into the pulmonary venous system and partly into the azygos veins, which are a part of the systemic venous system. The bronchial circulation normally constitutes about 1% of the cardiac output. Therefore, the fraction of the bronchial blood flow that returns to the left atrium (via the pulmonary veins) rather than to the right atrium (via the azygos veins) constitutes at most 1% of the venous return to the heart. This small quantity of bronchial venous blood, plus a small amount of coronary venous blood that drains directly into the left atrium or left ventricle, "contaminates" the pulmonary venous blood, which is ordinarily fully saturated with O_2. Hence, the aortic blood is very slightly desaturated. This small quantity of venous drainage directly into the left side of the heart also accounts for the fact that, even under true equilibrium conditions, the output of the left ventricle slightly exceeds that of the right ventricle.

In certain pathological states, the bronchial circulation may become substantial, and the admixture of blood between the systemic and pulmonary circuits may be appreciable. Sustained abridgment of the pulmonary arterial blood supply to a lung, after pulmonary embolism, for example, usually increases the precapillary (arterial) communications between vessels of the systemic and pulmonary circuits. Conversely, inflammatory and degenerative diseases of the lung are often associated with an increased bronchial blood flow and significant admixtures of blood take place between the two systems.

Pulmonary Hemodynamics

Pressures in the Pulmonary Circulation. In normal individuals, the average systolic and diastolic pressures in the pulmonary artery are about 25 and 10 mm Hg, respectively, and the mean pressure is about 15 mm Hg (Fig. 11-8). These pressures are much lower than those in systemic arteries (see Fig. 11-8), because the pulmonary vascular resistance is only about one tenth the resistance of the systemic vascular bed. The mean pressure in the left atrium is normally about 5 mm Hg, and so the total pulmonary arteriovenous pressure gradient is only about 10 mm Hg. The mean hydrostatic pressure in the pulmonary capillaries lies between the pulmonary arterial and pulmonary venous values, but somewhat closer to the latter.

The mean left atrial pressure is an index of the left ventricular filling pressure. To determine whether a patient is in left heart failure, it is desirable but difficult to measure the left atrial pressure directly. However, a flexible, balloon-tipped catheter can easily be guided into the pulmonary artery. If the catheter is advanced until the tip is wedged into a small branch of the pulmonary artery, the **pulmonary artery wedge pressure** serves as a useful estimate of the pressure in the left atrium. The wedged catheter halts flow in the small vessels distal to the catheter. These vessels serve as an extension of the catheter, allowing it in effect to communicate with the pulmonary veins and left atrium.

Pulmonary Blood Flow. At equilibrium, the pulmonary and systemic blood flows are equal, except for the small disparity ascribable to the bronchial circulation. Because of the low pressures in the pulmonary blood vessels and their great distensibility, gravity affects the regional distribution of blood flow in the lungs.

Three distinct flow patterns may be found at different hydrostatic levels in the lung, as illustrated in Fig. 11-9. Consider that the pulmonary artery delivers blood at a steady pressure of 15 mm Hg and that the pulmonary venous pressure remains constant at 5 mm Hg. In those pulmonary arterial and venous branches

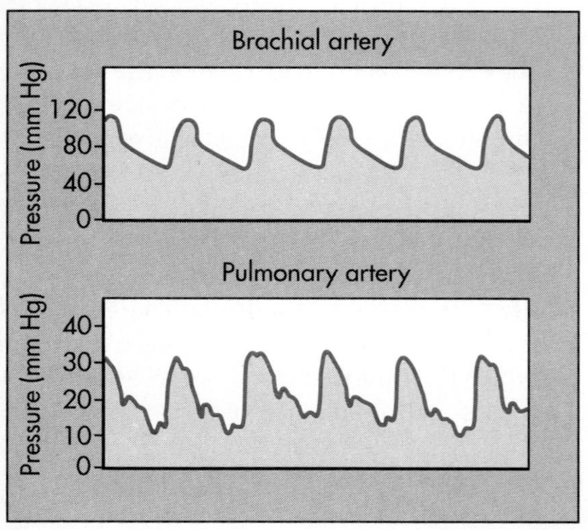

Fig. 11-8 ■ Pressures recorded in the brachial and pulmonary arteries of a normal human subject. (Modified from Harris, P., and Heath D.: Human pulmonary circulation, Edinburgh, 1962, E and S Livingstone Ltd.)

that are 13 cm below (zone *C*) the hydrostatic level of the main pulmonary vessels, the respective pressures will be 10 mm Hg (equivalent of 13 cm of blood) greater than those in the main vessels, by virtue of gravitational effects. Conversely, in pulmonary arterial and venous branches that are 13 cm above (zone *A*) the main vessels, the respective pressures will be 10 mm Hg less than those in the main vessels. At the same hydrostatic level (zone *B*) as the main vessels, the respective pressures in the branches will be approximately equal to those in the main vessels.

Consider that the alveolar pressure equals 7 mm Hg in all alveoli. Such an alveolar pressure might exist in an individual receiving positive-pressure ventilation. In zone *A,* the alveolar pressure would exceed the local arterial and venous pressures (see Fig. 11-9). The pulmonary capillary pressures lie between those of the arteries and veins, and therefore alveolar pressure would also exceed capillary pressure. Capillaries lying between adjacent alveoli would be collapsed. Those alveoli would not be perfused, and gas would not be exchanged.

Ordinarily the mean pressure in the alveoli is atmospheric. Therefore, the conditions depicted in zone *A* do not ordinarily prevail in any region of the lungs. In hypovolemic states, however, the mean pulmonary artery pressure is often very low. Therefore, vascular pressures in the lung apices might be subatmospheric. The atmospheric pressure in the alveoli would then compress the apical capillaries, so that virtually no blood would flow to that region from the pulmonary circulation. However, the bronchial circulation, which operates at much higher pressures, would be unaffected.

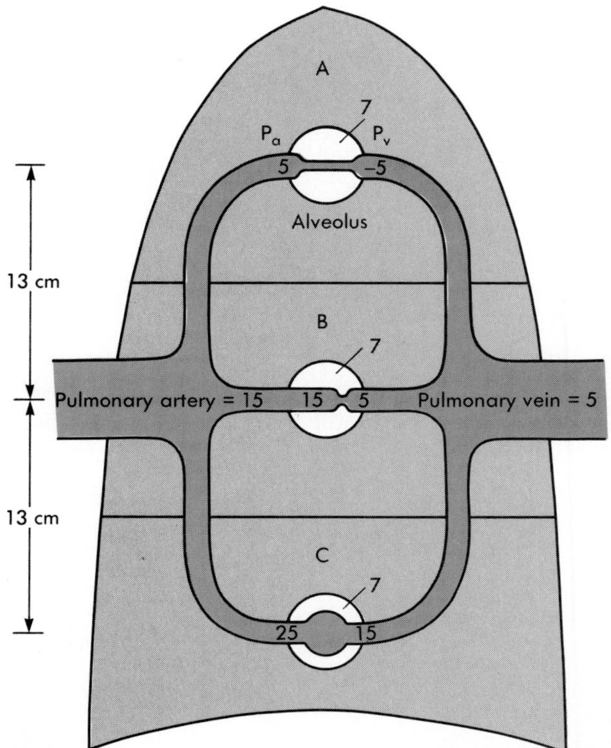

Fig. 11-9 ■ Schematic representation of the three types of flow regimens that might exist in the pulmonary circulation. In zone *A,* alveolar pressure exceeds intravascular pressures. Pulmonary capillaries in this zone will not be perfused. In zone *B,* alveolar pressure is intermediate between pulmonary arterial and venous pressures. Pulmonary capillaries will flutter between the open and closed states. In zone *C,* intravascular pressures exceed alveolar pressure. The pulmonary capillaries are always open, but the flow resistances in individual vessels vary with the hydrostatic pressure in the vessel.

In zone *B,* the alveolar pressure lies between the local arterial and venous pressures (see Fig. 11-9). Again, if alveolar pressure equals 7 mm Hg, a capillary in that region will flutter between the open and closed state. When the capillary is open, blood will flow through it, and the capillary pressure will decrease progressively from the arterial to the venous end. The pressure at the venous end will be less than the alveolar pressure, and therefore the capillary will collapse at that end. With the cessation of flow, the arterial and capillary pressures at a given hydrostatic level will equalize. Thus, the capillary pressure will quickly rise to that in the local small arteries, which exceeds the prevailing alveolar pressure. Hence, the capillary will then be forced open. With the restitution of flow, however, the pressure will drop along the length of the capillary. As the pressure at the venous end drops below the ambient alveolar pressure, the capillary will again close. Hence, the capillary will flutter between the open and closed states.

The critical pressure gradient for flow in zone *B* is the arterioalveolar pressure difference; it is not the arteriovenous pressure difference, as it is for most vessels in the body. As long as the venous pressure is less than the alveolar pressure, the venous pressure does not influence the flow. Such a flow condition is called a **waterfall effect,** because the height of a waterfall has no influence on the flow.

In zone *C,* the arterial and venous pressures both exceed the alveolar pressure. Hence, the pressure everywhere along the capillary exceeds the alveolar pressure, and the capillary remains permanently open. In this zone, the flow is determined by the arteriovenous pressure gradient, and the resistance may be calculated by the conventional analog of Ohm's law. The large and small pulmonary vessels, including the capillaries, are very distensible, as noted above. The pressure difference that determines the caliber of a distensible tube is the **transmural pressure,** that is, the difference between the internal and external pressures. In an erect individual the intravascular pressures in the lungs increase from apex to base. The transmural pressures increase accordingly, and the diameter of the pulmonary vessels increases from apex to base. Because resistance to flow varies inversely with vessel caliber, resistance decreases and flow increases in zone *C* in the apex-to-base direction. Such predicted changes in flow have been verified in humans.

Regulation of the Pulmonary Circulation

The total volume of blood pumped by the heart passes through the pulmonary circulation. Therefore, the various cardiac and vascular factors that determine cardiac output in general also determine the total pulmonary blood flow. These factors have been discussed in Chapter 9.

The autonomic nervous system innervates the pulmonary blood vessels. Although the small pulmonary vessels contain little smooth muscle, small changes in smooth muscle tone may alter vascular resistance substantially, because the pulmonary circulation is such a low-pressure system. Baroreceptor stimulation can dilate the pulmonary resistance vessels reflexly. Conversely, peripheral chemoreceptor stimulation constricts the pulmonary vessels. The importance of such neural regulation remains to be established, however.

Hypoxia is the most important influence on pulmonary vasomotor tone. Acute and chronic hypoxia both increase pulmonary vascular resistance (Fig. 11-10). Regional reductions in alveolar O_2 tension constrict the nearby arterioles. This response helps maintain an optimum ventilation-perfusion ratio. The O_2 tension in poorly ventilated alveoli will fall toward the Po_2 in the pulmonary arterial blood. Blood flowing by such alveoli will not be well oxygenated, and therefore the O_2 tension of the blood returning to the left atrium will de-

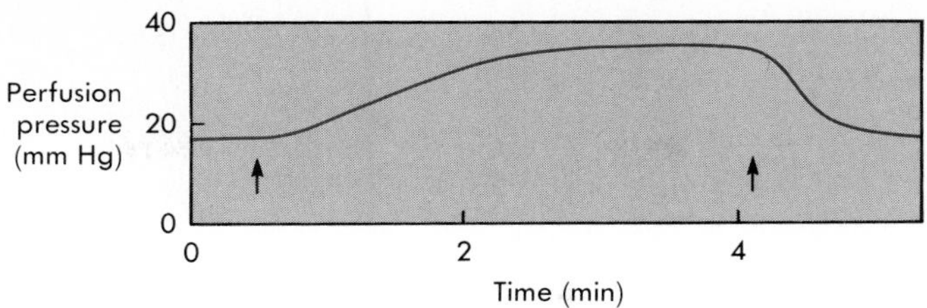

Fig. 11-10 ■ The effect of hypoxia on vascular resistance of an isolated rat lung. The lung was perfused with blood at a constant flow. When the O_2 tension of the inspired air was reduced (between the arrows), the pulmonary resistance vessels constricted, as indicated by the substantial rise in perfusion pressure. (Modified from Grover, R.F., Wagner, W.W., Jr., McMurtry, I.F., and Reeves, J.T.: In Handbook of physiology; Section 2: The cardiovascular system—peripheral circulation and organ blood flow, vol. III, Bethesda, Md., 1983, American Physiological Society.)

crease. Arteriolar vasoconstriction reduces the blood flow to such poorly ventilated alveoli, and it thereby reduces the contamination of the pulmonary venous blood with poorly oxygenated blood. Thus, this mechanism shunts the pulmonary blood flow from the poorly ventilated regions to the better ventilated regions of the lungs, and it thereby improves the O_2 saturation of the systemic arterial blood. The mechanism by which hypoxia raises pulmonary vascular resistance is still obscure, despite considerable investigation.

■ RENAL CIRCULATION

Anatomy

The primary branches of the **renal artery** divide into a number of **interlobar arteries.** These interlobar branches (Fig. 11-11) proceed radially from the hilus toward the corticomedullary junction, between adjacent medullary pyramids. As an interlobar artery approaches the corticomedullary junction (horizontal dashed line, Fig. 11-11), it branches into a number of **arcuate arteries,** which travel in various directions over the bases of the adjacent medullary pyramids, in the zone between the cortex and medulla. The arcuate branches that arise from adjacent interlobar arteries do not interconnect. Hence occlusion of an interlobar artery destroys a pyramidal-shaped region of the kidney.

From the arcuate arteries, a number of **interlobular branches** travel toward the capsular surface of the kidney (see Fig. 11-11). The **afferent arterioles** to the **glomeruli** are branches of these interlobular arteries. Each human kidney has approximately 1 million glomeruli. The afferent arteriole to each glomerulus divides into several vessels that form discrete capillary loops (Fig. 11-12). The proximal and distal limbs of each loop are interconnected by many smaller capillaries. The distal limbs of each capillary loop within a glomerulus rejoin to form the **efferent arteriole,** the diameter of which is usually less than that of the afferent arteriole. The entire glomerular capillary tuft is enveloped by **Bowman's capsule,** which collects the glomerular filtrate.

The efferent arterioles divide into another capillary network, the **peritubular capillaries.** The architecture of the peritubular capillary network varies, depending on whether the efferent arteriole arises from glomeruli close to the medullary border (the **juxtamedullary glomeruli**) or from glomeruli in the more peripheral regions of the renal cortex (see Fig. 11-11).

Capillaries that originate from the regular

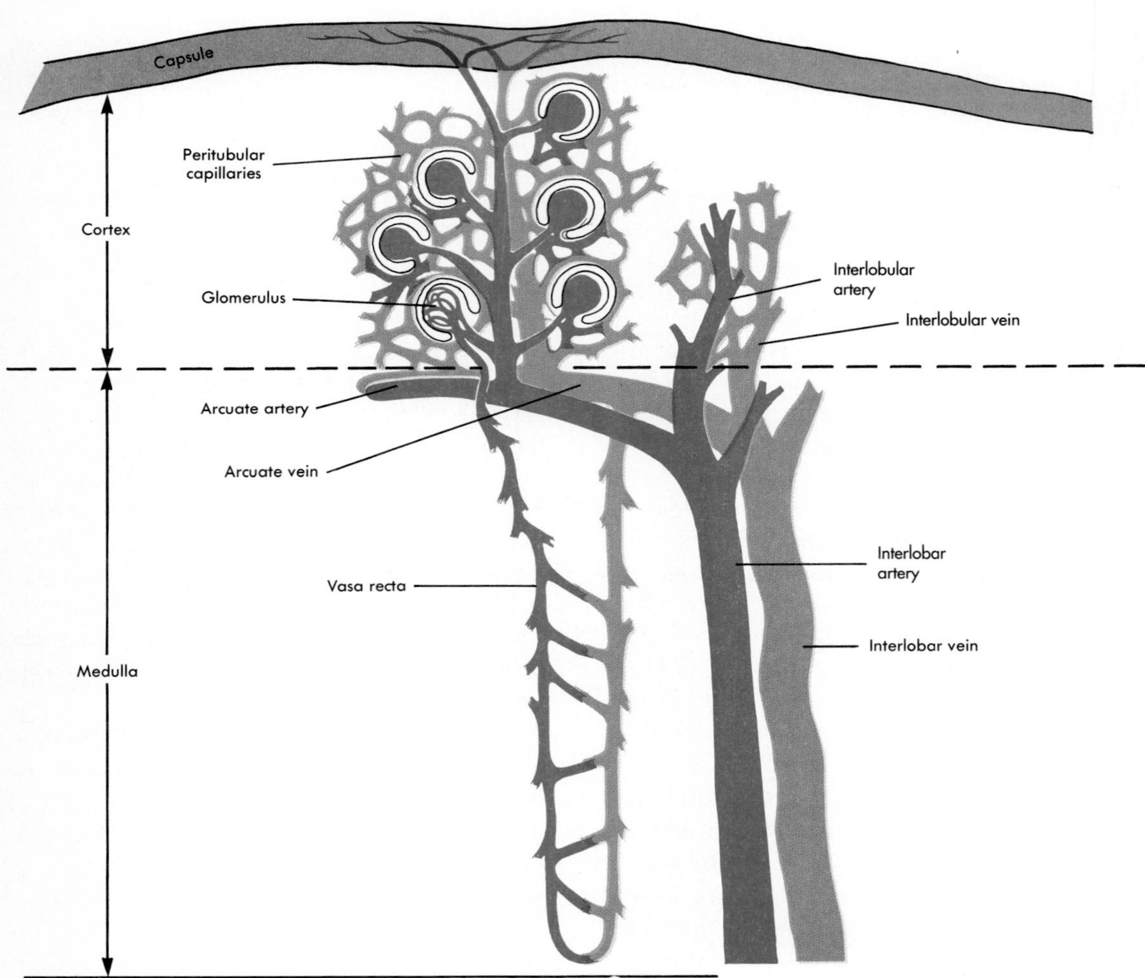

Fig. 11-11 ■ Anatomy of the vasculature to one lobe of the kidney.

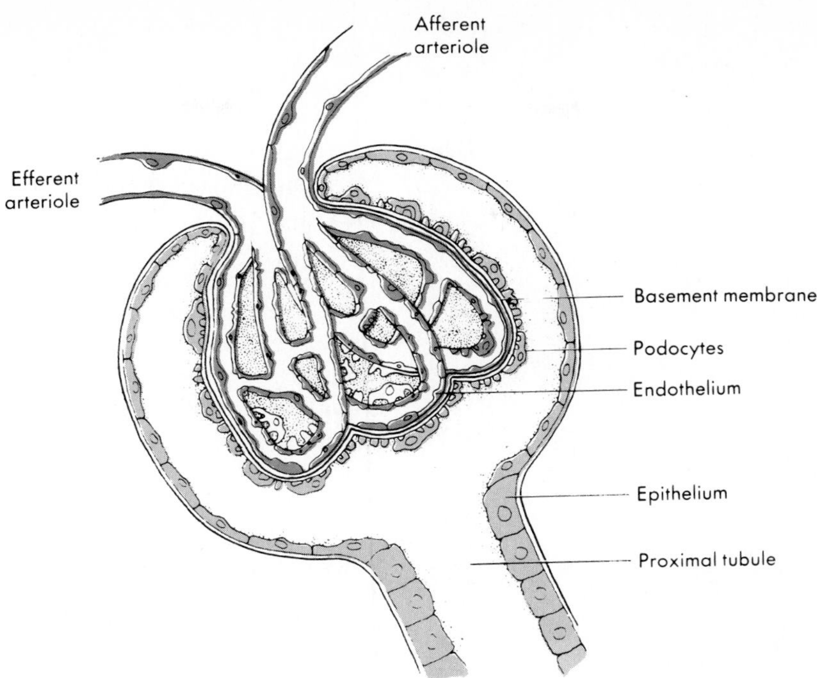

Fig. 11-12 ■ Anatomy of the mammalian glomerulus.

cortical glomeruli surround relatively short renal tubules, which are located almost entirely in the cortex itself. The capillary networks of neighboring cortical nephrons freely communicate with one another. Most of the capillaries arising from the efferent arterioles of juxtamedullary glomeruli form long hairpin loops **(vasa recta)** that accompany the loops of Henle deep into the renal medulla, sometimes to the tips of the renal papillae. The vasa recta participate in the countercurrent exchange system responsible for concentrating the urine. In general, the renal venous system parallels the arterial distribution to the renal tissues (see Fig. 11-11).

Renal Hemodynamics

Segmental Resistance. The pressure drops only slightly in the interlobar, arcuate, and interlobular arteries; the main preglomerular resistance resides in the afferent arterioles (Fig. 11-13). The pressure in the glomerular capillaries is normally about 50 to 60 mm Hg. Thus, the net balance of forces across the capillary wall favors the outward filtration of plasma water along the entire length of the capillary loop. Furthermore, the filtration coefficient of the glomerular capillaries exceeds that of most other capillaries in the body. Hence, about 20% of the plasma water that enters the glomerular capillaries is filtered into Bowman's capsule. The greatest hydraulic resistance in the renal circulation is in the efferent arterioles. Consequently, the pressure in the peritubular capillaries is normally about 10 to 20 mm Hg. Such pressures favor the net reabsorption of the large quantities of fluid that pass from the renal tubules to the interstitial spaces of the

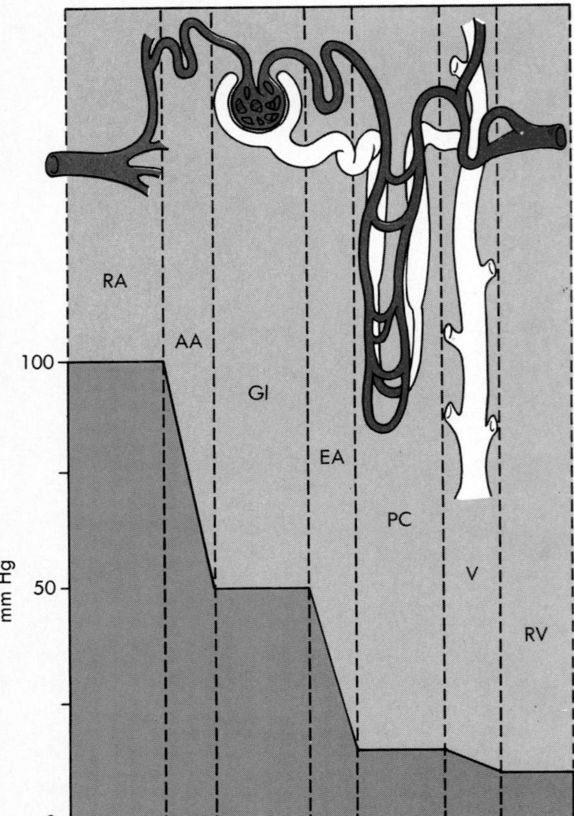

Fig. 11-13 ■ Intravascular pressures in the renal artery *(RA),* afferent arterioles *(AA),* glomerular capillaries *(Gl),* efferent arterioles *(EA),* peritubular capillaries *(PC),* venules *(V),* and renal vein *(RV).* (From Frohnert, P.P.: In Knox, F.G., editor: Textbook of renal pathophysiology, Hagerstown, Md., 1978, Harper & Row Publishers, Inc.; based on data from Brenner, B.M.: J. Clin. Invest. 50:1776, 1971.)

kidney. The peritubular capillaries also are considerably more permeable than most of the other capillaries in the body.

Renal Blood Flow. The weight of the kidneys comprises only about 0.5% of the total body weight, and yet the kidneys receive about 20% of the cardiac output. Most of this rich blood supply perfuses the renal cortex; the inner medulla and papillae receive only about one tenth of the blood flow per unit weight that perfuses the cortex. Nevertheless, even these medullary tissues receive as much blood per unit weight as does the brain.

The kidney has one of the highest metabolic rates in the body. The large renal blood flow does not subserve the great metabolic rate, however. The kidney extracts less than 10% of the O_2 present in the renal arterial blood. Therefore, the renal blood flow is at least ten times greater than that needed to deliver the required O_2 and nutrients. The excessively high renal blood flow delivers large volumes of blood to the glomeruli for the process of ultrafiltration.

Regulation of the Renal Circulation

Autoregulation. Renal blood flow tends to remain constant, despite fluctuations in the arterial perfusion pressure. In the experiment represented in Fig. 11-14, for example, the arterial pressure was suddenly raised from 140 to 190 mm Hg. This stepwise change in pressure rapidly increased the renal blood flow, from 135 to 155 ml/min. This rise in renal blood flow was transitory, however, and flow returned close to the control level in less than 1 minute. Over a pressure range of about 75 to 160 mm Hg, the steady-state level of renal blood flow is relatively insensitive to changes in arterial pressure. Beyond this range, however, renal blood flow varies directly with perfusion pressure.

This ability of the renal blood flow to remain constant, despite fluctuations in perfusion pressure, is a process intrinsic to the kidney itself; it has been demonstrated even in isolated kidney preparations (see Fig. 11-14). Concomitant measurement of glomerular filtration rate (GFR) reveals that the tendency for GFR to be autoregulated is equally pronounced. Therefore, the resistance change induced by an alteration in perfusion pressure must occur mainly

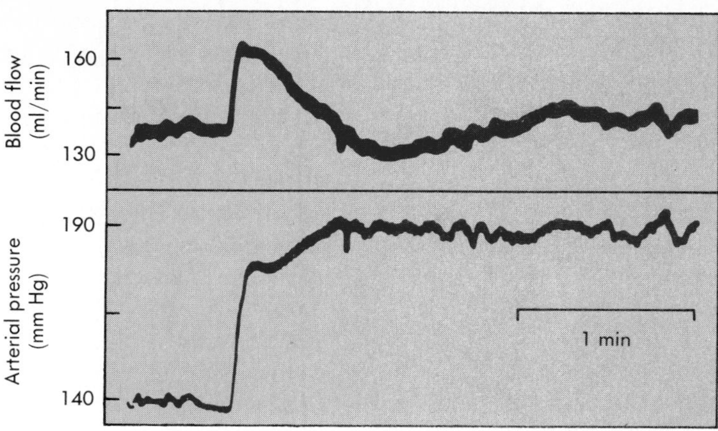

Fig. 11-14 ■ Changes in renal blood flow evoked by a sudden increase in arterial perfusion pressure from 140 to 190 mm Hg in an isolated dog kidney. The kidney was perfused from a peripheral artery of another dog. (Modified from Semple, S.J.G., and deWardener, H.E.: Circ. Res. 7:643, 1959. With permission of the American Heart Association.)

in the afferent arteriole. As the perfusion pressure is raised, for example, afferent arteriolar constriction not only limits the increase in renal blood flow but also restricts the rise in glomerular capillary pressure and the concomitant increment in GFR.

Renal autoregulation has been studied extensively, but the mechanism remains controversial. Many mechanisms have been proposed, including the tissue pressure, myogenic, and metabolic hypotheses (see Chapter 8). None of these mechanisms accounts entirely for the autoregulatory process in the kidneys, although each mechanism may contribute.

Considerable attention also has been directed toward the **juxtaglomerular apparatus,** which is involved in the release of **renin** by the kidneys. Renin is an enzyme that acts on a substrate circulating in the blood, and it releases a peptide, **angiotensin,** which is a potent vasoconstrictor. Investigators have proposed that a rise in renal perfusion pressure initially increases GFR. The consequent increase in fluid flow in the renal tubules is somehow sensed by the juxtaglomerular apparatus, which responds by releasing renin. The angiotensin thus generated constricts the afferent arterioles and thereby attenuates the increases in GFR and renal blood flow.

Neural Regulation. Stimulation of the renal sympathetic nerves decreases renal blood flow substantially, but reduces GFR only slightly. The neural activity constricts the afferent and efferent arterioles and the proximal segments of the vasa recta. Presumably, the reduction of renal blood flow exceeds the reduction of GFR because the postglomerular constriction is greater than the preglomerular constriction.

In resting subjects, the basal level of renal sympathetic tone is low; abolition of that tone scarcely affects renal blood flow. The arterial baroreceptor reflexes only influence the renal vasculature slightly. Activation of low-pressure receptors elicits much larger reflex effects on the renal circulation. A reduction in left atrial pressure, for example, increases renal nerve activity and renal vascular resistance greatly. Emotional reactions, such as anxiety, fear, and rage, also curtail renal blood flow dramatically.

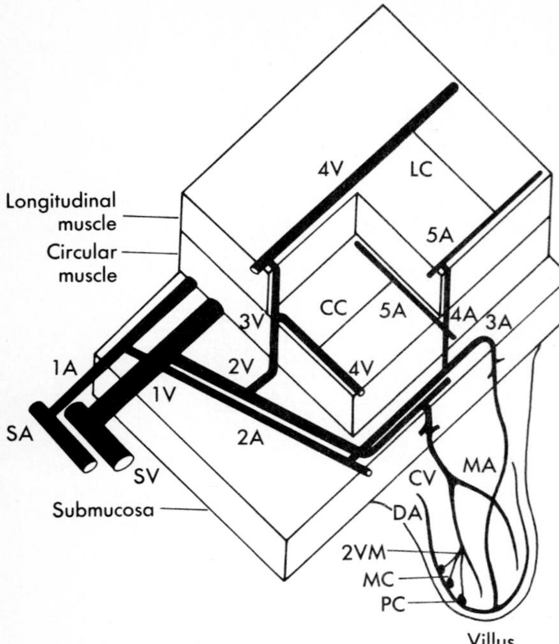

Fig. 11-15 ■ The distribution of small blood vessels to the rat intestinal wall. *SA,* Small artery; *SV,* small vein; *1A* to *5A,* first- to fifth-order arterioles; *1V* to *4V,* first- to fourth-order venules; *CC* and *LC,* capillaries in circular and longitudinal muscle layers; *MA* and *CV,* main arteriole and collecting venule of a villus; *DA,* distribution arteriole; *2VM,* second-order mucosal venule; *PC,* precapillary sphincter; *MC,* mucosal capillary. (From Gore, R.W., and Bohlen, H.G.: Am. J. Physiol. 233:H685, 1977.)

■ SPLANCHNIC CIRCULATION

The splanchnic circulation consists of the blood supply to the gastrointestinal tract, liver, spleen, and pancreas. Several features distinguish the splanchnic circulation, the most noteworthy of which is that two large capillary beds are partially in series with one another. The small splanchnic arterial branches supply the capillary beds in the gastrointestinal tract, spleen, and pancreas. From these capillary beds, the venous blood ultimately flows into the portal vein, which normally provides most of the blood supply to the liver. However, the hepatic artery also supplies blood to the liver.

Intestinal Circulation

Anatomy. The gastrointestinal tract is supplied by the celiac, superior mesenteric, and inferior mesenteric arteries. The superior mesenteric artery is the largest of all the aortic branches and carries over 10% of the cardiac output. Small mesenteric arteries form an extensive vascular network in the submucosa (Fig. 11-15). Their branches penetrate the longitudinal and circular muscle layers and give rise to third- and fourth-order arterioles. Some third-order arterioles in the submucosa become the main arterioles to the tips of the villi.

The direction of the blood flow in the capillaries and venules in a villus is opposite to that in the main arteriole (Fig. 11-16). This arrangement constitutes a countercurrent exchange system. An effective countercurrent multiplier in the villus facilitates the absorption of sodium and water. The countercurrent exchange also permits diffusion of O_2 from arterioles to venules. At low flow rates, a substantial fraction of the O_2 may be shunted from arterioles to venules near the base of the villus, thereby curtailing the supply of O_2 to the mucosal cells at the tip of the villus. When intestinal blood flow is reduced, the shunting of O_2 is exaggerated, which may cause extensive necrosis of the intestinal villi.

Neural Regulation. The neural control of the mesenteric circulation is almost exclusively sympathetic. Increased sympathetic activity constricts the mesenteric arterioles, precapillary sphincters, and capacitance vessels. These responses are mediated by alpha-receptors, which are prepotent in the mesenteric circulation; however, beta-receptors are also present. Infusion of a beta-receptor agonist,

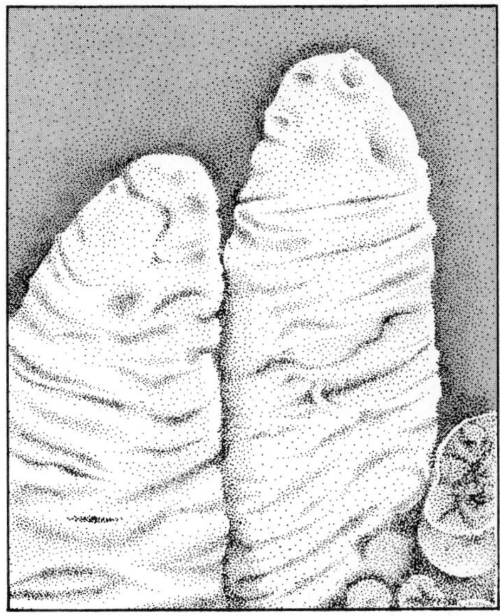

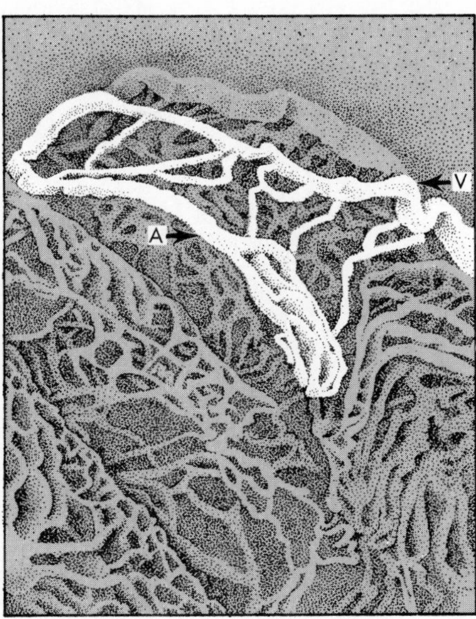

Fig. 11-16 ■ Scanning electron micrographs of rabbit intestinal villi *(left panel)* and corrosion cast of the microcirculation in the villus *(right panel)*. *A,* Arteriole; *V,* venule. (From Gannon, B.J., Gore, R.W., and Rogers, P.A.W.: Biomed. Res. 2(Suppl.):235, 1981.)

such as isoproterenol, causes vasodilation.

During fighting or in response to artificial stimulation of the hypothalamic "defense" area, pronounced vasoconstriction occurs in the mesenteric vascular bed. This shifts blood flow from the temporarily less important intestinal circulation to the more crucial skeletal muscles, heart, and brain.

Autoregulation. Autoregulation in the intestinal circulation is not as well developed as it is in certain other vascular beds, such as those in the brain and kidney. The principal mechanism responsible for autoregulation is metabolic, although a myogenic mechanism probably also participates. The adenosine concentration in the mesenteric venous blood rises fourfold after brief arterial occlusion. Adenosine is a potent vasodilator in the mesenteric vascular bed and may be the principal metabolic mediator of autoregulation. However, potassium and altered osmolality may also contribute to the overall response.

The O_2 consumption of the small intestine is more rigorously controlled than is the blood flow. In one series of experiments, the O_2 uptake of the small intestine remained constant when the arterial perfusion pressure was varied between 30 and 125 mm Hg.

Functional Hyperemia. Food ingestion increases intestinal blood flow. The secretion of certain gastrointestinal hormones contributes to this hyperemia. Gastrin and cholecystokinin augment intestinal blood flow, and they are secreted when food is ingested. The absorption of food affects the intestinal blood flow. Undigested food has no vasoactive influence, whereas several products of digestion are potent vasodilators. Among the various

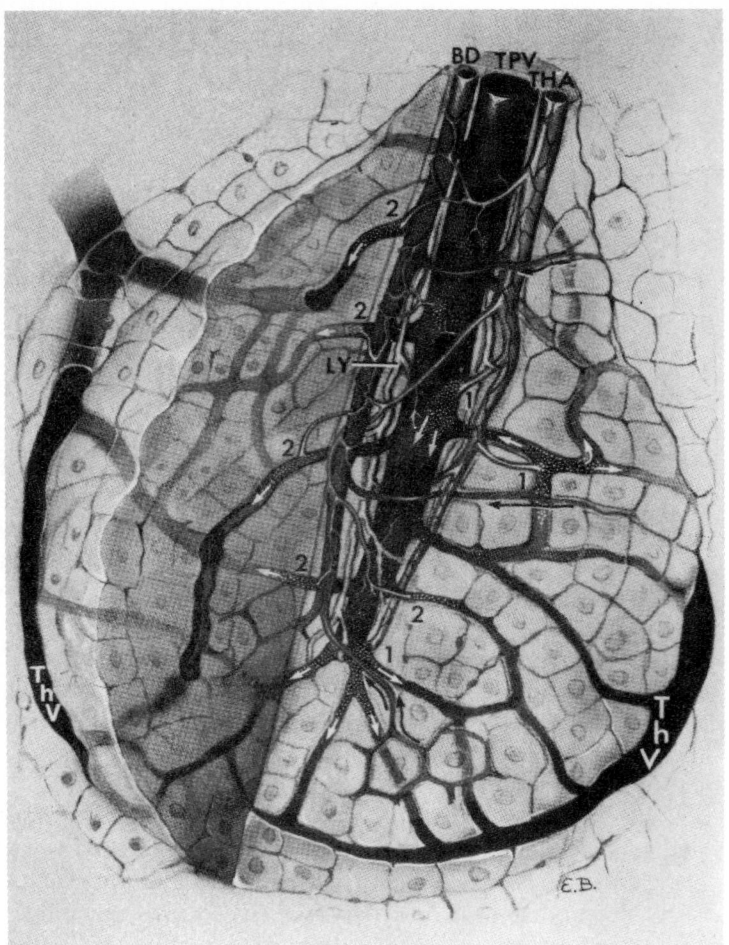

Fig. 11-17 ■ Microcirculation to a hepatic acinus. *THA,* Terminal hepatic arteriole; *TPV,* terminal portal venule; *BD,* bile ductule; *THV,* terminal hepatic venule; *LY,* lymphatic. The hepatic arterioles empty either directly *(1)* or through the peribiliary plexus *(2)* into the sinusoids that run from the terminal portal venule to the terminal hepatic venules. (From Rappaport, A.M.: Microvasc. Res. 6:212, 1973.)

constituents of chyme, the principal mediators of mesenteric hyperemia are glucose and fatty acids.

Hepatic Circulation

Anatomy. The blood flow to the liver normally is about 25% of the cardiac output. The flow is derived from two sources, the portal vein and the hepatic artery. Ordinarily, the portal vein provides about three fourths of the blood flow. The portal venous blood already has passed through the gastrointestinal capillary bed, and therefore much of the O_2 already has been extracted. The hepatic artery delivers the remaining one fourth of the blood, which is fully saturated with O_2. Hence, about three fourths of the O_2 used by the liver is derived from the hepatic arterial blood.

The small branches of the portal vein and hepatic artery give rise to terminal portal venules and hepatic arterioles (Fig. 11-17). These terminal vessels enter the hepatic acinus (the functional unit of the liver) at its center. Blood flows from these terminal vessels into the sinusoids, which constitute the capillary network of the liver. The sinusoids radiate toward the periphery of the acinus, where they connect with the terminal hepatic venules. Blood from these terminal venules drains into progressively larger branches of the hepatic veins, which are tributaries of the inferior vena cava.

Hemodynamics. The mean blood pressure in the portal vein is about 10 mm Hg and that in the hepatic artery is about 90 mm Hg. The resistance of the vessels upstream to the hepatic sinusoids is considerably greater than that of the downstream vessels. Consequently, the pressure in the sinusoids is only 2 or 3 mm Hg greater than that in the hepatic veins and inferior vena cava. The ratio of presinusoidal to postsinusoidal resistance in the liver is much greater than is the ratio of precapillary to postcapillary resistance for almost any other vascular bed. Hence, drugs and other interventions that alter the presinusoidal resistance usually affect the pressure in the sinusoids only slightly. Such changes in presinusoidal resistance have little effect on the fluid exchange across the sinusoidal wall. Conversely, changes in hepatic venous (and in central venous) pressure are transmitted almost quantitatively to the hepatic sinusoids and profoundly affect the transsinusoidal exchange of fluids. When central venous pressure is elevated, as in congestive heart failure, plasma water transudes from the liver into the peritoneal cavity, leading to **ascites.**

Regulation of Flow. Blood flows in the portal venous and hepatic arterial systems vary reciprocally. When blood flow is curtailed in one system, the flow increases in the other system. However, the resultant increase in flow in one system usually does not fully compensate for the initiating reduction in flow in the other system.

The portal venous system does not autoregulate. As the portal venous pressure and flow are raised, resistance either remains constant or it decreases. The hepatic arterial system does autoregulate, however.

The liver tends to maintain a constant O_2 consumption, because the extraction of O_2 from the hepatic blood is very efficient. As the rate of O_2 delivery to the liver is varied, the liver compensates by an appropriate change in the fraction of O_2 extracted from the blood. This extraction is facilitated by the distinct separation of the presinusoidal vessels at the acinar center from the postsinusoidal vessels at the periphery of the acinus (see Fig. 11-17). The substantial distance between these types of vessels prevents the countercurrent exchange of O_2, contrary to the condition that exists in an intestinal villus (see Fig. 11-16).

The sympathetic nerves constrict the presinusoidal resistance vessels in the portal venous and hepatic arterial systems. Neural effects on the capacitance vessels are more important, however. The effects are mediated mainly by alpha-receptors.

Capacitance Vessels. The liver contains about 15% of the total blood volume of the body. Under appropriate conditions, such as in response to hemorrhage, about half of the hepatic blood volume can be rapidly expelled. Hence, the liver constitutes an important blood reservoir in humans. In certain other species, such as the dog, the spleen is a more important blood reservoir. Smooth muscle in the capsule and trabeculae of the spleen contract in response to increased sympathetic

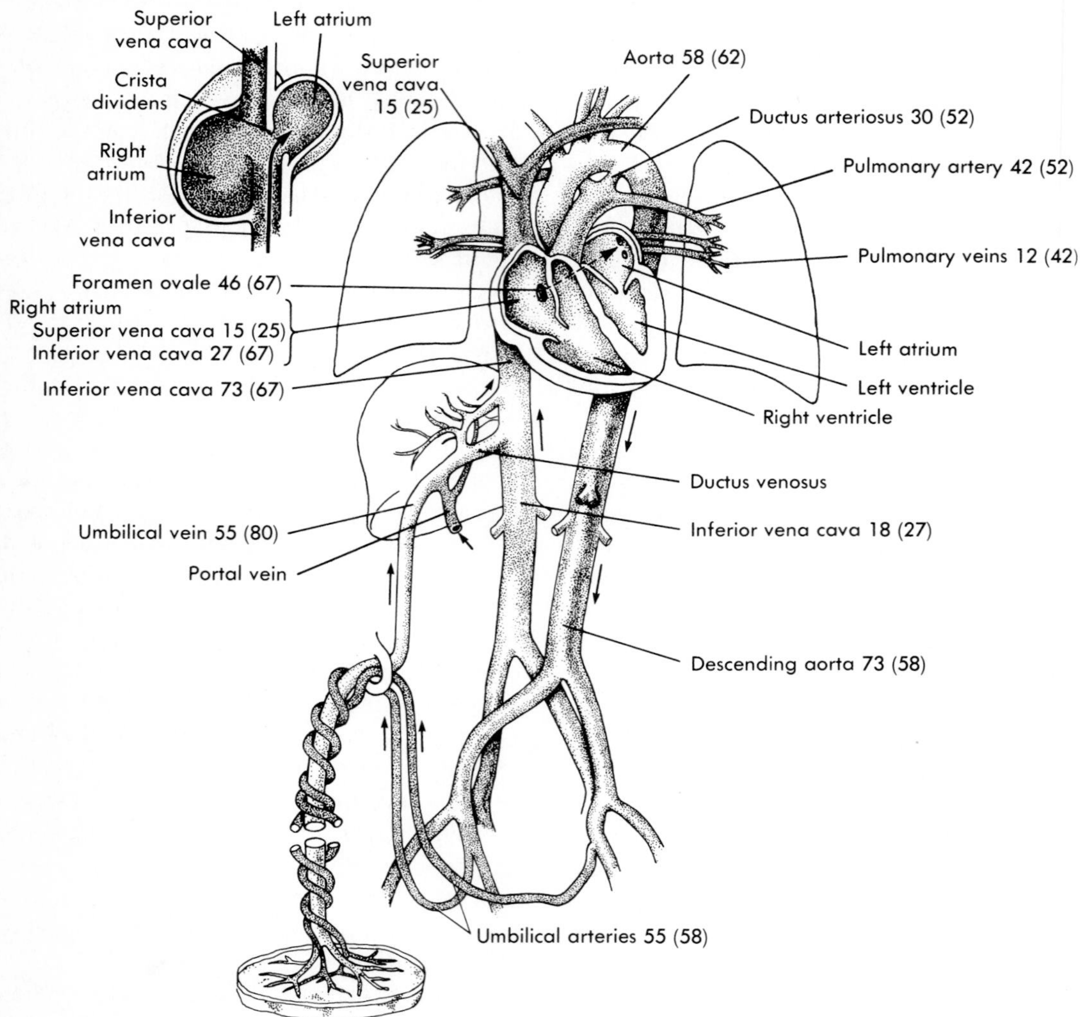

Fig. 11-18 ■ Schematic diagram of the fetal circulation. The numbers without parentheses represent the distribution of cardiac output as a percentage of the sum of the right and left ventricular outputs, and the numbers within parentheses represent the percentage of O_2 saturation of the blood flowing in the indicated blood vessel. The insert at the upper left illustrates the direction of flow of a major portion of the inferior vena cava blood through the foramen ovale to the left atrium. (Values for percentage distribution of blood flow and O_2 saturations are from Dawes, G.S., Mott, J.C., and Widdicombe, J.G.: J. Physiol. 126:563, 1954.)

neural activity, such as occurs during exercise or hemorrhage. However, this mechanism does not exist in humans.

■ FETAL CIRCULATION

The circulation of the fetus shows a number of differences from that of the postnatal infant. The fetal lungs are functionally inactive, and the fetus depends completely on the placenta for O_2 and nutrient supply. Oxygenated fetal blood from the placenta passes through the umbilical vein to the liver. A major fraction passes through the liver, and a small fraction bypasses the liver to the inferior vena cava through the **ductus venosus** (Fig. 11-18). In the inferior vena cava, blood from the ductus venosus joins blood returning from the lower trunk and extremities and this combined stream is in turn joined by blood from the liver through the hepatic veins. The streams of blood tend to maintain their identity in the inferior vena cava and are divided into two streams of unequal size by the edge of the interatrial septum **(crista dividens).** The larger stream, which is primarily blood from the umbilical vein, is shunted to the left atrium through the **foramen ovale,** which lies between the inferior vena cava and the left atrium (inset, Fig. 11-18). The other stream passes into the right atrium, where it is joined by superior vena caval blood returning from the upper parts of the body and by blood from the myocardium. In contrast to the adult, in whom the right and left ventricles pump in series, in the fetus the ventricles operate essentially in parallel. Because of the large pulmonary resistance, less than one third of the right ventricular output goes through the lungs. The remainder passes through the **ductus arteriosus** from the pulmonary artery to the aorta at a point distal to the origins of the arteries to the head and upper extremities. Flow from pulmonary artery to aorta occurs because pulmonary artery pressure is about 5 mm Hg higher than aortic pressure in the fetus. The large volume of blood coming through the foramen ovale into the left atrium is joined by blood returning from the lungs and is pumped out by the left ventricle into the aorta. About one third of the aortic blood goes to the head, upper thorax, and arms and the remaining two thirds go to the rest of the body and the placenta. The amount of blood pumped by the left ventricle is about 20% greater than that pumped by the right ventricle, and the major fraction of the blood that passes down the descending aorta flows by way of the two umbilical arteries to the placenta.

In Fig. 11-18 the distribution of fetal blood flow is given in a percentage of the combined right and left ventricular outputs. Note that over half of the combined cardiac output is returned directly to the placenta without passing through any capillary bed. Also indicated in Fig. 11-18 are the O_2 saturations of the blood (numbers in parentheses) at various points of the fetal circulation. Fetal blood leaving the placenta is 80% saturated, but the saturation of the blood passing through the foramen ovale is reduced to 67% by mixing with desaturated blood returning from the lower part of the body and the liver. Addition of the desaturated blood from the lungs reduces the O_2 saturation of left ventricular blood to 62%, which is the level of saturation of the blood reaching the head and upper extremities. The blood in the right ventricle, a mixture of desaturated superior vena caval blood, coronary venous blood, and inferior vena caval blood, is only 52% saturated with O_2. When the major portion of this blood traverses the ductus arteriosus and joins that pumped out by the left ventricle, the resultant O_2 saturation of blood traveling to the lower part of the body and back to the placenta is 58% saturated. Thus it is apparent that the tissues receiving blood of the highest O_2 saturation are the liver, heart, and upper parts of the body, including the head.

At the placenta the chorionic villi dip into the maternal sinuses, and O_2, CO_2, nutrients, and metabolic waste products exchange across the membranes. The barrier to exchange is quite large, and the equilibrium of O_2 tension between the two circulations is not reached at normal rates of blood flow. Therefore, the O_2 tension of the fetal blood leaving the placenta is very low. Were it not for the fact that fetal hemoglobin has a greater affinity for O_2 than does adult hemoglobin, the fetus would not receive an adequate O_2 supply. The fetal oxyhemoglobin dissociation curve is shifted to the left so that at equal pressures of O_2 fetal blood will carry significantly more O_2 than will maternal blood. If the mother is subjected to hypoxia, the reduced blood O_2 tension is reflected in the fetus by tachycardia and an increase in blood flow through the umbilical vessels. If the hypoxia persists or if flow through the umbilical vessels is impaired, fetal distress occurs and is first manifested as bradycardia. In early fetal life the high cardiac glycogen levels that prevail (which gradually decrease to adult levels by term) may protect the heart from acute periods of hypoxia.

Circulatory Changes That Occur at Birth

The umbilical vessels have thick muscular walls that are very reactive to trauma, tension, sympathomimetic amines, bradykinin, angiotensin, and changes in O_2 tension. In animals in which the umbilical cord is not tied, hemorrhage of the newborn is prevented by constriction of these large vessels in response to one or more of these stimuli. Closure of the umbilical vessels produces an increase in total peripheral resistance and of blood pressure. When blood flow through the umbilical vein ceases, the ductus venosus, a thick-walled vessel with a muscular sphincter, closes. What initiates closure of the ductus venosus is still unknown. The asphyxia, which starts with constriction or clamping of the umbilical vessels, plus the cooling of the body activate the respiratory center of the newborn infant. With the filling of the lungs with air, pulmonary vascular resistance decreases to about one tenth of the value existing before lung expansion. This resistance change is not caused by the presence of O_2 in the lungs, because the change is just as great if the lungs are filled with nitrogen. However, filling the lungs with liquid does not reduce pulmonary vascular resistance.

The left atrial pressure is raised above that in the inferior vena cava and right atrium by (1) the decrease in pulmonary resistance, with the resulting large flow of blood through the lungs to the left atrium, (2) the reduction of flow to the right atrium caused by occlusion of the umbilical vein, and (3) the increased resistance to left ventricular output produced by occlusion of the umbilical arteries. This reversal of the pressure gradient across the atria abruptly closes the valve over the foramen ovale, and fusion of the septal leaflets occurs over a period of several days.

With the decrease in pulmonary vascular resistance, the pressure in the pulmonary artery falls to about one half its previous level (to about 35 mm Hg), and this change in pressure, coupled with a slight increase in aortic pressure, reverses the flow of blood through the ductus arteriosus. However, within several minutes the large ductus arteriosus begins to constrict, producing turbulent flow, which is manifest as a murmur in the newborn. Constriction of the ductus arteriosus is progressive and usually is complete within 1 to 2 days after birth. Closure of the ductus arteriosus appears to be initiated by the high O_2 tension of the arterial blood passing through it, because pulmonary ventilation with O_2 or with air low in O_2 induces, respectively, closure and opening of this shunt vessel. Whether O_2 acts directly on the ductus or through the release of a vasoconstrictor substance is not known. Similarly, in a heart-lung preparation made from a newborn lamb, the ductus arteriosus may be made to close with high Pa_{O_2} and to open with low Pa_{O_2}. The mechanism whereby increases in Pa_{O_2} produce closure of the ductus arteriosus is unknown, but changes in the concentrations of bradykinin, prostaglandins, and adenosine in blood or ductal tissue may be involved.

At birth the walls of the two ventricles are approximately of the same thickness, with a possibly slight preponderance of the right ventricle. Also present in the newborn is thickening of the muscular levels of the pulmonary arterioles, which is apparently responsible in part for the high pulmonary vascular resistance of the fetus. After birth the thickness of the walls of the right ventricle diminishes, as does the muscle layer of the pulmonary arterioles; the left ventricular walls increase in thickness. These changes are progressive over a period of weeks after birth.

Failure of the foramen ovale or ductus arteriosus to close after birth is occasionally observed and constitutes two of the more common congenital cardiac abnormalities that are now amenable to surgical correction.

■ SUMMARY

Skin Circulation

1. Most of the resistance vessels in the skin are under dual control of the sympathetic nervous system and local vasodilator metabolites, but the arteriovenous anastomoses found in the hands, feet, and face are solely under neural control.
2. The main function of skin blood vessels is to aid in the regulation of body temperature by constricting to conserve heat and dilating to lose heat.
3. Skin blood vessels dilate directly and reflexly in response to heat and constrict directly and reflexly in response to cold.

Skeletal Muscle Circulation

1. Skeletal muscle blood flow is regulated centrally by the sympathetic nerves and locally by the release of vasodilator metabolites.
2. At rest, neural regulation of blood flow is paramount, but it yields to metabolic regulation during muscle contractions.

Cerebral Circulation

1. Cerebral blood flow is predominantly regulated by metabolic factors, especially CO_2, K^+, and adenosine.
2. Increased regional cerebral activity produced by stimuli such as touch, pain, hand motion, talking, reading, reasoning, and problem solving are associated with enhanced blood flow in the activated areas of the contralateral cerebral cortex.

Pulmonary Circulation

1. The pulmonary circulation consists of the pulmonary vasculature, whose function is to promote the exchange of O_2 and CO_2 across the pulmonary capillaries, and the bronchial vasculature, whose function is to deliver O_2 and nutrients to the airways.
2. The pulmonary vasculature is a low resistance system, and because of the low pulmonary vascular pressures the distribution of blood flow to different regions of the lungs is affected by the body's position in space.
3. The smooth muscles in the pulmonary arterioles constrict in response to hypoxia. This response tends to shift blood flow to the well-ventilated alveoli and away from the poorly ventilated alveoli.

Renal Circulation

1. Renal blood flow is very high (about 20% of cardiac output), and the chief resistance to blood flow in the kidneys resides in the afferent and efferent arterioles.
2. Glomerular capillary pressure is high (about 50 to 60 mm Hg), and the glomerular capil-

laries are very permeable to water; these two factors favor the filtration of large quantities of water from the blood to Bowman's capsule.

Intestinal Circulation

1. The microcirculation in the intestinal villi constitutes a countercurrent exchange system for O_2. This places the villi in jeopardy in states of low blood flow.
2. The splanchnic resistance and capacitance vessels are very responsive to changes in sympathetic neural activity.

Hepatic Circulation

1. The liver receives about 25% of the cardiac output; about three fourths of this comes via the portal vein and about one fourth via the hepatic artery. When flow is diminished in either the portal or hepatic systems, flow in the other system usually increases, but not proportionately.
2. The liver tends to maintain a constant O_2 consumption, in part because its mechanism for extracting O_2 from the blood is so efficient.
3. The liver normally contains about 15% of the total blood volume. It serves as an important blood reservoir for the body.

Fetal Circulation

1. In the fetus a large percent of the right atrial blood passes through the foramen ovale to the left atrium, and a large percent of the pulmonary artery blood passes through the ductus arteriosus to the aorta.
2. At birth, the umbilical vessels, ductus venosus, and ductus arteriosus close by contraction of their muscle layers. The reduction in the pulmonary vascular resistance caused by lung inflation is the main factor that reverses the pressure gradient between the atria, thereby closing the foramen ovale.

■ BIBLIOGRAPHY

Journal articles

Abboud, F.M., editor: Regulation of the cerebral circulation (symposium), Fed. Proc. 40:2296, 1981.

Berne, R.M., Winn, H.R., and Rubio, R.: The local regulation of cerebral blood flow, Prog. Cardiovasc. Dis. 24:243, 1981.

Brunner, J.J., Greene, A.S., Frankle, A.E., and Shoukas, A.A.: Carotid sinus baroreceptor control of splanchnic resistance and capacity, Am. J. Physiol. 255:H1305, 1988.

Bshouty, Z., and Younes, M.: Distensibility and pressure-flow relationship of the pulmonary circulation, I, II, J. Appl. Physiol. 68:1501, 1514, 1990.

Butler, J: Bronchial circulation, News Physiol. Sci. 6:21, 1991.

Farrukh, I.S., Gurtner, G.H., Terry, P.B., Tohidi, W., Yang, J., Adkinson, N.F., Jr., and Michael, J.R.: Effect of pH on pulmonary vascular tone, reactivity, and arachidonate metabolism, J. Appl. Physiol. 67:445, 1989.

Greenway, C.V., and Lautt, W.W. Distensibility of hepatic venous resistance sites and consequences on portal pressure, Am. J. Physiol. 254:H452, 1988.

Heymann, M.A., Iwamoto, H.S., and Rudolf, A.M.: Factors affecting changes in the neonatal systemic circulation. Ann. Rev. Physiol. 43:371, 1981.

Heymann, M.A., and Rudolph, A.M.: Control of the ductus arteriosus, Physiol. Rev. 55:62, 1975.

Hyman, A.L., and Kadowitz, P.J.: Analysis of responses to sympathetic nerve stimulation in the feline pulmonary vascular bed, J. Appl. Physiol. 67:371, 1989.

Kontos, H.A.: Regulation of the cerebral circulation, Ann. Rev. Physiol. 43:397, 1981.

Laughlin, M.H.: Skeletal muscle blood flow capacity: role of muscle pump in exercise hyperemia, Am. J. Physiol. 253:H993, 1987.

Lautt, W.W.: Hepatic nerves: a review of their functions and effects, Can. J. Physiol. Pharmacol. 58:105, 1980.

Marshall, C., and Marshall, B.: Site and sensitivity for stimulation of hypoxic pulmonary vasoconstriction, J. Appl. Physiol. 55:711, 1983.

Olsson, R.A.: Local factors regulating cardiac and skeletal muscle blood flow, Ann. Rev. Physiol. 43:385, 1981.

Persson, P., Ehmke, H., and Kirchheim, H.: Influence of the renin-angiotensin system on the autoregulation of renal blood flow and glomerular filtration rate in conscious dogs, Acta Physiol. Scand. 134:1, 1988.

Schwartz, L.M., and McKenzie, J.E.: Adenosine and active hyperemia in soleus and gracilis muscle of cats, Am. J. Physiol. 259:H1295, 1990.

Shepherd, A.P., and Riedel, G.L.: Intramural distribution of intestinal blood flow during sympathetic stimulation, Am. J. Physiol. 255:H1091, 1988.

Wanner, A.: Circulation of the airway mucosa, J. Appl. Physiol. 67:917, 1989.

Wright, F.S., and Briggs, J.P.: Feedback control of glomerular blood flow, pressure, and filtration rate, Physiol. Rev. 59:958, 1979.

Books and monographs

Berne, R.M., Winn, H.R., and Rubio, R.: Metabolic regulation of cerebral blood flow. In Mechanisms of vasodilation—Second Symposium, New York, 1981, Raven Press.

Donald, D.E.: Splanchnic circulation. In Handbook of physiology; Section 2: The cardiovascular system—peripheral circulation and organ blood flow, vol. III, Bethesda, Md., 1983, American Physiological Society.

Faber, J.J., and Thornburg, K.L.: Placental physiology, New York, 1983, Raven Press.

Fishman, A.P.: The pulmonary circulation, Philadelphia, 1990, University of Pennsylvania Press.

Gootman, N., and Gootman, P.M., editors: Perinatal cardiovascular function, New York, 1983, Marcel Dekker, Inc.

Granger, D.N., Kvietys, P.R., Korthuis, R.J., and Premen, A.J.: Microcirculation of the intestinal mucosa. In Handbook of physiology, gastrointestinal system, vol. I, Bethesda, Md., 1989, American Physiological Society.

Greenway, C.V., and Lautt, W.W.: Hepatic circulation. In Handbook of physiology, gastrointestinal System; motility and circulation, vol. I, Bethesda, Md., 1989, American Physiological Society.

Grover, R.F., Wagner, W.W., Jr., McMurtry, I.F., and Reeves, J.T.: Pulmonary circulation. In Handbook of physiology; Section 2: The cardiovascular system—peripheral circulation and organ blood flow, vol. III, Bethesda, Md., 1983, American Physiological Society.

Guth, P.H., Leung, F.W., and Kauffman, G.L., Jr.: Physiology of gastric circulation. In Handbook of physiology, gastrointestinal system, vol. I, Bethesda, Md., 1989, American Physiological Society.

Heistad, D.D., and Kontos, H.A.: Cerebral circulation. In Handbook of physiology; Section 2: The cardiovascular system—peripheral circulation and organ blood flow, vol. III, Bethesda, Md., 1983, American Physiological Society.

Hellon, R.: Thermoreceptors. In Handbook of physiology; Section 2: The cardiovascular system—peripheral circulation and organ blood flow, vol. III, Bethesda, Md., 1983, American Physiological Society.

Knox, F.G., and Spielman, W.S.: Renal circulation. In Handbook of physiology; Section 2: The cardiovascular system—peripheral circulation and organ blood flow, vol. III, Bethesda, Md., 1983, American Physiological Society.

Lewis, T.: Blood vessels of the human skin and their responses, London, 1927, Shaw & Son, Ltd.

Longo, L.D., and Reneau, D.D., editors: Fetal and newborn cardiovascular physiology, vol. 1, Developmental aspects, New York, 1978, Garland STPM Press.

Mott, J.C., and Walker, D.W.: Neural and endocrine regulation of circulation in the fetus and newborn. In Handbook of physiology; Section 2: The cardiovascular system—peripheral circulation and organ blood flow, vol. III, Bethesda, Md., 1983, American Physiological Society.

Owman, C., and Edvinsson, L., editors: Neurogenic control of the brain circulation, Oxford, 1977, Pergamon Press.

Roddie, E.C.: Circulation to skin and adipose tissue. In Handbook of physiology; Section 2: The cardiovascular system—peripheral circulation and organ blood flow, vol. III, Bethesda, Md., 1983, American Physiological Society.

Shepherd, J.T.: Circulation to skeletal muscle. In Handbook of physiology; Section 2: The cardiovascular system—peripheral circulation and organ blood flow, vol. III, Bethesda, Md., 1983, American Physiological Society.

12 Interplay of Central and Peripheral Factors in the Control of the Circulation

The primary function of the circulatory system is to deliver the supplies needed for tissue metabolism and growth and to remove the products of metabolism. To explain how the heart and blood vessels serve this function, it has been necessary to analyze the system morphologically and functionally and to discuss the mechanisms of action of the component parts in their contribution to maintaining adequate tissue perfusion under different physiological conditions. Once the functions of the various components are understood, it is essential that their interrelationships in the overall role of the circulatory system be considered. Tissue perfusion depends on arterial pressure and local vascular resistance, and arterial pressure in turn depends on cardiac output and total peripheral resistance (TPR). Arterial pressure is maintained within a relatively narrow range in the normal individual, a feat that is accomplished by reciprocal changes in cardiac output and TPR. However, cardiac output and peripheral resistance are each influenced by a number of factors, and it is the interplay among these factors that determines the level of these two variables. The autonomic nervous system and the baroreceptors play the key role in regulating blood pressure. However, from the long-range point of view the control of fluid balance by the kidney, adrenal cortex, and central nervous system, with maintenance of a constant blood volume, is of the greatest importance.

In a well-regulated system one way to study the extent and sensitivity of the regulatory mechanism is to disturb the system and observe its response to restore the preexisting steady state. Disturbances in the form of physical exercise and hemorrhage will be used to illustrate the effects of the various factors that go into regulation of the circulatory system.

■ EXERCISE

The cardiovascular adjustments in exercise comprise a combination and integration of neural and local (chemical) factors. The neural factors consist of (1) **central command,** (2) reflexes originating in the contracting muscle, and (3) the baroreceptor reflex. Central command is the cerebrocortical activation of the sympathetic nervous system that produces cardiac acceleration, increased myocardial contractile force, and peripheral vasoconstriction. Reflexes can be activated intramuscularly by stimulation of mechanoreceptors (stretch, tension) and "chemoreceptors" (products of metabolism) in response to muscle contraction. Impulses from these receptors travel centrally via small myelinated (group III) and unmyelinated (group IV) afferent nerve fibers. The group IV unmyelinated fibers may represent the muscle chemoreceptors; no morphological chemoreceptor has been identified. The central connections of this reflex are unknown, but the efferent limb is the sympathetic nerve fibers to the heart and peripheral blood vessels. The baroreceptor reflex has been described on p. 184, and the local factors that influence skeletal muscle blood flow (metabolic vasodilators) are described on p. 178, 239. Vascular chemoreceptors do not play a significant role in regulation of the cardiovascular system in exercise. The pH, Pco_2, and Po_2 of arterial blood are normal during exercise, and the vascular chemoreceptors are located on the arterial side of the circulatory system.

Mild to Moderate Exercise

In humans or in trained animals, anticipation of physical activity inhibits the vagal nerve impulses to the heart and increases sympathetic discharge. The concerted inhibition of parasympathetic areas and activation of sympathetic areas of the medulla on the heart result in an increase in heart rate and myocardial contractility. The tachycardia and the enhanced contractility increase cardiac output.

Peripheral Resistance. At the same time that cardiac stimulation occurs, the sympathetic nervous system also elicits vascular resistance changes in the periphery. In skin, kidneys, splanchnic regions, and inactive muscle, sympathetic-mediated vasoconstriction increases vascular resistance, which diverts blood away from these areas (Fig. 12-1). This increased resistance in vascular beds of inactive tissues persists throughout the period of exercise.

As cardiac output and blood flow to active muscles increase with progressive increments in the intensity of exercise, blood flow to the splanchnic and renal vasculatures decreases. Blood flow to the myocardium increases,

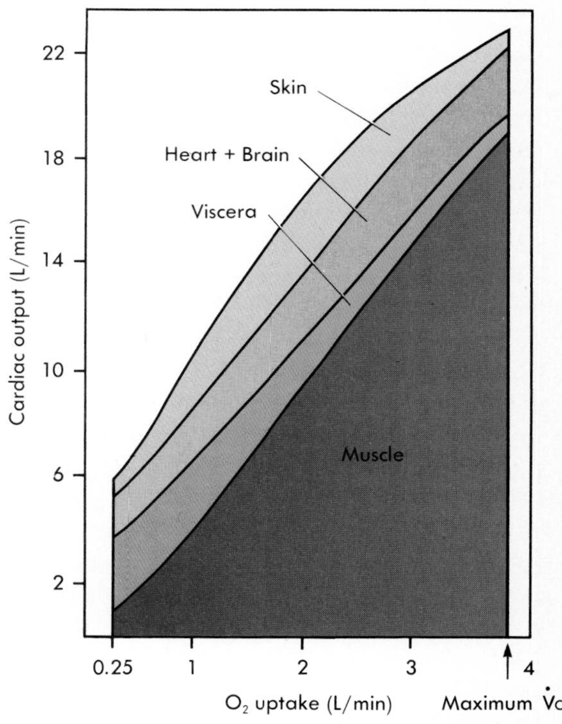

Fig. 12-1 ■ Approximate distribution of cardiac output at rest and at different levels of exercise up to the maximum O_2 consumption ($\dot{V}o_{2max}$) in a normal young man. Viscera refers to splanchnic and renal blood flow. (Redrawn from Ruch, H.P., and Patton, T.C.: Physiology and biophysics, ed. 12, 1974, W.B. Saunders Co.)

whereas that to the brain is unchanged. Skin blood flow initially decreases during exercise and then increases as body temperature rises with increments in duration and intensity of exercise. Skin blood flow finally decreases when the skin vessels constrict as the total body O_2 consumption nears maximum (see Fig. 12-1).

The major circulatory adjustment to prolonged exercise involves the vasculature of the active muscles. Local formation of vasoactive metabolites induces marked dilation of the resistance vessels, which progresses with increases in the intensity level of exercise. Potassium is one of the vasodilator substances released by contracting muscle, and it may be in part responsible for the initial decrease in vascular resistance in the active muscles. Other contributing factors may be the release of adenosine and a decrease in pH during sustained exercise. The local accumulation of metabolites relaxes the terminal arterioles. Blood flow through the muscle may increase fifteen to twenty times above the resting level. This metabolic vasodilation of the precapillary vessels in active muscles occurs very soon after the onset of exercise, and the decrease in TPR enables the heart to pump more blood at a lesser load and more efficiently (less pressure work, p. 228) than if TPR were unchanged. Only a small percentage of the capillaries is perfused at rest, whereas in actively contracting muscle all or nearly all of the capillaries contain flowing blood **(capillary recruitment).** The surface available for exchange of gases, water, and solutes is increased manyfold. Furthermore, the hydrostatic pressure in the capillaries is increased because of the relaxation of the resistance vessels. Hence, there is a net movement of water and solutes into the muscle tissue. Tissue pressure rises and remains elevated during exercise as fluid continues to move out of the capillaries and is carried away by the lymphatics. Lymph flow is increased as a result of the increase in capillary hydrostatic pressure and the massaging effect of the contracting muscles on the valve-containing lymphatic vessels.

The contracting muscle avidly extracts O_2 from the perfusing blood (increased AV-O_2 difference, Fig. 12-2), and the release of O_2 from the blood is facilitated by the nature of oxyhe-

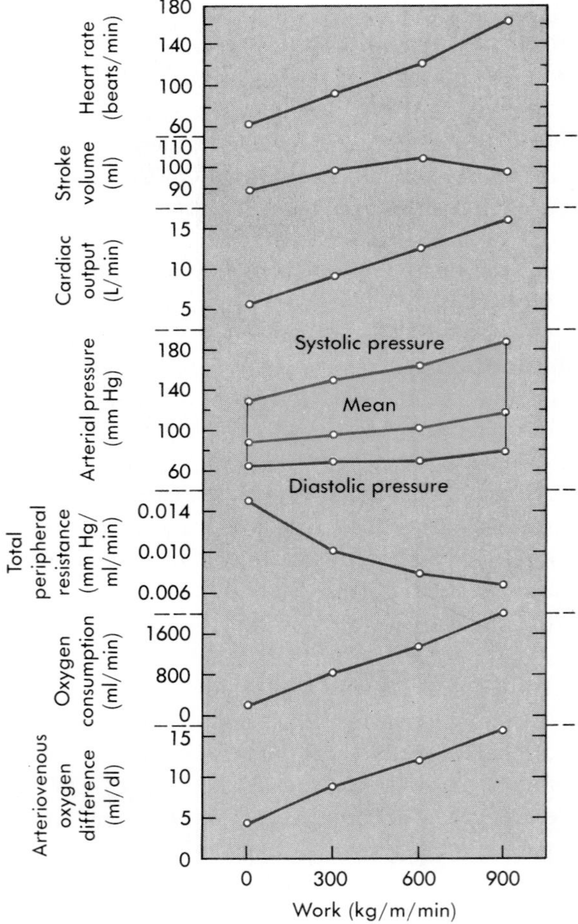

Fig. 12-2 ■ Effect of different levels of exercise on several cardiovascular variables. (Data from Carlsten, A., and Grimby, G.: The circulatory response to muscular exercise in man, Springfield, Ill., 1966, Charles C Thomas, Publisher.)

moglobin dissociation. The reduction in pH caused by the high concentration of CO_2 and the formation of lactic acid and the increase in temperature in the contracting muscle contribute to shifting the oxyhemoglobin dissociation curve to the right. At any given partial pressure of O_2, less O_2 is held by the hemoglobin in the red cells, and consequently there is a more effective O_2 removal from the blood. Oxygen consumption may increase as much as sixtyfold with only a fifteenfold increase in muscle blood flow. Muscle myoglobin may serve as a limited O_2 store in exercise and can release attached O_2 at very low partial pressures. However, it can facilitate O_2 transport from capillaries to mitochondria by serving as an O_2 carrier.

Cardiac Output. The enhanced sympathetic drive and the reduced parasympathetic inhibition of the sinoatrial node continue during exercise, and consequently tachycardia persists. If the work load is moderate and constant, the heart rate will reach a certain level and remain there throughout the period of exercise. However, if the work load increases, a concomitant increase in heart rate occurs until a plateau is reached in severe exercise at about 180 beats per minute (see Fig. 12-2). In contrast to the large increment in heart rate, the increase in stroke volume is only about 10% to 35% (see Fig. 12-2), the larger values occurring in trained individuals. (In very well-trained distance runners, whose cardiac outputs can reach six to seven times the resting level, stroke volume reaches about twice the resting value.)

Thus it is apparent that the increase in cardiac output observed with exercise is achieved principally by an increase in heart rate. If the baroreceptors are denervated, the cardiac output and heart rate responses to exercise are sluggish when compared to the changes in animals with normally innervated baroreceptors. However, in the absence of autonomic innervation of the heart, as produced experimentally in dogs by total cardiac denervation, exercise still elicits an increment in cardiac output comparable to that observed in normal animals, but chiefly by means of an elevated stroke volume. However, if a beta-adrenergic receptor blocking agent is given to dogs with denervated hearts, exercise performance is impaired. The beta-adrenergic receptor blocker apparently prevents the cardiac acceleration and enhanced contractility caused by increased amounts of circulating catecholamines and hence limits the increase in cardiac output necessary for maximum exercise performance.

Venous Return. In addition to the contribution made by sympathetically mediated constriction of the capacitance vessels in both exercising and nonexercising parts of the body, venous return is aided by the working skeletal muscles and the muscles of respiration. The intermittently contracting muscles compress the vessels that course through them, and in the case of veins with their valves oriented toward the heart, pump blood back toward the right atrium. The flow of venous blood to the heart is also aided by the increase in the pressure gradient developed by the more negative intrathoracic pressure produced by deeper and more frequent respirations. In humans, with the exception of the skin, lungs, and liver, there is little evidence that blood reservoirs contribute much to the circulating blood volume. In fact, blood volume is usually reduced slightly during exercise, as evidenced by a rise in the hematocrit ratio, because of water loss externally by sweating and enhanced ventilation, and fluid movement into the contracting muscle. The fluid loss from the vascular compartment into contracting muscle reaches a plateau as interstitial fluid pressure rises and opposes the increased hydrostatic pressure in the capillaries of the active muscle. The fluid loss is partially offset by movement of fluid from the splanchnic regions and inactive muscle into the bloodstream. This influx of fluid occurs as a result of a decrease of hydrostatic pressure in the capillaries of these tissues and of an increase in plasma osmolarity because of movement of osmotically active particles into the blood from the contracting muscle. In addition, reduced urine formation by the kidneys helps to conserve body water.

The large volume of blood returning to the heart is so rapidly pumped through the lungs and out into the aorta that central venous pressure remains essentially constant. Thus the Frank-Starling mechanism of a greater initial fiber length does not account for the greater stroke volume in moderate exercise. Chest x-ray films of individuals at rest and during exercise reveal a decrease in heart size in exercise, which is in harmony with the observations of a constant ventricular filling pressure. However, in maximum or near-maximum exercise, right atrial pressure and end-diastolic ventricular volume do increase. Thus, the Frank-Starling mechanism contributes to the enhanced stroke volume in very vigorous exercise.

Arterial Pressure. If the exercise involves a large proportion of the body musculature, such as in running or swimming, the reduction in total vascular resistance can be considerable (see Fig. 12-2). Nevertheless, arterial pressure starts to rise with the onset of exercise, and the increase in blood pressure roughly parallels the severity of the exercise performed (see Fig. 12-2). Therefore, the increase in cardiac output is proportionally greater than the decrease in TPR. The vasoconstriction produced in the inactive tissues by the sympathetic nervous system (and to some extent by the release of catecholamines from the adrenal medulla) is important for maintaining normal or increased blood pressure, because sympathectomy or drug-induced block of the adrenergic sympathetic nerve fibers results in a decrease in arterial pressure **(hypotension)** during exercise.

Sympathetic-mediated vasoconstriction also occurs in active muscle when additional muscles are activated after about half of the total skeletal musculature is contracting. In experiments in which one leg is working at maximum levels and then the other leg starts to work, blood flow decreases in the first working leg. Furthermore, blood levels of norepinephrine rise significantly in exercise, and most of it comes from sympathetic nerves in the active muscles.

As body temperature rises during exercise, the skin vessels dilate in response to thermal stimulation of the heat-regulating center in the hypothalamus, and TPR decreases further. This would result in a decline in blood pressure were it not for the increasing cardiac output and constriction of arterioles in the renal, splanchnic, and other tissues.

In general, mean arterial pressure rises during exercise as a result of the increase in cardiac output. However, the effect of enhanced cardiac output is offset by the overall decrease in TPR so that the mean blood pressure increase is relatively small. Vasoconstriction in the inactive vascular beds contributes to the maintenance of a normal arterial blood pressure for adequate perfusion of the active tissues. The actual pressure attained represents a balance between cardiac output and TPR (p. 144). Systolic pressure usually increases more than diastolic pressure, which results in an increase in pulse pressure (see Fig. 12-2). The larger pulse pressure is primarily attributable to a greater stroke volume and to a lesser degree to a more rapid ejection of blood by the left ventricle with less peripheral runoff during the brief ventricular ejection period.

Severe Exercise

In severe exercise taken to the point of exhaustion, the compensatory mechanisms begin to fail. Heart rate attains a maximum level of about 180 beats per minute, and stroke volume reaches a plateau and often decreases, re-

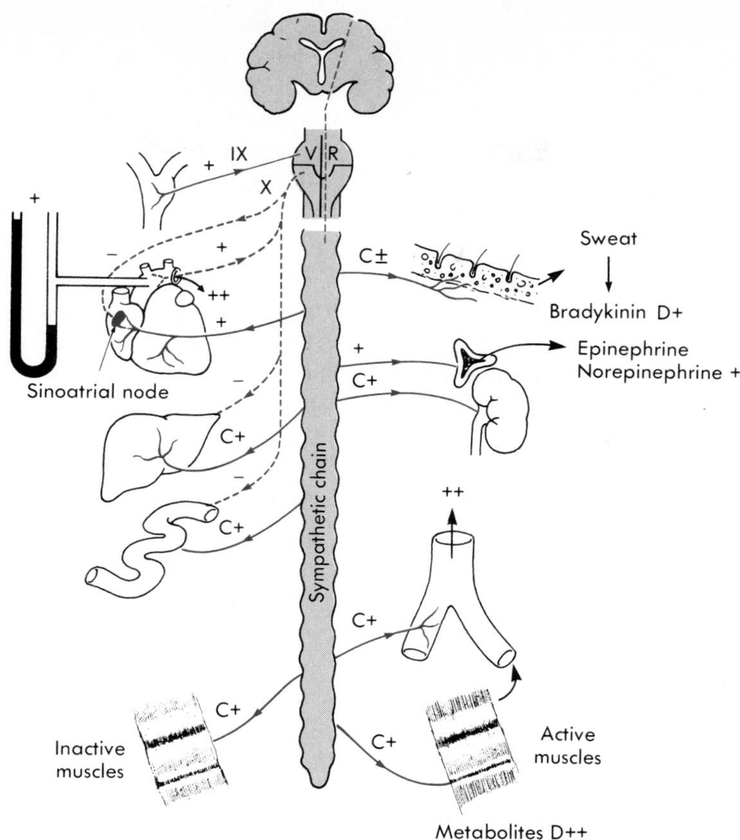

Fig. 12-3 ■ Cardiovascular adjustments in exercise. *VR,* Vasomotor region; *C,* vasoconstrictor activity; *D,* vasodilator activity; *IX,* glossopharyngeal nerve; *X,* vagus nerve; +, increased activity; −, decreased activity.

sulting in a fall in blood pressure. Dehydration occurs. Sympathetic vasoconstrictor activity supersedes the vasodilator influence on the cutaneous vessels and has the hemodynamic effect of a slight increase in effective blood volume. However, cutaneous vasoconstriction also decreases the rate of heat loss. Body temperature is normally elevated in exercise, and reduction in heat loss through cutaneous vasoconstriction can, under these conditions, lead to very high body temperatures with associated feelings of acute distress. The tissue and blood pH decrease, as a result of increased lactic acid and CO_2 production, and the reduced pH is probably the key factor that determines the maximum amount of exercise a given individual can tolerate because of muscle pain, subjective feeling of exhaustion, and inability or loss of will to continue. A summary of the neural and local effects of exercise on the cardiovascular system is schematized in Fig. 12-3.

Postexercise Recovery

When exercise stops, an abrupt decrease in heart rate and cardiac output occurs—the sympathetic drive to the heart is essentially removed. In contrast, TPR remains low for some time after the exercise is ended, presumably because of the accumulation of vasodilator metabolites in the muscles during the exercise period. As a result of the reduced cardiac output and persistence of vasodilation in the muscles, arterial pressure falls, often below preexercise levels, for brief periods. Blood pressure is then stabilized at normal levels by the baroreceptor reflexes.

Limits of Exercise Performance

The two main forces that could limit skeletal muscle performance in the human body are the rate of O_2 utilization by the muscles and the O_2 supply to the muscles. Muscle O_2 usage is probably not critical, because during exercise maximum O_2 consumption ($\dot{V}o_{2max}$) by a large percentage of the body muscle mass is not increased when additional muscles are activated. If muscle O_2 utilization were limiting, recruitment of more contracting muscle would use additional O_2 to meet the enhanced O_2 requirements and would thereby increase total body O_2 consumption. Limitation of O_2 supply could be caused by inadequate oxygenation of blood in the lungs or limitation of the supply of O_2-laden blood to the muscles. Failure to fully oxygenate blood by the lungs can be excluded, because even with the most strenuous exercise at sea level, arterial blood is fully saturated with O_2. Therefore, O_2 delivery (or blood flow, because arterial blood O_2 content is normal) to the active muscles appears to be the limiting factor in muscle performance. This limitation could be caused by the inability to increase cardiac output beyond a certain level as a result of a limitation of stroke volume, because heart rate reaches maximum levels before $\dot{V}o_{2max}$ is reached. However, blood pressure provides the energy for muscle perfusion, and blood pressure depends on peripheral resistance, as well as on cardiac output. With increasing levels of exercise at peak $\dot{V}o_{2max}$ and peak cardiac output, blood pressure would fall as more muscle vascular beds dilate in response to locally released vasodilator metabolites if some degree of centrally mediated vasoconstriction (baroreceptor reflex) did not occur in the resistance vessels of the active muscles. Hence, the adjustment of resistance in the active muscles appears to be a contributing factor in the limitation of whole body exercise. *The major factor is the pumping capacity of the heart.* With exercise of a small group of muscles, such as the hand, when the cardiovascular system is not severely taxed, the limiting factor is unknown but lies within the muscle.

Physical Training and Conditioning

The response of the cardiovascular system to regular exercise is to increase its capacity to deliver O_2 to the active muscles and to improve the ability of the muscle to utilize O_2. The $\dot{V}o_{2max}$ is quite reproducible in a given individual and varies with the level of physical conditioning. Training progressively increases the $\dot{V}o_{2max}$, which reaches a plateau at the highest level of conditioning. Highly trained athletes have a lower resting heart rate, greater stroke volume, and lower peripheral resistance than they had before training or after deconditioning (becoming sedentary). The low resting heart rate is due to a higher vagal tone and a lower sympathetic tone. With exercise, the maximum heart rate of the trained individual is the same as that in the untrained, but is attained at a higher level of exercise. The trained person also exhibits a low vascular resistance that is inherent in the muscle. For example, if an individual exercises one leg regularly over an extended period and does not exercise the other leg, the vascular resistance is lower and the $\dot{V}o_{2max}$ is higher in the "trained" leg than in the "untrained" leg. Also, the well-trained athlete has a lower resting sympathetic outflow to the viscera than does a sedentary counterpart.

Physical conditioning is also associated with greater extraction of O_2 from the blood (greater AV-O_2 difference) by the muscles but not with an improvement in cardiac contractility. With long-term training capillary density in skeletal muscle increases. One can speculate that the number of arterioles also increases and can account for the decrease in muscle vascular resistance. The number of mitochondria increases, as do the oxidative enzymes in the mitochondria. Also, it appears that ATPase activity, myoglobin, and enzymes involved in lipid metabolism increase with physical conditioning. Endurance training, such as running or swimming, produces an increase in left ventricular volume without an increase in left ventricular wall thickness. In contrast, strength exercises, such as weight lifting, appear to produce some increase in left ventricular wall thickness (hypertrophy) with little effect on ventricular volume. However, this increase in wall thickness is small relative to that observed in hypertension in which there is a persistent elevation of afterload because of the high peripheral resistance.

■ HEMORRHAGE

In an individual who has lost a large quantity of blood, the principal findings are related to the cardiovascular system. The arterial systolic, diastolic, and pulse pressures diminish and the pulse is rapid and feeble. The cutaneous veins are collapsed and fill slowly when compressed centrally. The skin is pale, moist, and slightly cyanotic. Respiration is rapid, but the depth of respiration may be shallow or deep.

Course of Arterial Blood Pressure Changes

Cardiac output decreases as a result of blood loss (p. 207). The changes in mean arterial pressure evoked by an acute hemorrhage in experimental animals are illustrated in Fig. 12-4. If sufficient blood is withdrawn rapidly to bring mean arterial pressure to 50 mm Hg, the pressure tends to rise spontaneously toward control over the subsequent 20 or 30 minutes. In some animals (curve *A*, Fig. 12-4) this trend continues, and normal pressures are regained within a few hours. In other animals (curve *B*), after an initial pressure rise, the pressure be-

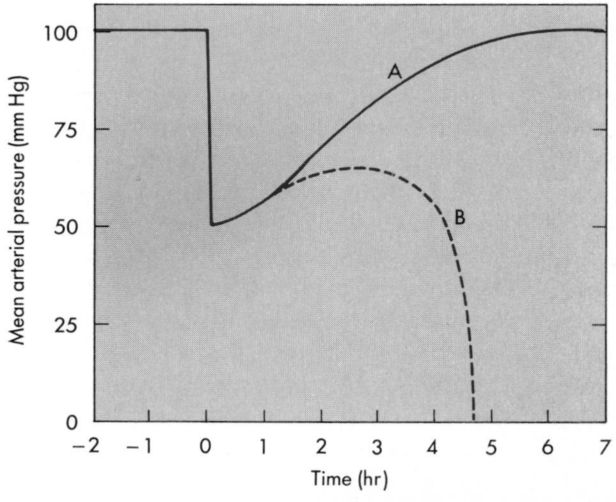

Fig. 12-4 ■ The changes in mean arterial pressure after a rapid hemorrhage. At time zero, the animal is bled rapidly to a mean arterial pressure of 50 mm Hg. After a period in which the pressure returns toward the control level, some animals will continue to improve until the control pressure is attained (curve *A*). However, in other animals the pressure will begin to decline until death ensues (curve *B*).

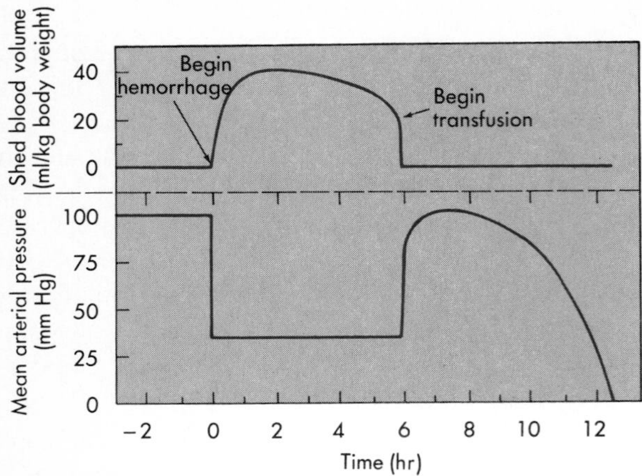

Fig. 12-5 ■ Changes in shed blood volume and mean arterial pressure during and after a 6-hour period of hemorrhage sufficient to hold mean arterial pressure at 35 mm Hg. The shed blood was reinfused after 6 hours.

gins to decline and it continues to fall at an accelerating rate until death ensues.

In other experiments, animals are bled to a given hypotensive level, for example, to 35 mm Hg, by connecting a peripheral artery to a reservoir elevated to an appropriate height (Fig. 12-5). The arterial blood runs rapidly into the reservoir until the pressures become equilibrated and then continues to flow into the reservoir at a progressively slower rate for about 2 hours. This gradual increase in shed blood volume reflects the same compensatory mechanisms that produced the rise in arterial blood pressure after transitory hemorrhage in the experiment depicted in Fig. 12-4. However, in the experiment represented in Fig. 12-5, as the arterial pressure tends to rise higher than the pressure established by the reservoir, blood flows from the cannulated vessel into the reservoir.

About 2 hours after the beginning of hemorrhage, the arterial pressure tends to fall below the established level, and blood begins to flow from the reservoir to the animal (Fig. 12-5). Once about 50% of the maximum shed volume has returned to the animal, rapid reinfusion of the remaining shed blood improves arterial pressure only transiently. The arterial pressure then falls progressively until the animal dies. This progressive deterioration of cardiovascular function is termed **shock.** At some point the deterioration becomes irreversible; a lethal outcome can be retarded only temporarily by any known therapy, including massive transfusions of donor blood.

Compensatory Mechanisms

The changes in arterial pressure immediately after an acute blood loss (see Fig. 12-4) and in shed blood volume during the initial stages of sustained hemorrhage (see Fig. 12-5) indicate that certain compensatory mechanisms must be operating. Any mechanism that raises the arterial pressure toward normal in response to the reduction in pressure may be designated a **negative feedback mechanism.** It is termed "negative" because the secondary change in pressure is opposite to the initiating change. The following negative feedback responses are evoked: (1) the baroreceptor reflexes, (2) the chemoreceptor reflexes, (3) cerebral ischemia responses, (4) reabsorption of tissue fluids, (5) release of endogenous vasoconstrictor substances, and (6) renal conservation of salt and water.

Baroreceptor Reflexes. The reduction in mean arterial pressure and in pulse pressure during hemorrhage decreases the stimulation

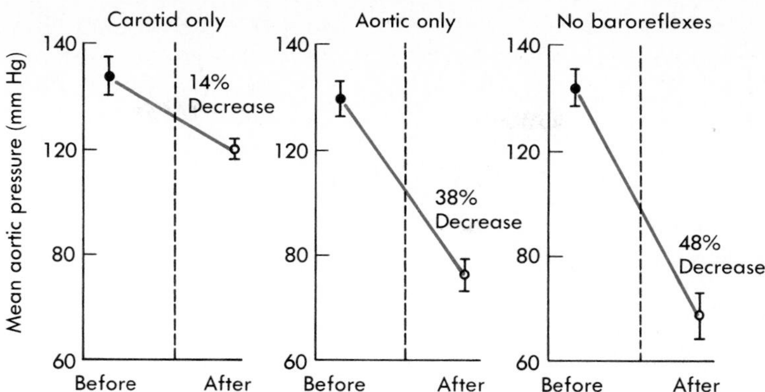

Fig. 12-6 ■ The changes in mean aortic pressure in response to an 8% blood loss in a group of eight dogs. *Left panel,* The carotid sinus baroreceptor reflexes were intact, and the aortic reflexes were interrupted. *Middle panel,* The aortic reflexes were intact, and the carotid sinus reflexes were interrupted. *Right panel,* All sinoaortic reflexes were abrogated. (From Shepherd, J.T.: Circulation 50:418, 1974. By permission of the American Heart Association, Inc.; derived from the data of Edis, A.J.: Am. J. Physiol. 221:1352, 1971.)

of the baroreceptors in the carotid sinuses and aortic arch (see Chapter 8). Several cardiovascular responses are thus evoked, all of which tend to return the arterial pressure toward normal. Reduction of vagal tone and enhancement of sympathetic tone increase heart rate and enhance myocardial contractility.

The increased sympathetic discharge also produces generalized venoconstriction, which has the same hemodynamic consequences as a transfusion of blood (p. 202). Sympathetic activation constricts certain blood reservoirs, which provides an autotransfusion of blood into the circulating bloodstream. In the dog considerable quantities of blood are mobilized by contraction of the spleen. In humans the spleen is not an important blood reservoir. Instead, the cutaneous, pulmonary, and hepatic vasculatures probably constitute the principal blood reservoirs.

Generalized arteriolar vasoconstriction is a prominent response to the diminished baroreceptor stimulation during hemorrhage. The reflex increase in peripheral resistance minimizes the fall in arterial pressure resulting from the reduction of cardiac output. Fig. 12-6 shows the effect of an 8% blood loss on mean aortic pressure in a group of dogs. If both vagi are cut to eliminate the influence of the aortic arch baroreceptors and only the carotid sinus baroreceptors are operative (left panel), this hemorrhage decreases mean aortic pressure by 14%. This pressure change did not differ significantly from the pressure decline (12%) evoked by the same hemorrhage before vagotomy (not shown). When the carotid sinuses are denervated and the aortic baroreceptor reflexes are intact, the 8% blood loss decreases mean aortic pressure by 38% (middle panel). Hence, the carotid sinus baroreceptors are more effective than the aortic baroreceptors in attenuating the fall in pressure. The aortic baroreceptors must also be operative, however, because when both sets of afferent baroreceptor pathways are interrupted, an 8% blood loss reduces arterial pressure by 48%.

Although the arteriolar vasoconstriction is widespread during hemorrhage, it is by no means uniform. Vasoconstriction is most severe in the cutaneous, skeletal muscle, and splanchnic vascular beds and is slight or absent in the cerebral and coronary circulations. In many instances the cerebral and coronary vascular resistances are diminished. Thus the reduced cardiac output is redistributed to favor flow through the brain and the heart.

The severe cutaneous vasoconstriction accounts for the characteristic pale, cold skin of patients suffering from blood loss. Warming the skin of such patients improves their appearance considerably, much to the satisfaction of well-meaning individuals rendering first aid. However, it also inactivates an effective, natural compensatory mechanism—to the possible detriment of the patient.

In the early stages of mild to moderate hemorrhage, the changes in renal resistance are usually slight. The tendency for increased sympathetic activity to constrict the renal vessels is counteracted by autoregulatory mechanisms (p. 252). With more-prolonged and severe hemorrhages, however, renal vasoconstriction becomes intense. The reductions in renal circulation are most severe in the outer layers of the renal cortex. The inner zones of the cortex and outer zones of the medulla are spared.

The severe renal and splanchnic vasoconstriction during hemorrhage favors the heart and brain. However, if such constriction persists too long, it may be harmful. Frequently patients survive the acute hypotensive period only to die several days later from kidney failure resulting from renal ischemia. Intestinal ischemia also may have dire effects. In the dog, for example, intestinal bleeding and extensive sloughing of the mucosa occur after only a few hours of hemorrhagic hypotension. Furthermore, the low splanchnic flow swells the centrilobular cells in the liver. The resultant obstruction of the hepatic sinusoids raises the portal venous pressure, which intensifies the intestinal blood loss. Fortunately, the pathological changes in the liver and intestine are usually much less severe in humans than in dogs.

Chemoreceptor Reflexes. Reductions in arterial pressure below about 60 mm Hg do not evoke any additional responses through the baroreceptor reflexes, because this pressure level constitutes the threshold for stimulation (see Chapter 8). However, low arterial pressure may stimulate peripheral chemoreceptors because of hypoxia in the chemoreceptor tissue consequent to inadequate local blood flow. Chemoreceptor excitation enhances the already existent peripheral vasoconstriction evoked by the baroreceptor reflexes. Also, respiratory stimulation assists venous return by the auxiliary pumping mechanism described on p. 214.

Cerebral Ischemia. When the arterial pressure is below about 40 mm Hg, the resulting cerebral ischemia activates the sympathoadrenal system. The sympathetic nervous discharge is several times greater than the maximum activity that occurs when the baroreceptors cease to be stimulated. Therefore, the vasoconstriction and facilitation of myocardial contractility may be pronounced. With more severe degrees of cerebral ischemia, however, the vagal centers also become activated. The resulting bradycardia may aggravate the hypotension that initiated the cerebral ischemia.

Reabsorption of Tissue Fluids. The arterial hypotension, arteriolar constriction, and reduced venous pressure during hemorrhagic hypotension lower the hydrostatic pressure in the capillaries. The balance of these forces promotes the net reabsorption of interstitial fluid into the vascular compartment. The rapidity of this response is displayed in Fig. 12-7. In a group of cats, 45% of the estimated blood volume was removed over a 30-minute period. The mean arterial blood pressure declined rapidly to about 45 mm Hg. The pressure then returned rapidly, but only temporarily, to near the control level. The plasma colloid osmotic pressure declined markedly during the bleeding and continued to decrease more gradually for several hours. The reduction in colloid osmotic pressure reflects the dilution of the blood by tissue fluids.

Considerable quantities of fluid thus may be

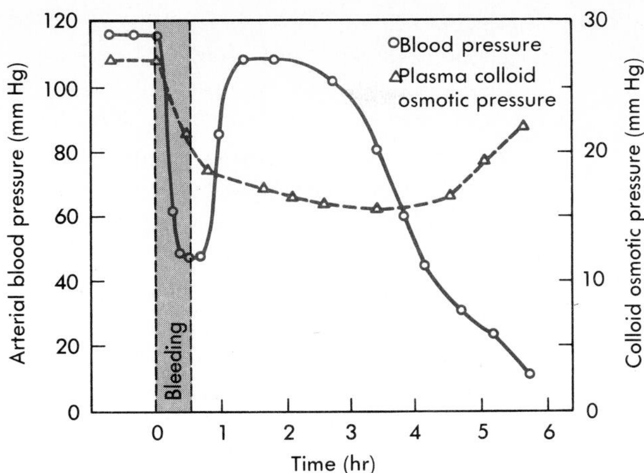

Fig. 12-7 ■ The changes in arterial blood pressure and plasma colloid osmotic pressure in response to withdrawal of 45% of the estimated blood volume over a 30-minute period, beginning at time zero. The data are the average values for twenty-three cats. (Redrawn from Zweifach, B.W.: Anesthesiology 41:157, 1974.)

drawn into the circulation during hemorrhage. About 0.25 ml of fluid per minute per kilogram of body weight may be reabsorbed. Approximately 1 liter of fluid per hour might be autoinfused into the circulatory system of an average individual from the interstitial spaces after an acute blood loss.

Considerable quantities of fluid also may be slowly shifted from intracellular to extracellular spaces. This fluid exchange is probably mediated by the secretion of cortisol from the adrenal cortex in response to hemorrhage. Cortisol appears to be essential for a full restoration of the plasma volume after hemorrhage.

Endogenous Vasoconstrictors. The **catecholamines,** epinephrine and norepinephrine, are released from the adrenal medulla in response to the same stimuli that evoke widespread sympathetic nervous discharge. Blood levels of catecholamines are high during and after hemorrhage. When animals are bled to an arterial pressure level of 40 mm Hg, the catecholamines increase as much as fifty times.

Epinephrine comes almost exclusively from the adrenal medulla, whereas norepinephrine is derived both from the adrenal medulla and the peripheral sympathetic nerve endings. These humoral substances reinforce the effects of sympathetic nervous activity listed previously.

Vasopressin, a potent vasoconstrictor, is actively secreted by the posterior pituitary gland in response to hemorrhage. Removal of about 20% of the blood volume in experimental animals increases vasopressin secretion about fortyfold. The receptors responsible for the augmented release are the sinoaortic baroreceptors and the receptors in the left atrium.

The diminished renal perfusion during hemorrhagic hypotension leads to the secretion of **renin** from the juxtaglomerular apparatus. This enzyme acts on a plasma protein, **angiotensinogen,** to form **angiotensin,** a very powerful vasoconstrictor.

Renal Conservation of Water. Fluid and electrolytes are conserved by the kidneys during hemorrhage in response to various stimuli, including the increased secretion of vasopressin (antidiuretic hormone) noted previously. The lower arterial pressure decreases the glomerular filtration rate, and thus curtails the excretion of water and electrolytes. Also the diminished renal blood flow raises the blood levels of angiotensin, as described above. This polypeptide accelerates the release of **aldosterone** from the adrenal cortex. Aldosterone in turn stimulates sodium reabsorption by the renal tubules, and water accompanies the sodium that is actively reabsorbed.

Decompensatory Mechanisms

In contrast to the negative feedback mechanisms just described, latent **positive feedback mechanisms** are also evoked by hemorrhage. Such mechanisms exaggerate any primary change initiated by the blood loss. Specifically, positive feedback mechanisms aggravate the hypotension induced by blood loss and tend to initiate **vicious cycles,** which may lead to death. The operation of positive feedback mechanisms is manifest in curve *B* of Fig. 12-4.

Whether a positive feedback mechanism will lead to a vicious cycle depends on the **gain** of that mechanism. Gain is defined as the ratio of the secondary change evoked by a given mechanism to the initiating change itself. A gain greater than 1 induces a vicious cycle; a gain less than 1 does not. For example, consider a positive feedback mechanism with a gain of 2. If, for any reason, mean arterial pressure decreases by 10 mm Hg, the positive feedback mechanism would then evoke a secondary pressure reduction of 20 mm Hg, which in turn would cause a further decrement of 40 mm Hg; that is, each change would induce a subsequent change that was twice as great. Hence mean arterial pressure would decline at an ever-increasing rate until death supervened, much as is depicted by curve *B* in Fig. 12-4.

Conversely, a positive feedback mechanism with a gain of 0.5 would indeed exaggerate any change in mean arterial pressure but would not necessarily lead to death. For example, if arterial pressure suddenly decreased by 10 mm Hg, the positive feedback mechanism would initiate a secondary, additional fall of 5 mm Hg. This in turn would provoke a further decrease of 2.5 mm Hg. The process would continue in ever-diminishing steps, with the arterial pressure approaching an equilibrium value asymptotically.

Some of the more important positive feedback mechanisms include (1) cardiac failure, (2) acidosis, (3) inadequate cerebral blood

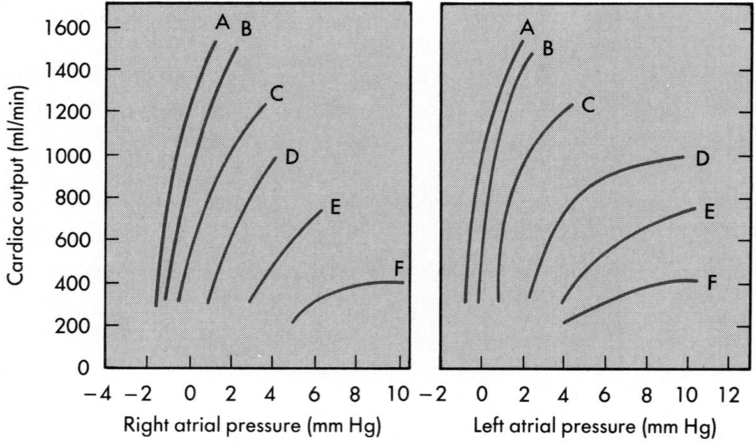

Fig. 12-8 ■ Ventricular function curves for the right and left ventricles during the course of hemorrhagic shock. Curves *A* represent the control function curve; curves *B,* 117 min; curves *C,* 247 min; curves *D,* 380 min; curves *E,* 295 min; and curves *F,* 310 min after the initial hemorrhage. (Redrawn from Crowell, J.W., and Guyton, A.C.: Am. J. Physiol. 203:248, 1962.)

flow, (4) aberrations of blood clotting, and (5) depression of the reticuloendothelial system.

Cardiac Failure. The role of cardiac failure in the progression of shock during hemorrhage is controversial. All investigators agree that the heart fails terminally, but opinions differ concerning the importance of cardiac failure during earlier stages of hemorrhagic hypotension. Shifts to the right in ventricular function curves (Fig. 12-8) constitute experimental evidence of a progressive depression of myocardial contractility during hemorrhage.

The hypotension induced by hemorrhage reduces the coronary blood flow and therefore depresses ventricular function. The consequent reduction in cardiac output leads to a further decline in arterial pressure, a classical example of a positive feedback mechanism. Furthermore, the reduced tissue blood flow leads to an accumulation of vasodilator metabolites, which decreases peripheral resistance and therefore aggravates the fall in arterial pressure.

Acidosis. The inadequate blood flow during hemorrhage affects the metabolism of all cells in the body. The resultant stagnant anoxia accelerates the production of lactic acid and other acid metabolites by the tissues. Furthermore, impaired kidney function prevents adequate excretion of the excess H^+, and generalized metabolic acidosis ensues (Fig. 12-9). The resulting depressant effect of acidosis on the heart further reduces tissue perfusion and thus aggravates the metabolic acidosis. Acidosis also diminishes the reactivity of the heart and resistance vessels to neurally released and circulating catecholamines, thereby intensifying the hypotension.

Central Nervous System Depression. The hypotension in shock reduces cerebral blood flow. Moderate degrees of cerebral ischemia induce a pronounced sympathetic nervous stimulation of the heart, arterioles, and veins, as stated previously. With severe degrees of hypotension, however, the cardiovascular centers in the brainstem eventually be-

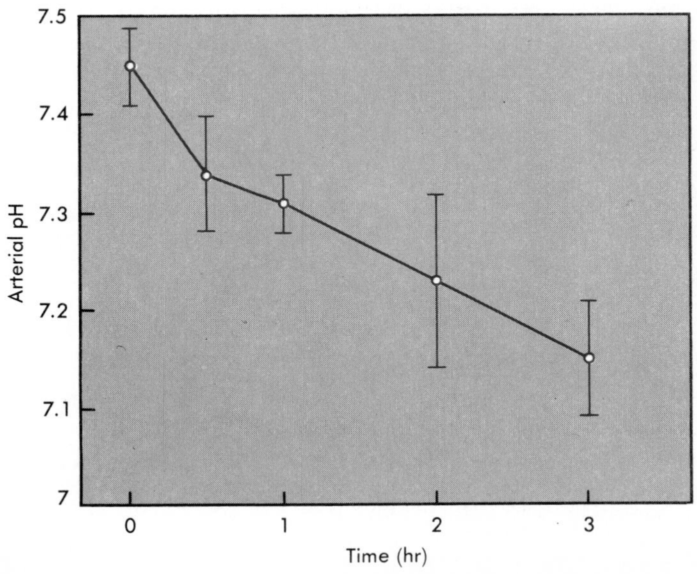

Fig. 12-9 ■ The reduction in arterial blood pH (mean ± SD) in a group of eleven dogs whose blood pressure had been held at a level of 35 mm Hg by bleeding into a reservoir, beginning at time zero. (Modified from Markov, A.K., Oglethorpe, N., Young, D.B., and Hellems, H.K.: Circ. Shock 8:9, 1981.)

come depressed because of inadequate blood flow to the brain. The resultant loss of sympathetic tone then reduces cardiac output and peripheral resistance. The resulting reduction in mean arterial pressure intensifies the inadequate cerebral perfusion.

Various endogenous **opioids,** such as **enkephalins** and **beta-endorphin,** may be released into the brain substance or into the circulation in response to the same stresses that provoke circulatory shock. Enkephalins exist along with catecholamines in secretory granules in the adrenal medulla, and they are released together in response to stress. Similar stimuli release beta-endorphin and adrenocorticotrophic hormone (ACTH) from the anterior pituitary gland. These opioids depress the centers in the brainstem that mediate some of the compensatory autonomic adaptations to blood loss, endotoxemia, and other shock-provoking stresses. Conversely, the opioid antagonist, **naloxone,** improves cardiovascular function and survival in various forms of shock.

Aberrations of Blood Clotting. The alterations of blood clotting after hemorrhage are typically biphasic—an initial phase of hypercoagulability followed by a secondary phase of hypocoagulability and fibrinolysis. In the initial phase intravascular clots, or **thrombi,** develop within a few minutes of the onset of severe hemorrhage, and coagulation may be extensive throughout the minute blood vessels.

Thromboxane A_2 may be released from various ischemic tissues. It aggregates platelets, and more thromboxane A_2 is released from the trapped platelets, which serves to trap additional platelets. This form of positive feedback intensifies and prolongs the clotting tendency. The mortality from certain standard shock-provoking procedures has been reduced considerably by anticoagulants such as heparin.

In the later stages of hemorrhagic hypotension, the clotting time is prolonged and fibrinolysis is prominent. It was mentioned previously that in the dog, hemorrhage into the intestinal lumen is common after several hours of hemorrhagic hypotension. Blood loss into the intestinal lumen would, of course, aggravate the hemodynamic effects of the original hemorrhage.

Reticuloendothelial System. During the course of hemorrhagic hypotension, reticuloendothelial system (RES) function becomes depressed. The phagocytic activity of the RES is modulated by an opsonic protein. The opsonic activity in plasma diminishes during shock, which may account in part for the depression of RES function. As a consequence, the antibacterial and antitoxic defense mechanisms are impaired. Endotoxins from the normal bacterial flora of the intestine constantly enter the circulation. Ordinarily they are inactivated by the RES, principally in the liver. When the RES is depressed, these endotoxins invade the general circulation. Endotoxins produce a form of shock that resembles in many respects that produced by hemorrhage. Therefore, depression of the RES aggravates the hemodynamic changes caused by blood loss.

In addition to their role in inactivating endotoxin, the macrophages release many of the mediators that are associated with shock: acid hydrolases, neutral proteases, certain coagulation factors, and the arachidonic acid derivatives—prostaglandins, thromboxanes, and leukotrienes. Macrophages also release certain regulatory proteins, called **monokines,** that modulate temperature regulation, intermediary metabolism, hormone secretion, and the immune system.

Interactions of Positive and Negative Feedback Mechanisms

Hemorrhage provokes a multitude of circulatory and metabolic derangements. Some of these changes are compensatory; others are decompensatory. Some of these feedback mechanisms possess a high gain, others, a low gain. Furthermore, the gain of any specific mechanism varies with the severity of the hemorrhage. For example, with only a slight loss of blood, mean arterial pressure is within the range of normal and the gain of the baroreceptor reflexes is high. With greater losses of blood, when mean arterial pressure is below about 60 mm Hg (that is, below the threshold for the baroreceptors), further reductions of pressure will have no additional influence through the baroreceptor reflexes. Hence below this critical pressure the baroreceptor reflex gain will be zero or near zero.

As a general rule, with minor degrees of blood loss, the gains of the negative feedback mechanisms are high, whereas those of the positive feedback mechanisms are low. The converse is true with more severe hemorrhages. The gains of the various mechanisms are additive algebraically. Therefore, whether a vicious cycle develops depends on whether the sum of the various gains exceeds 1. Total gains in excess of 1 are, of course, more likely with severe losses of blood. Therefore, to avert a vicious cycle, serious hemorrhages must be treated quickly and intensively, preferably by whole blood transfusions, before the process becomes irreversible.

■ SUMMARY

Exercise

1. In anticipation of exercise the vagus nerve impulses to the heart are inhibited and the sympathetic nervous system is activated by central command. The result is an increase in heart rate, myocardial contractile force, and regional vascular resistance.
2. With exercise, vascular resistance increases in skin, kidneys, splanchnic regions, and inactive muscles and decreases in active muscles. The increase in cardiac output is mainly caused by the increase in heart rate. Stroke volume increases only slightly. Total peripheral resistance decreases, oxygen consumption, and blood oxygen extraction increase, and systolic and mean blood pressure increase slightly.
3. As body temperature rises during exercise, the skin blood vessels dilate. However, when heart rate becomes maximal during severe exercise, the skin vessels constrict. This increases the effective blood volume but causes greater increases in body temperature and a feeling of exhaustion.
4. The limiting factor in exercise performance is the delivery of blood to the active muscles.

Hemorrhage

1. Acute blood loss induces the following hemodynamic changes: tachycardia, hypotension, generalized arteriolar vasoconstriction, and generalized venoconstriction.
2. Acute blood loss invokes a number of negative feedback (compensatory) mechanisms, such as baroreceptor and chemoreceptor reflexes, responses to moderate cerebral ischemia, reabsorption of tissue fluids, release of endogenous vasoconstrictors, and renal conservation of water and electrolytes.
3. Acute blood loss also induces a number of positive feedback (decompensatory) mechanisms, such as cardiac failure, acidosis, central nervous system depression, aberrations of blood coagulation, and depression of the reticuloendothelial system.
4. The outcome of an acute blood loss depends on the gains of the various feedback mechanisms and on the interactions between the positive and negative feedback mechanisms.

■ BIBLIOGRAPHY

Journal articles

Abel, F.L.: Myocardial function in sepsis and endotoxin shock, Am. J. Physiol. 257:R1265, 1989.

Averill, D.B., Scher, A.M., and Feigl, E.O.: Angiotensin causes vasoconstriction during hemorrhage in baroreceptor-denervated dogs, Am. J. Physiol. 245:H667, 1983.

Bernton, E.W., Long, J.B., and Holaday, J.W.: Opioids and neuropeptides: mechanisms in circulatory shock, Fed. Proc. 44:290, 1985.

Bevegåard, B.S., and Shepherd, J.T.: Regulation of the circulation during exercise in man, Physiol. Rev. 47:178, 1967.

Blomqvist, C.G., and Saltin, B.: Cardiovascular adaptations to physical training, Ann. Rev. Physiol. 45:169, 1983.

Bond, R.F., and Johnson, G., III: Vascular adrenergic interactions during hemorrhagic shock, Fed. Proc. 44:281, 1985.

Brengelmann, G.L.: Circulatory adjustments to exercise and heat stress, Ann. Rev. Physiol. 45:191, 1983.

Briand, R., Yamaguchi, N., and Gagne, J.: Plasma catecholamine and glucose concentrations during hemorrhagic hypotension in anesthetized dogs, Am. J. Physiol. 257:R317, 1989.

Christensen, N.J., and Galbo, H.: Sympathetic nervous activity during exercise, Ann. Rev. Physiol. 45:139, 1983.

Clausen, J.P.: Effect of physical training on cardiovascular adjustments to exercise in man, Physiol. Rev. 57:779, 1977.

Connett, R.J., Pearce, F.J., and Drucker, W.R.: Scaling of physiological responses: a new approach for hemorrhagic shock, Am. J. Physiol. 250:R951, 1986.

Cornish, K.G., Gilmore, J.P., and McCulloch, T.: Central blood volume and blood pressure in conscious primates, Am. J. Physiol. 254:H693, 1988.

Eldridge, F.L. et al.: Stimulation by central command of locomotion, respiration, and circulation during exercise, Resp. Physiol. 59:313, 1985.

Filkins, J.P.: Monokines and the metabolic pathophysiology of septic shock, Fed. Proc. 44:300, 1985.

Hosomi, H., Katsuda, S., Morita, H., Nishida, Y., and Koyama, S.: Interactions among reflex compensatory systems for posthemorrhage hypotension, Am. J. Physiol. 250:H944, 1986.

Laughlin, M.H., and Armstrong, R.B.: Muscle blood flow during locomotory exercise, Exerc. Sport Sci. Rev. 13:95, 1985.

Lefer, A.M.: Eicosanoids as mediators of ischemia and shock, Fed. Proc. 44:275, 1985.

Liard, J.F.: Vasopressin in cardiovascular control: role of circulating vasopressin, Clin. Sci. 67:473, 1984.

Ludbrook, J.: Reflex control of blood pressure during exercise, Ann. Rev. Physiol. 45:155, 1983.

Ludbrook, J., and Graham, W.F.: The role of cardiac receptor and arterial baroreceptor reflexes in control of the circulation during acute change of blood volume in the conscious rabbit, Circ. Res. 54:424, 1984.

Mitchell, J.H., Kaufman, M.P., and Iwamoto, G.A.: The exercise pressor reflex: its cardiovascular effects, afferent mechanisms, and central pathways, Ann. Rev. Physiol. 45:229, 1983.

Saltin, B., and Rowell, L.B.: Functional adaptations to physical activity and inactivity, Fed. Proc. 39:1506, 1980.

Sanders, J.S., Mark, A.L., and Ferguson, D.W.: Importance of aortic baroreflex in regulation of sympathetic responses during hypotension, Circ. 79:83, 1989.

Schadt, J.C., and Ludbrook, J.: Hemodynamic and neurohumoral responses to acute hypovolemia in conscious mammals, Am. J. Physiol. 260:H305, 1991.

Share, L.: Role of vasopressin in cardiovascular regulation, Physiol. Rev. 68:1248, 1988.

Shen, Y.-T., Knight, D.R., Thomas, J.X., Jr., and Vatner, S.F.: Relative roles of cardiac receptors and arterial baroreceptors during hemorrhage in conscious dogs, Circ. Res. 66:397, 1990.

Vatner, S.F., and Pagani, M.: Cardiovascular adjustments to exercise: hemodynamics and mechanisms, Prog. Cardiovasc. Dis. 19:91, 1976.

Books and monographs

Altura, B.M., Lefer, A.M., and Schumer, W.: Handbook of shock and trauma, vol. 1, Basic science, New York, 1983, Raven Press.

Bond, R.F., Adams, H.R., and Chaudry, I.H., associate editors: Perspectives in shock research, New York, 1988, Alan R. Liss, Inc.

Brooks, G.A., and Fahey, T.D.: Exercise physiology—human bioenergetics and its applications, New York, 1984, John Wiley & Sons, Inc.

Carlsten, A., and Grimby, G.: The circulatory response to muscular exercise in man, Springfield, Ill., 1966, Charles C Thomas, Publisher.

Janssen, H.F., and Barnes, C.D., editors: Circulatory shock: basic and clinical implications, New York, 1985, Academic Press, Inc.

Lind, A.R.: Cardiovascular adjustments to isometric contractions: static effort. In Handbook of physiology; Section 2: The cardiovascular system—peripheral circulation and organ blood flow, vol. III, Bethesda, Md., 1983, American Physiological Society.

Mitchell, J.H., and Schmidt, R.F.: Cardiovascular reflex control by afferent fibers from skeletal muscle receptors. In Handbook of physiology; Section 2: The cardiovascular system—peripheral circulation and organ blood flow, vol. III, Bethesda, Md., 1983, American Physiological Society.

Roth, B.L., Nielsen, T.B., and McKee, A.E., editors: Molecular and cellular mechanisms of septic shock. In: Progress in clinical and biological research, vol. 286, New York, 1988, Alan R. Liss, Inc.

Rowell, L.B.: Integration of body systems in exercise. In Principles of physiology, Berne, R.M., and Levy, M.N., editors: St. Louis, 1990, The C.V. Mosby Co.

Rowell, L.B.: Human circulation: regulation during physical stress, New York, 1986, Oxford University Press.

Index

Q

R